Hemodynamics and Immune Defense

Discoveries in Pharmacology

Volume 3

Hemodynamics and Immune Defense

Second Edition

Edited by

Michael J. Parnham
Professor, Faculty of Biochemistry,
Chemistry and Pharmacy,
Goethe University Frankfurt,
Frankfurt am Main, Germany

Clive P. Page
Professor of Pharmacology, King's College London and
Director of the Sackler Institute of Pulmonary
Pharmacology, King's College London, United Kingdom

Jacques Bruinvels
Professor Emeritus of Pharmacology,
Department of Pharmacology,
Erasmus University Rotterdam, Rotterdam,
The Netherlands

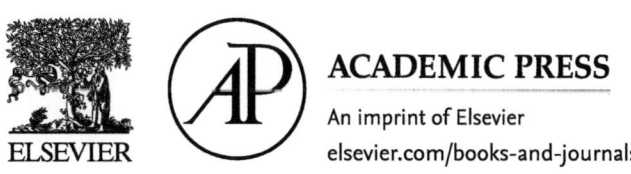

ACADEMIC PRESS

An imprint of Elsevier
elsevier.com/books-and-journals

ELSEVIER

Academic Press is an imprint of Elsevier

125 London Wall, London EC2Y 5AS, United Kingdom
525 B Street, Suite 1650, San Diego, CA 92101, United States
50 Hampshire Street, 5th Floor, Cambridge, MA 02139, United States
The Boulevard, Langford Lane, Kidlington, Oxford OX5 1GB, United Kingdom

Notices
Knowledge and best practice in this field are constantly changing. As new research and experience broaden our
understanding, changes in research methods, professional practices, or medical treatment may become necessary.

Practitioners and researchers must always rely on their own experience and knowledge in evaluating and using any
information, methods, compounds, or experiments described herein. In using such information or methods they
should be mindful of their own safety and the safety of others, including parties for whom they have a professional
responsibility.

To the fullest extent of the law, neither the Publisher nor the authors, contributors, or editors, assume any liability
for any injury and/or damage to persons or property as a matter of products liability, negligence or otherwise, or
from any use or operation of any methods, products, instructions, or ideas contained in the material herein.

ISBN: 978-0-443-18442-0

For Information on all Academic Press publications visit our
website at https://www.elsevier.com/books-and-journals

Publisher: Stacy Masucci
Acquisitions Editor: Andre G. Wolff
Editorial Project Manager: Sam Young
Production Project Manager: Sajana Devasi P K
Cover Designer: Miles Hitchen

Typeset by Aptara, New Delhi, India

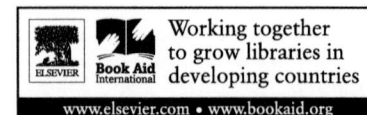

Working together
to grow libraries in
developing countries

www.elsevier.com • www.bookaid.org

Contents

Chapter 2A: Can drugs be devised to lower elevated blood pressure by blocking sympathetic autonomic traffic? Commentary on Ganglion and adrenergic neurone-blocking agents by Alan L.A. Boura and Alan F. Green....................................41

John Christie McGrath

Chapter 2B: Peripheral anti-hypertensives: Ganglion and adrenergic neurone-blocking agents...47

Alan L.A. Boura and Alan F. Green

Chapter 3A: Commentary on The proliferation of non-steroidal anti-inflammatory drugs (NSAIDs) by T.Y. Shen 77

Kim D. Rainsford

Contents

Contributors

Peter J. Barnes, National Heart & Lung Institute, Imperial College London, London, United Kingdom

Robert Behnisch, Pahlkestrasse 3, Wuppertal, Germany

Alan L.A. Boura, Department of Pharmacology, Monash University, Clayton, Victoria, Australia

Walter E. Brocklehurst, Lilly Research Centre Ltd., Windlesham, Surrey, United Kingdom

Richard W. Burg, Merck, Sharp & Dohme Research Laboratories, Rahway, NJ, United States

Karen Bush, Indiana University, Bloomington, IN, United States

Søren Brøgger Christensen, Department of Drug Design and Pharmacology, University of Copenhagen, Copenhagen, Denmark

Harry O.J. Collier, Department of Pharmacology, Chelsea College, London University, London, United Kingdom

Madeleine Ennis, Centre for Infection and Immunity, The Wellcome-Wolfson Building, School of Medicine, Dentistry and Biomedical Sciences, The Queen's University Belfast, United Kingdom

Roderick J. Flower, The William Harvey Research Institute, Queen Mary University of London, London, United Kingdom

Alan F. Green, The Wellcome Research Laboratories, Beckenham, United Kingdom

Wilfried Lorenz, Department of Theoretical Surgery, Centre for Operative Medicine 1, Klinikum-Lahnberge, Marburg, Germany

John Christie McGrath, Autonomic Physiology Unit, School of Cardiovascular & Metabolic Health, University of Glasgow, Glasgow, Scotland

Martin C. Michel, Department of Pharmacology, University Medical Center, Johannes Gutenberg University, Mainz, Germany

Heinz Moser, Novartis Institutes for Biomedical Research, Emeryville, CA, United States

Kim D. Rainsford, Department of Biosciences and Chemistry, Sheffield Hallam University, Sheffield, United Kingdom

Sydney Selwyn, Department of Medical Microbiology, Charing Cross and Westminster Medical School, London, United Kingdom

Robert G. Shanks, Department of Therapeutics and Pharmacology, The Queen's University of Belfast, Belfast, United Kingdom

T.Y. Shen, Merck, Sharp & Dohme Research Laboratories, Rahway, NJ, United States

Katerina Tiligada, Department of Pharmacology, Medical School, National and Kapodistrian University of Athens, Athens, Greece

H. Boyd Woodruff, Soil Microbiology Associates, Inc., Watchung, NJ, United States

Preface

Blood circulation, as the transport system of the body, has to be maintained within carefully regulated limits to ensure the supply of oxygen and nutrients as well as delivering cells and mediators for host defense and repair to the tissues and preventing the failure of the heart or of the functions of the blood vessels. While pulmonary circulation was recognized by the ancient Greek physician Galen and the circulation of the blood from and to the heart described by William Harvey in 1628, little was known about the effects of drugs. Ergot from *Claviceps purpurea*, the parasitic fungus on rye, was known to exert multiple effects, but not understood till the early 20th century, thanks to the studies of Henry H. Dale on the blood pressure changes caused by ergot alkaloids. Subsequent research led to the crucial discoveries of drugs controlling blood pressure and two chapters on important anti-hypertensives are included in this volume.

Effective blood clotting processes and induced permeability of blood vessels to leukocytes and plasma are essential for wound healing and host defense, but when these reactions become excessive or infection is uncontrolled they result in tissue injury. It was again Galen who described the cardinal signs of inflammation while the emigration of blood cells was observed by Rudolf Virchow and Elie Metchnikoff in the 19th century. The role of inflammatory mediators was first understood by Dale and others in the 20th century. In contrast, the traditional usefulness of salicylate-containing plant materials in treating pain and inflammation had become clear several centuries earlier. Yet it was the discovery of inflammatory mediators which provided explanations for the pharmacology of these early and subsequently developed anti-inflammatory drugs, as described in several chapters in this volume.

The availability of leukocytes, lymphocytes, and their precursors in the blood is also crucial to defense against infection. Edward Jenner was unaware of this in 1796 when he demonstrated that a cowpox vaccine would provide immunity against smallpox and it was not until 1900 that Paul Ehrlich proposed the existence of antibodies that could circulate in the blood. Ehrlich also discovered the first antibacterial drug, arsphenamine (Salvarsan) which was used to treat syphilis, caused by the bacterium, *Treponema pallidum*. The final three chapters in this volume relate the stories behind the development of antibiotics and some of the issues that have resulted.

With the publication of this third volume on *Hemodynamics and Immune Defense* in the *Discoveries in Pharmacology* series, we complete the reprinting of selected chapters from the original edition, published nearly 40 years ago. As with the previous two volumes on the *Nervous System* and on *Standardizing Pharmacology: Assays and Hormones*, this latest volume continues the reprinting of selected original chapters which are placed into today's context together with commentaries by current experts for whose contributions we are very grateful. We also thank Andre Wolff, Sam Young, Stalin Viswanathan, Sajana Devasi, and Selvaraj Raviraj at Elsevier for their support, patience, and persistence in putting the contributions together for publication. (The original books were printed at a time when digital publishing was not possible, so typing errors could not be detected so readily. The reproduction of these chapters means that some printing errors are also carried over from 40 years ago).

We hope you enjoy reading the historical accounts provided and gain a greater understanding of the people and research that have made pharmacology what it is today.

—Michael J. Parnham

—Clive P. Page

—Jacques Bruinvels

Septembert, 2023

Commentary on The discovery of beta adrenoceptor blocking drugs by Robert G. Shanks

Martin C. Michel

Department of Pharmacology, University Medical Center, Johannes Gutenberg University, Mainz, Germany

Introduction

When Shanks reviewed the discovery of β-adrenoceptor antagonists in 1984 (Shanks, 1984), the world appears to have been much simpler than today—not only for β-adrenoceptors. At the time, four subtypes of adrenoceptors were recognized, grouped into two subfamilies of α- and β-adrenoceptors, i.e., α_1-, α_2-, β_1-, and β_2-adrenoceptors. However, pharmacological evidence had started to emerge for the existence of more than these. Following the molecular cloning of the hamster β_2-adrenoceptor in 1986 (Dixon et al., 1986), nine mammalian adrenoceptor subtypes have been cloned. They are now classified into three subfamilies of α_1-adrenoceptors (α_{1A}, α_{1B}, and α_{1D}), α_2-adrenoceptors (α_{2A}, α_{2B}, and α_{2C}) and β-adrenoceptors (β_1, β_2, and β_3) (Bylund et al., 1994; Hieble et al., 1995). Starting with the human β_2-adrenoceptor (Cherezov et al., 2007), the crystal structures of various adrenoceptor subtypes were determined in various states of binding to agonist and antagonist ligands. Some additionally proposed subtypes have turned out to be variations of these nine subtypes: The α_{1L}-adrenoceptor (characterized by an unusually low affinity for prazosin) apparently is a state of the α_{1A}-adrenoceptor that can be observed in some cellular contexts (White et al., 2019). The proposed β_4-adrenoceptor is explained by an allosteric site on the β_1-adrenoceptor that has a distinct ligand recognition and activation profile as compared to the orthotopic ligand recognition site used by the endogenous catecholamines (Kaumann and Molenaar, 2008). Interestingly, ligands such as CGP 12,177 can be antagonists at the orthotopic and (partial) agonists at the heterotopic site. Ligands at some of the newly discovered adrenoceptor subtypes such as the β_3-adrenoceptor agonist mirabegron (Chapple et al., 2014) have become guideline-recommended drugs for the treatment of certain diseases because their subtype selectivity has led to much-improved benefit/risk ratio for some conditions by avoiding side effects mediated by other adrenoceptor subtypes.

Discoveries in Pharmacology, Volume 3, Hemodynamics and
Immune Defense.
DOI: https://doi.org/10.1016/B978-0-443-18442-0.00002-1

Selective β-adrenoceptor antagonists

The initially reported β-adrenoceptor antagonists such as propranolol were considered to be selective for this subfamily but not for individual subtypes. While the data at the time supported this concept, propranolol and all other clinically used β-adrenoceptor antagonists have much lower affinity for β_3- when compared with β_1- and β_2-adrenoceptors (Cernecka et al., 2014). Nonetheless, the dichotomous classification of β-adrenoceptors was rooted too deeply in the minds of pharmacologists, so the authors kept referring incorrectly to propranolol as a non-specific β-adrenoceptor antagonist until very recently. At the time of Shanks' review (Shanks, 1984), only very limited steps had been made to develop subtype-selective β-adrenoceptor antagonists, practolol being an example. Moreover, most texts at the time did not describe them mechanistically as β_1-selective but rather as cardio-selective. This turned out to be a well-intended but false concept as β_2-adrenoceptors (and in rodents β_3-adrenoceptors) contribute to a degree to the regulation of cardiac function (Brodde and Michel, 1999). Meanwhile, many more β_1-selective antagonists such as bisoprolol have been developed, and selectivity for β_1- over β_2-adrenoceptors has become a characteristic defining suitability for certain indications. The only β_2-selective antagonist ever tested in humans, ICI 118,551, was not developed further due to compound-specific toxicity issues and lack of commercial interest; β_3-adrenoceptor antagonists have not yet been introduced into clinical medicine. Other than selectivity among the β-adrenoceptor subtypes, selectivity toward other drug targets has become an issue. For instance, pindolol also has activity on some subtypes of serotonin receptors, and various β-adrenoceptor agonists and antagonists intentionally or unintentionally have a relevant affinity for α_1-adrenoceptors (Michel, 2020). The latter may not be surprising considering that all adrenoceptors share a pharmacophore for adrenaline and noradrenaline.

It became clear rapidly after the cloning of the adrenoceptor subtypes, that the genes encoding them exhibit polymorphisms. While some of the polymorphisms of β_1- and β_2-adrenoceptors apparently have some degree of clinical relevance (Engelhardt and Ahles, 2014), those of β_3-adrenoceptors apparently do not (Michel, 2023). However, the field of adrenoceptor gene polymorphism research is plagued by the problem that the existing literature often is controversial. Accordingly, none of the reported adrenoceptor gene polymorphisms led to genotype-specific therapeutic recommendations.

Inverse agonism

It was already recognized in 1984 that some β-adrenoceptor antagonists can have a moderate degree of agonistic activity, a phenomenon called intrinsic sympathomimetic activity at the time (Shanks, 1984), now more precisely described as weak partial agonism. We now have an armamentarium of compounds for experimental and clinical use at our disposal that covers the entire spectrum from full agonism via strong and weak partial agonism to antagonism, the latter now called neutral antagonism. However, it also became clear that some compounds not only block activation of β-adrenoceptor activation by agonists but also can stabilize the inactive state of the receptor in the absence of agonists, a phenomenon called inverse agonism. Many adrenoceptor ligands exhibit such inverse agonism (Michel et al., 2020). Of note, the degree of agonism or inverse agonism exhibited by a ligand not only depends on its intrinsic properties but also on the cellular context in which it is expressed. Thus, the same compound can act as an inverse agonist, neutral antagonist, or as partial agonist depending on the cell expressing the receptor.

Biased signaling

Another phenomenon not foreseen in 1984 is what is now called biased signaling. This refers to the fact that some compounds preferentially stimulate one signaling pathway of a receptor over another. In theory, knowledge of biased agonism could lead drug development to favor a pathway mediating a desired response over another signaling pathway of the same receptor which mediates an adverse event. However, whether this is a promising reality in drug research and development is under debate (Kenakin, 2018; Michel and Charlton, 2018). Some of this controversy stems from the problem that biased agonism is partially a ligand property and partially, similar to inverse agonism, a property of the cell in which the receptor is expressed; a cellular property defining this can be the stoichiometric ratio of the receptor relative to the signaling pathway components in that cell. Moreover, this ratio is not fixed and can undergo dynamic changes in the context of disease or drug treatment, a phenomenon dubbed dynamic bias (Michel et al., 2014). Accordingly, it is very difficult to robustly determine the most promising target profile for a given indication during compound selection for further preclinical and clinical development.

Expanded clinical uses

When Sir James Black initially developed propranolol, it was primarily for the indication of coronary heart disease (Shanks, 1984); however, it became clear soon thereafter that β-adrenoceptor antagonists also had the potential for the treatment of arterial hypertension. Meanwhile, β-adrenoceptor antagonists have been approved for 20 distinct indications by the US Food and Drug Administration; moreover, they are used as an evidence-backed, off-label treatment for another 11 indications, even including certain malignancies (Bond et al., 2022) (Table 1.1). The possible use of β-adrenoceptor antagonist in other malignant tumors is currently under investigation (Dal Monte et al., 2019). Ironically, arterial hypertension was one of the first indications to be pursued for β-adrenoceptor antagonists and these drugs were guideline recommended as 1st line treatment for many years. However, other drug classes have exhibited a superior benefit/risk ratio in hypertension, relegating β-adrenoceptor antagonists to 2nd and 3rd line treatment of hypertension (Williams et al., 2018).

Table 1.1: Indications of β-adrenoceptor antagonists.

FDA-approved indications	Off-label uses
Angina	Anxiety
Hypertension	Public speaking
Congestive heart failure	Post-traumatic stress
Myocardial infarction prophylaxis	Hypotension induction
Atrial fibrillation	Portal hypertension
Open-angle glaucoma	Ethanol withdrawal
Migraine prophylaxis	Esophageal varices
Tremor	Hypertensive emergency
Thyrotoxicosis	Variceal bleeding prophylaxis
Atrial flutter	Perioperative hypertension
Ventricular arrhythmias (ventricular premature beats)	Infantine hemangiomas
Myocardial infarction	
Pheochromocytoma	
Ocular hypertension	
Paroxysmal supraventricular tachycardia	
Idiopathic hypertrophic subaortic stenosis	
Scleroderma renal crisis	
Hypertrophic subaortic stenosis	
Supraventricular tachycardia of non-compensatory sinus tachycardia	
Intraoperative and postoperative tachycardia and hypertension	

From: Bond et al. (2022).

Perhaps the most surprising development in β-adrenoceptor antagonist research has been for heart failure. Based on the positive inotropic effects of acute administration of β-adrenoceptor agonists, heart failure was long seen as a contraindication for the use of β-adrenoceptor antagonists. However, it later turned out that chronic administration of such agonists may have adverse effects on survival. On the other hand, slowly titrated β-adrenoceptor antagonists have been shown to improve the survival of heart failure patients (Bond et al., 2022). Nevertheless, such beneficial effects of β-adrenoceptor antagonists in heart failure are not universal but only apply to some members of this drug class. It has been speculated that biased agonism may be the reason for this clinical observation (Thanawala et al., 2014). Based on the beneficial effects of β$_2$-adrenoceptor agonists in asthma, obstructive airway disease has been a contraindication for the use of β-adrenoceptor antagonists. Inspired by the findings in heart failure patients and supported by evidence from animal models (Thanawala et al., 2015), the idea emerged that some slowly titrated β-adrenoceptor antagonists may not be harmful but therapeutically useful in asthma (Dickey et al., 2010). This concept is currently undergoing clinical evaluation and has provided promising initial results.

In conclusion, over the almost 40 years since the publication of the historical review by Shanks (Shanks, 1984), there has been major progress, in many ways in directions that were and could not have been foreseen by Shanks. The use of β-adrenoceptor antagonists has broadened from cardiovascular diseases into a much larger range of other conditions (Table 1.1). Most intriguing is the concept that the chronic use of antagonists may have effects that mimic the acute use of agonists, e.g., in heart failure and, at least in experimental animals, in asthma.

References

Bond, R.A., Michel, M.C., Parra, S., 2022. Cardiovascular, hematopoietic, urinary and respiratory pharmacology. In: Michel, M.C. (Ed.), Comprehensive Pharmacology, Vol. 4. Elsevier, Amsterdam, pp. 497–506.

Brodde, O.E., Michel, M.C., 1999. Adrenergic and muscarinic receptors in the human heart. Pharmacol. Rev. 51 (4), 651–689.

Bylund, D.B., Eikenberg, D.C., Hieble, J.P., Langer, S.Z., Lefkowitz, R.J., Minneman, K.P., et al., 1994. International union of pharmacology nomenclature of adrenoceptors. Pharmacol. Rev. 46 (2), 121–136.

Cernecka, H., Sand, C., Michel, M.C., 2014. The odd sibling: features of β_3-adrenoceptor pharmacology. Mol. Pharmacol. 86 (5), 479–484.

Chapple, C.R., Cardozo, L., Nitti, V.W., Siddiqui, E., Michel, M.C., 2014. Mirabegron in overactive bladder: a review of efficacy, safety, and tolerability. Neurourol. Urodyn. 33 (1), 17–30.

Cherezov, V., Rosenbaum, D.M., Hanson, M.A., Rasmussen, S.G.F., Thian, F.S., Kobilka, T.S., et al., 2007. High-resolution crystal structure of an engineered human β_2-adrenergic G protein-coupled receptor. Science 318, 1258–1265.

Dal Monte, M., Calvani, M., Cammalleri, M., Favre, C., Filippi, L., Bagnoli, P., 2019. β-adrenoceptors as drug targets in melanoma: novel preclinical evidence for a role of β_3-adrenoceptors. Br. J. Pharmacol. 176 (14), 2496–2508.

Dickey, B.F., Walker, J.K.L., Hanania, N.A., Bond, RA., 2010. β-adrenoceptor inverse agonists in asthma. Curr. Opin. Pharmacol. 10 (3), 254–259.

Dixon, R.A.F., Kobilka, B.K., Strader, D.J., Benovic, J.L., Dohlman, H.G., Frielle, T., et al., 1986. Cloning of the gene and cDNA for mammalian β-adrenergic receptor and homology with rhodopsin. Nature 321, 75–79.

Engelhardt, S., Ahles, A., 2014. Polymorphic variants of adrenoceptors: physiology, pharmacology and role in disease. Pharmacol. Rev. 66 (2), 598–637.

Hieble, J.P., Bylund, D.B., Clarke, D.E., Eikenburg, D.C., Langer, S.Z., Lefkowitz, R.J., et al., 1995. International union of pharmacology X. Recommendation for nomenclature of α_1-adrenoceptors: consensus update. Pharmacol. Rev. 47, 267–270.

Kaumann, A.J., Molenaar, P., 2008. The low affinity site of the β_1-adrenoceptor and its relevance to cardiovascular pharmacology. Pharmacol. Ther. 118, 303–336.

Kenakin, T., 2018. Is the quest for signaling bias worth the effort? Mol. Pharmacol. 93 (4), 266–269.

Michel, M.C., 2020. α_1-adrenoceptor activity of β-adrenoceptor ligands: an expected drug property with limited clinical relevance. Eur. J. Pharmacol. 889, 173632.

Michel, M.C., 2023. Are β3-adrenoceptor gene polymorphisms relevant for urology? Neurourol. Urodyn. 42 (1), 33 39.

Michel, M.C., Charlton, S.J., 2018. Biased agonism in drug discovery: is it too soon to choose a path? Mol. Pharmacol. 93 (4), 259–265.

Michel, M.C., Michel-Reher, M.B., Hein, P., 2020. A systematic review of inverse agonism at adrenoceptor subtypes. Cells 9, 1923.

Michel, M.C., Seifert, R., Bond, R.A., 2014. Dynamic bias and its implications for GPCR drug discovery. Nat. Rev. Drug Discov. 13 (11), 869 870.

Shanks, R.G., 1984. The discovery of beta adrenoceptor blocking drugs. In: Parnham M.J., Bruinvels J., (Eds.), Discoveries in Pharmacology, Vol. 2. Elsevier, Amsterdam, pp. 38–72.

Thanawala, V.J., Forkuo, G.S., Stallaert, W., Leff, P., Bouvier, M., Bond, R., 2014. Ligand bias prevents class equality among beta-blockers. Curr. Opin. Pharmacol. 16 (1), 50–57.

Thanawala, V.J., Valdez, D.J., Joshi, R., Forkuo, G.S., Parra, S., Knoll, B.J., et al., 2015. ß-Blockers have differential effects on the murina asthma phenotype. Br. J. Pharmacol. 172, 4833–4846.

White, C.W., da Silva Junior, E.D., Lim, L., Ventura, S., 2019. What makes the α_{1A}-adrenoceptor gene product assume a α_{1L}-adrenoceptor phenotype? Br. J. Pharmacol. 176 (14), 2358–2365.

Williams, B., Mancia, G., Spiering, W., Agabiti Rosei, E., Azizi, M., Burnier, M., et al., 2018. 2018 ESC/ESH guidelines for the management of arterial hypertension: The task force for the management of arterial hypertension of the European Society of Cardiology (ESC) and the European Society of Hypertension (ESH). Eur. Heart J. 39 (33), 3021–3104.

The control of blood pressure: The discovery of beta adrenoceptor blocking drugs

Robert G. Shanks

Contents

Disclaimer: The original text that follows is reproduced from the first edition and carries errors and omissions from it. The editors and publisher agreed to retain them and honor the original authors and challenges they had to deal with in publishing back in those times.

Discoveries in Pharmacology, Volume 3, Hemodynamics and Immune Defense.

DOI: https://doi.org/10.1016/B978-0-443-18442-0.00061-6

1.1 Introduction

Beta adrenoceptor blocking drugs have been one of the most important group of drugs discovered during the past 25 years. They have been of value as investigative tools in many aspects of basic and applied biological science and clinical medicine and been an important advance in the treatment of several diseases some of which are extremely common. An enormous literature has accumulated on many aspects of beta adrenoceptor blocking drugs including a large number of excellent reviews but no publication has yet described the discovery of these drugs.

There are many aspects to the discovery of beta adrenoceptor blocking drugs and it has been a major problem defining the interpretation and application of 'discovery' to these drugs. It could be applied only to the pharmacological studies and chemical synthesis which led to the discovery of the compounds which block beta adrenoceptors. On the other hand it could also include the pharmacological studies and controversies which preceded the classification of adrenoceptors and the extensive studies in many diseases which have established the position of these drugs in the treatment of many diseases. I have tried to reach a compromise and have started with Ahlquist's classification of adrenoceptors and ended with a brief description of the early studies which indicated that beta adrenoceptor blocking drugs have a role in clinical medicine.

Many people have contributed to all aspects of the discovery of these drugs although the signal contributions were made by Dr. R.P. Ahlquist and by Sir James Black but important roles were played by Dr. N.C. Moran, Mr. C.E. Powell and Dr. I.H. Slater in the description of dichloroisoprenaline, chemists at the Pharmaceuticals Division of Imperial Chemical Industries, who made many of the compounds, and the biologists at I.C.I. who tested them. The clinicians who made the initial observation with these new drugs and then performed the clinical trials to define their role were most important. It has been my pleasure to have worked with many of these people during the past 25 years and to have this opportunity to describe the discovery of these drugs. Unfortunately detailed records have not been kept or are not available for all parts of the story and people's memories for events which happened over 20 years ago may have faded slightly.

1.2 Classification of adrenoceptors

In 1948, Dr. R.P. Ahlquist published his classic paper, *A Study of the Adrenotropic Receptors,* in which he suggested that there were two distinct types of adrenotropic receptors, which he designated alpha and beta (Ahlquist, 1948). Ahlquist had not set out to classify adrenotropic receptors but was searching for a compound to relax the human uterus; the Chairman of his Department, Professor R.A. Woodbury, had proposed, on the basis of clinical studies, that a uterine relaxant would be a treatment for dysmenorrhoea (Ahlquist, 1980). As

Woodbury and Abreu (1944) had shown that adrenaline relaxed the human uterus, Ahlquist tested a series of catecholamines on a large variety of organs and systems in several species. The results are summarised as follows:

> 'There are two distinct types of adrenotropic receptors as determined by their relative responsiveness to the series of racemic sympathomimetic amines most closely related structurally to epinephrine. The *alpha* adrenotropic receptor is associated with most of the excitatory functions (vasoconstriction, and stimulation of the uterus, nictitating membrane, ureter and *dilator pupillae*) and one important inhibitory function (intestinal relaxation). The *beta* adrenotropic receptor is associated with most of the inhibitory functions (vasodilation, and inhibition of the uterine and bronchial musculature) and one excitatory function (myocardial stimulation)' (Ahlquist, 1948).

Ahlquist stated 'This concept of two fundamental types of receptors is directly opposed to the concept of two mediator substances (sympathin E and sympathin I) as propounded by Cannon and Rosenbleuth (Ahlquist, 1980) and now widely quoted as a 'law' of physiology' (see *Discoveries in Pharmacology,* Vol. 1, chapt. 2).

Ahlquist's paper was not accepted by the *Journal of Pharmacology and Experimental Therapeutics* and was only published in the *American Journal of Physiology* after the intervention of his friend and Professor of Physiology in Augusta, W.F. Hamilton. It is interesting to note that in this paper Ahlquist found epinephrine (adrenaline) to be the most active substance at alpha adrenoceptors and almost the most active on beta adrenoceptors and on this basis suggested that it was 'the most logical substance to be the sympathetic neuro-hormone . . .' (Ahlquist, 1948). About the same time Von Euler (1946) demonstrated that noradrenaline was the transmitter substance at sympathetic nerve endings. Ahlquist subsequently realised that he had been wrong in predicting that adrenaline was the sympathetic neurotransmitter (Ahlquist, 1980) but by this time his classification had been universally accepted.

In his 1948 paper Ahlquist does not refer to the effect of antagonists on the responses associated with these two adrenoceptors although it was known at that time that several compounds including ergotoxine, tolazoline and dibenamine would block excitatory responses, except in the heart, to adrenaline, without affecting the inhibitory response. This action was most clearly observed in the cardiovascular system where these drugs converted the normal pressor response to adrenaline to a depressor response – 'epinephrine reversal' (Nickerson, 1949).

There was, however, controversy over the effects of dibenamine and related drugs on the excitatory effects of adrenaline and other catecholamines on the heart. Early studies with dibenamine appeared to demonstrate a distinction between the effective blockade of excitatory responses of smooth muscle and failure to inhibit the positive inotropic and chronotropic responses of the myocardium to adrenergic stimulation (Nickerson, 1949). Conclusive studies could not be made in intact animals as no precise methods were available for determination of the inotropic responses to drugs. Moran and Cotten working at the National Heart Institute in the mid 1950s re-investigated this problem in anaesthetised dogs using a strain gauge arch sutured to the right ventricle to measure the force of cardiac contraction and a transducer to record arterial pressure in order to assess changes in peripheral vascular resistance. These techniques enabled them to assess simultaneously the effects of antagonists on the inotropic and vascular responses to catecholamines (Cotten, Moran and Stopp, 1957). They concluded that phenoxybenzamine and phentolamine specifically and completely blocked the cardiac effects of noradrenaline, adrenaline and isoprenaline but at doses higher than those needed to block the vasoconstrictor effects of noradrenaline and adrenaline. The vasodilator effects of adrenaline and isoprenaline were also 'blocked' with these high doses. They concluded that 'these findings do not conflict with the concept proposed by Ahlquist (1948) that different types of sympathetic receptors exist in heart muscle and arterial smooth muscle, but they do suggest that the differences may be only quantitative and not necessarily qualitative in nature' (Cotton et al., 1957). This situation was to change dramatically within two years. Although Moran was familiar with Ahlquist's paper he did not think of the possibility of a programme of systematic development of a second class of adrenergic blocking drug to fit Ahlquist's terminology (Moran, 1982).

1.3 Dichloroisoprenaline

1.3.1 Discovery

When Irwin Slater joined Lilly Research Laboratories in Indianapolis, Indiana in 1954, chemical compounds were being screened for bronchodilator activity using tracheal chains contracted with pilocarpine. Relaxation induced by candidate compounds was compared with adrenaline-induced relaxation. The technician (Mr. L. Le Compte) tested 3 or 4 compounds on each tracheal chain using recovery of the adrenaline-induced relaxation as an index of tissue responsiveness (Slater, 1982). Mr. Le Compte complained to his supervisor, Mr. C.E. Powell, that each time he tested compound 20522 (dichloroisoprenaline – DCI) the tissue lost the ability to relax on adrenaline exposure. This was discussed by members of the Cardiovascular Research Group but nobody was interested (Slater, 1982). At that time Slater was working in neuropharmacology but was asked by Powell in November 1956 to help him understand 20522. The compound was administered to anaesthetised cats and shown to enhance the pressor action of adrenaline and reduce the depressor action of isoprenaline. Further observations showed that 20522 reduced the vasodilator effect of isoprenaline in an anaesthetised dog. These results were communicated at the Federation Meetings in 1957 by Slater and Powell who concluded in their abstract that '. . . 20522 is combining with certain inhibitory adrenergic receptor sites . . .' (Slater and Powell, 1957). The complete results were published in April 1958 and showed that 20522 inhibited bronchodilator, vasodilator and other inhibitory actions of adrenaline (Powell and Slater, 1958). They commented that although compound

20522 combined with adrenergic inhibitory sites it did not 'trigger the series of reactions that lead to typical inhibitory effects'. No observations were made on the cardiac effects of 20522 and no reference is made to Ahlquist in the paper.

In retrospect Slater has said that 'we understood what we had found but underestimated the degree of intrinsic activity. We had few ideas for clinical utility and were not in a position to do detailed cardiovascular studies' (Slater, 1982).

Isoprenaline   Dichloroisoprenaline

1.3.2 Blockade of beta adrenoceptors

Neil Moran heard Irwin Slater give his paper on Lilly compound 20522 at the meeting in 1957, and 'was struck by the fact that this compound might fit into Ahlquist's scheme of *alpha* and *beta* adrenergic receptors and that the heart was the crucial item' (Moran, 1982). He even thought that 'DCI might be the *beta* adrenergic receptor blocking drug' (Moran, 1982).

Moran asked Slater for a sample of DCI after his talk, received it two weeks later and was able to test it immediately as he was doing experiments in which blood pressure, heart rate and cardiac contractile force were recorded in dogs.

> 'I used a protocol I had routinely used for screening drugs in a screening program we had at The National Heart Institute, namely after initial testing responses to agonists (in this instance, epinephrine, nor-epinephrine, isoproterenol, acetylcholine and tetramethylam-monium), the 'unknown' drug was given intravenously, usually at 1 mg/kg, and then at intervals given in geometrically increasing doses, with the standard agonists being tested between doses of the 'unknown'. I describe the protocol, because the blocking effect might have been obscured if only a single dose of DCI had been used – that is, the marked intrinsic sympathomimetic action of the first dose is inhibited by the subsequent larger doses and the cardiac blockade is fully revealed.

> My first experiment was one of those rare experiments that one could call exciting. I was convinced that DCI was a drug that blocked those adrenergic receptors Ahlquist called *beta*. I dropped the other projects I was working on and concentrated on DCI. I presented a paper at the Abel Centennial Meeting of the American Society for Pharmacology and Experimental Therapeutics at Johns Hopkins in Baltimore in September 1957 [*J. Pharm. Exp. Ther.* 122: 55A, 1957] in which I described the blockade by DCI of the cardiac effects of epinephrine, norepinephrine, isoproterenol and cardiac sympathetic nerve stimulation *at doses that blocked the vasodilator effects of isoproterenol* and emphasized the fact that vasoconstrictor responses were not blocked. I postulated that the myocardial sympathetic

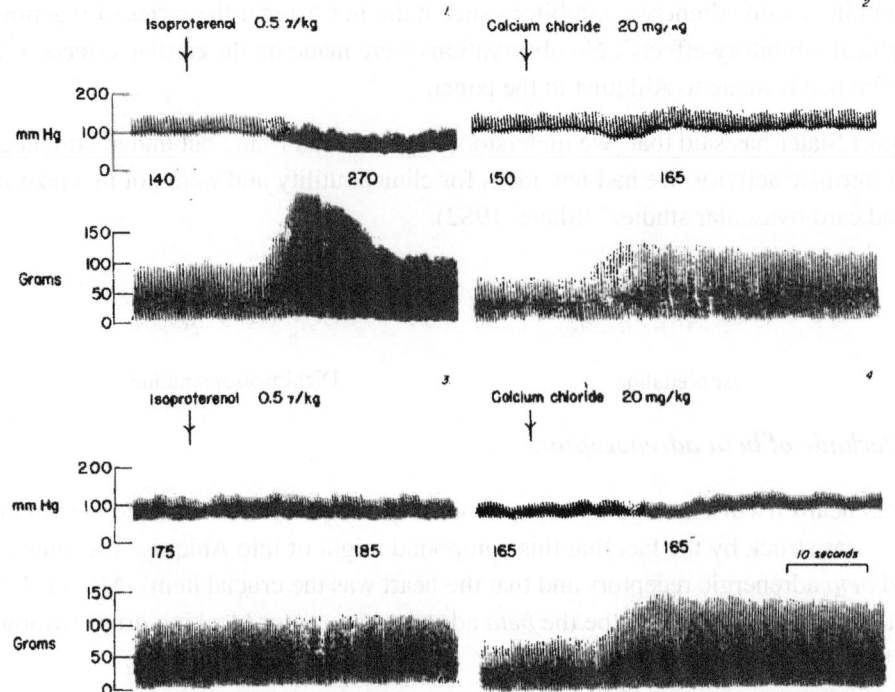

An example of the specificity of cardiac adrenergic blockade by DCI in a vagotomized, anesthetized dog.

Upper pair of tracings shows the effect of intravenous injections of isoproterenol, 0.5 μg/kg, and of calcium chloride, 20 mg/kg, on blood pressure and right ventricular contractile force and heart rate (numbers above contractile force tracings) before administration of DCI. Lower pair of tracings shows the effects of the same drugs after administration of a cumulative dose of DCI of 7 mg/kg.

Figure 1.1
Reproduced from the *Journal of Pharmacology and Experimental Therapeutics*, 1958, *124*, 232.
By permission of the authors and editor.

receptors and the adrenergic inhibitory receptors are functionally homologous, but I did not, at that juncture, propose that DCI was blocking beta adrenergic receptors. I don't remember why, perhaps caution and conservatism' (Moran, 1982).

The full account of this work was published in November 1958 (Moran and Perkins, 1958). They showed in anaesthetised dogs with bilateral cervical sympathectomy that the increase in right ventricular contractile force produced by the intravenous injection of small doses of adrenaline, noradrenaline and isoprenaline and by cardiac post-ganglionic sympathetic nerve stimulation was partially inhibited by small doses of DCI (0.25 mg/kg); complete or nearly complete abolition of the responses occurred with cumulative doses of 7 to 15 mg/kg. DCI also greatly reduced the increase in heart rate and the vasodepressor response produced by isoprenaline. This blocking action of DCI was specific as it did not inhibit the positive inotropic actions of digoxin or calcium chloride or the positive chronotropic action of theophylline (Fig. 1.1).

In vagotomised dogs the intravenous injection of DCI (0.25–2.0 mg/kg) produced slight to moderate increases in cardiac contractile force and heart rate lasting for more than 1 hour and transient decreases in blood pressure lasting less than 15 minutes. These effects indicate stimulation of beta adrenoceptors. Subsequent doses of DCI depressed contractile force and slowed heart rate. Similar effects were seen – stimulation followed depression – in isolated rabbit hearts.

Moran and Perkins (1958) concluded that:

> 'The inhibition of the positive inotropic and chronotropic effects of adrenergic stimuli by the dichloro analogue of isoproterenol appears to represent a specific cardiac adrenergic blockade. To our knowledge this represents the first description of specific adrenergic blockade of mammalian hearts with the exception of reports that several conventional adrenergic blocking agents, such as dibenamine, phenoxybenzamine, phentolamine and piperoxan (933F), inhibit the cardiac actions of sympathomimetic amines. However, these agents produce inconsistent cardiac blocking effects' (Moran and Perkins, 1958). 'The selective blockade of most inhibitory functions and the lack of blockade of vasoconstriction coupled with the present demonstration of blockade by DCI of cardiac positive inotropic and chronotropic effects of adrenergic stimuli support the postulate of Ahlquist (1948) that the adrenotropic inhibitory receptors and the cardiac chronotropic and inotropic adrenergic receptors are functionally identical, i.e. that both are beta type receptors. The concept of alpha and beta receptors represents, therefore, a useful classification of adrenergic receptors. It is suggested that this terminology be extended to the realm of adrenergic blocking drugs, e.g. that blocking drugs be designated according to the receptor for which they have the greatest affinity, as either alpha or beta adrenergic blocking drugs' (Moran and Perkins, 1958).

This appears to be the first use of the term 'beta adrenergic blocking drug' although Moran did not apply it to DCI at that time.

Moran and Perkins (1961) re-evaluated the effects of phenoxybenzamine, phentolamine, dihydroergotamine and DCI on the inotropic actions of catecholamines in anaesthetised dogs. The increase in right ventricular contractile force produced by adrenaline and noradrenaline was not selectively antagonised by the classical adrenergic blocking drugs but DCI selectively inhibited this response. The authors state:

> 'Thus, phenoxybenzamine, phentolamine, and other compounds with similar pharmacological properties would be classified as alpha adrenergic blocking drugs, capable of blocking such adrenergic responses as vasoconstriction and contraction of the nictitating membrane but not responses such as cardioacceleration, augmented cardiac contractile force, vasodilation and bronchodilation. DCI, on the other hand, as a beta adrenergic blocking drug, is capable of inhibiting these responses which the alpha blocking drugs are not and is not capable of blocking the responses inhibited by alpha blocking drugs'.

This would appear to be the first documented application of the terms alpha and beta adrenergic blocking drug to specific drugs.

Further observations on the effects of DCI were made by Dresel (1960) using isolated cat papillary muscles. DCI had considerable adrenaline-like activity as the strength of contraction of driven muscles was increased and the frequency of contraction of spontaneously beating muscles increased. Dresel described these effects as 'high intrinsic activity' and that this action will decrease its value in the elucidation of adrenergic mechanisms. Furchgott had earlier described this effect of DCI at a symposium on catecholamines held in Bethseda, Maryland, in October 1958. He found that DCI in concentrations greater than 10^{-6} M depressed tone and contraction amplitude and had some sympathomimetic activity at the receptors it blocked. He suggested that this latter action might be due in part to the action of DCI as a partial agonist for adrenergic receptors (Furchgott, 1959).

Slater and his colleagues continued to synthesise and test phenylethanolamines and examined about 100 compounds trying to find an agent with less intrinsic activity. Lilly filed a United States patent on nethalide (pronethalol) which was withdrawn because of an earlier filing date by Imperial Chemical Industries. Moran recalls a meeting convened by Lilly to discuss the future development of DCI but apparently no decisions were taken. It would appear that the therapeutic potential of this class of drugs was not appreciated by those present at the meeting or by Lilly.

1.3.3 Studies in man

DCI was reported to control a tachycardia and arrhythmia during excision of a phaechromocytoma (Riddell et al., 1963). This may be the only reported clinical use of a compound which was the forerunner of a most important group of drugs.

Henry Barcroft and David Greenfield had established venous occlusion plethysmography for the measurement of limb blood flow in the Departments of Physiology in St. Thomas's Hospital London and The Queen's University of Belfast in the period 1945–1955. In these Departments it had been demonstrated that the infusion of adrenaline into the brachial artery in man produced an initial large transient increase in flow through the forearm followed by a rapid return of flow to the resting level with small doses; with larger doses of adrenaline the transient increase in flow was followed by a reduction in blood flow to below the resting level (Duff and Swan, 1951). This biphasic response represents a balance between the vasodilator and vasoconstrictor actions of adrenaline. After the administration of phenoxybenzamine to the forearm, the vasoconstriction is reduced or abolished and a sustained dilator effect is unmasked (de La Lande and Whelan, 1959). The intravenous infusion of adrenaline in man, in doses corresponding to those given intra-arterially, produces an initial transient increase in flow followed by a smaller and sustained increase in flow (Allen et al., 1946). The reason for the difference between the responses of the forearm blood vessels to intra-arterial and intravenous infusions of adrenaline was not fully understood when I was appointed to the staff of the Department of Physiology in The Queen's University of Belfast in September 1960. During discussions on this subject, I remembered a seminar which Neil Moran gave in March 1960 when I was a fellow in the Departments of Pharmacology and Physiology in the Medical College of Georgia, Augusta, where Ahlquist was Chairman of Pharmacology. Moran had described the effects of DCI in blocking the vasodilator action of isoprenaline and adrenaline. We wondered if DCI would block the vasodilator action of adrenaline in man and if there would be differences in its effects on adrenaline given intra-arterially and intravenously. I obtained several ampoules containing sterilised powder of DCI (Lilly 20522) from Lilly Research Laboratories. Observations were made in collaboration with A.D.M. Greenfield and W.E. Glover. Blood flow to the forearms was measured by venous occlusion plethysmography in healthy volunteers and a needle inserted into the brachial artery for the administration of drugs (Glover et al., 1962). In the first experiment which was carried out on Greenfield (Chairman of the Department) adrenaline (1.0 ug/min) infused into the brachial artery for 3 minutes produced a typical response consisting of an initial increase in flow followed by a fall to below the resting level. Glover et al. (1962) reported:

> 'Dichloroisoprenaline was then infused into the brachial artery at the rate of 8 mg/min for 4 min. This caused a large transient increase in forearm blood flow on the infused side, which was associated with a warm feeling in the forearm. Flow on this side returned quickly towards the resting level, but remained above it until the end of the infusion. Two minutes after the dichloroisoprenaline infusion commenced the subject complained of a feeling of apprehension, palpitations and an increase in respiration; he described the sensations as being similar to those accompanying an intravenous infusion of adrenaline. Blood flow to the control forearm increased rapidly at this time, but both this rise in flow and the symptoms subsided before the end of the infusion. Twenty-seven minutes after the end of the dichloroisoprenaline infusion the flow was the same on both sides and the intra-arterial infusion of adrenaline was repeated. This time the adrenaline produced no change in flow; dichloroisoprenaline had abolished both the dilator and constrictor actions of adrenaline' (Glover et al., 1962).

These results are shown in Fig. 1.2.

After several further experiments it was discovered that blockade of the vasodilator action of adrenaline could be maintained by the continuous infusion of DCI into the brachial artery at 0.05 mg/min. In these doses, DCI inhibited the vasodilator action of adrenaline given intra-arterially without affecting the vasoconstriction. It also blocked the initial large vasodilatation and subsequent sustained modest vasodilatation produced by the intravenous infusion of adrenaline. The vasodilator action of intra-arterial isoprenaline was also blocked. These results were presented at a meeting of the Physiological Society on November 3, 1961, (Bharadwaj and Shanks, 1962), and the full paper published in the *British Journal of Pharmacology and Chemotherapy* in October 1962 (Glover et al., 1962). These studies confirmed

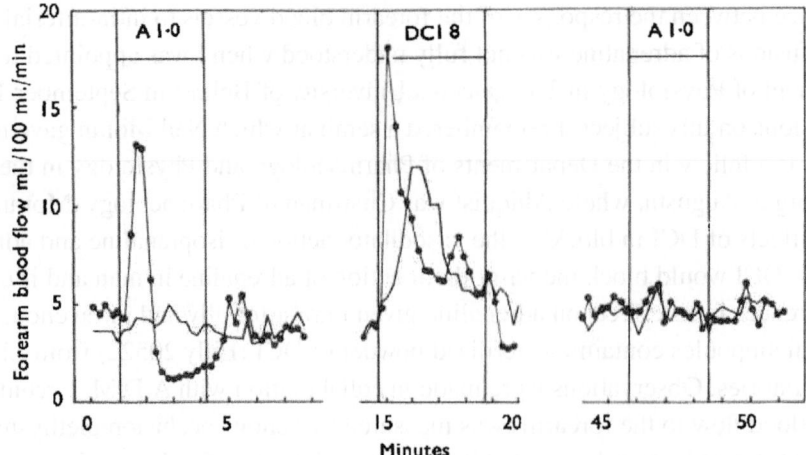

The response of forearm blood flow to intra-arterial adrenaline (1.0 μg/min) before and after the intra-arterial infusion of DCI (8 mg/min). —— Control side; ●——● infused side.

Figure 1.2
Reproduced from the *British Journal of Pharmacology and Chemotherapy*, 1962, *19*, 236. By permission of the authors and editor.

the presence of beta adrenoceptors in the blood vessels of the human forearm and that the sustained vasodilatation with intravenous adrenaline was due to stimulation of these receptors. These studies were the first to demonstrate the activity of a beta adrenoceptor blocking drug in man. The tachycardia and vasodilatation in the first experiment were manifestations of the intrinsic sympathomimetic activity (partial agonist activity) of DCI.

We made no observations of the effects of DCI on heart rate and blood pressure changes produced by the intravenous infusion of adrenaline. In retrospect this probably occurred for several reasons. In the first experiment a large dose (32 mg) of DCI was infused into the brachial artery and had marked systemic effects although 8 mg had no such effect. We were probably concerned that intravenous administration might lead to systemic effects, e.g. a tachycardia. At that time the main interest of the Department was in the peripheral vascular effects of drugs; changes in heart rate and blood pressure were not routinely measured and we saw no reason to include such observations in our studies. Although isoprenaline was given by infusion into the brachial artery we had no experience of intravenous infusion of this drug. At no time did we envisage any therapeutic role for DCI.

1.4 Beta adrenoceptor blocking drugs in treatment of angina

Bilateral cervical sympathectomy in which the upper three or four dorsal ganglia of the sympathetic chain were excised was introduced in the 1940s for the relief of refractory anginal pain as cardiac pain is transmitted by afferent fibres which accompany the sympathetic nerves to the heart (White, 1943). In 1960, Apthorp et al. (1960) using treadmill exercise, showed that objective improvement in myocardial performance was produced by cervical sympathectomy. These findings were extended by showing that the increase in effort tolerance after sympathectomy was associated with improvement in the electrocardiogram during effort (Apthorp et al., 1964). Exercise heart rate was reduced in 7 out of 8 patients after sympathectomy.

Dr. D.A. Chamberlain was a Medical Registrar at St. Bartholomew's Hospital when these observations were being made (1961–1964) and realised that the beneficial effects of cervical sympathectomy may have resulted from division of the sympathetic nerves to the heart and not from interruption of the afferent pain fibres. He was of the opinion that a similar effect could be obtained by the administration of a drug to block the effects of the sympathetic on the heart. He was familiar with the studies by Moran on DCI and tried for some time to obtain supplies of this drug from Lilly. The drug arrived the day before a paper was published in the *Lancet* by Black and Stephenson (1962) describing the properties of pronethalol. Instead of using DCI, he made studies with pronethalol which had effects on effort tolerance, the exercise electrocardiogram and exercise heart rate similar to cervical sympathectomy (Apthorp et al., 1964). They concluded that the objective improvement in angina following sympathectomy and beta adrenergic blockade were due principally to the reduction in tachycardia and oxygen-wasting increase in contractility which are the normal responses to excitement and exercise. Chamberlain (1966) subsequently showed that propranolol and cervical sympathectomy reduced an exercise tachycardia to the same extent.

It is probable that if Black had not commenced his quest for a drug to improve exercise tolerance by inhibiting cardiac sympathetic drive that Chamberlain would have demonstrated this effect with DCI and possibly encouraged Lilly to develop a drug which had less intrinsic sympathomimetic activity.

1.5 The hypothesis of J.W. Black

The discovery of beta adrenoceptor blocking drugs has been attributed to J.W. Black (now Sir James Black) but this is probably too simplistic a belief. Black's contribution was to appreciate that drugs which would block the beta adrenoceptor might be of value in the treatment of disease, in the first instance angina. This was the crucial step that was not made or appreciated by anyone who had worked with DCI with the exception of Chamberlain and in the end he made no observations with this drug in man.

Black qualified in medicine at St. Andrews University, Scotland, in 1946, and after a period in Malaya returned in 1950 to the University of Glasgow to a lectureship in veterinary physiology.

At that time, the drug treatment of angina pectoris was directed towards coronary vasodilatation to increase the supply of oxygen to the ischaemic myocardium. The only reliably effective drug for the relief of angina pectoris was glyceryl trinitrate which was thought to act through dilatation of the coronary vessels. Other drugs which were potent coronary vasodilators in animals were not effective in patients. While it was being realised that coronary vasodilator drugs were not increasing the supply of oxygen to the heart, other methods were being developed for this purpose. These involved patients breathing hyperbaric oxygen (Smith and Lawson, 1958) or having additional arteries implanted into the myocardium (Beck, 1957). Black worked with Smith in Glasgow and became familiar with the problems of increasing blood supply to the heart and appreciated that coronary artery disease – either angina pectoris or acute myocardial infarction – arose when the supply of oxygen did not meet the demand from the heart.

Black appreciated that many factors including age, sex, nutritional state, heredity, physical exercise and emotional stress were associated in the aetiology of coronary artery disease. In particular he was impressed by the crucial role of stress either emotional or exercise in precipitating an anginal attack. The intravenous injection of adrenaline was known to produce all the electrocardiographic signs of acute coronary insufficiency, and was even used as a diagnostic test.

Black had tested a commercial extract of bovine heart muscle, for which a variety of therapeutic claims relating to coronary artery disease had been made, and showed that the administration of this extract to rabbits for 2 weeks protected the rabbit hearts against the coronary vasoconstrictor effects of pitressin (Black, 1960). Other studies with this extract had shown the presence of 'anti-adrenaline activity' with respect to heart muscle but not with respect to blood vessels.

Black speculated that the treatment of coronary artery disease would be advanced by reducing cardiac oxygen consumption rather than trying to increase coronary blood flow. As increased catecholamine secretion during stress leads to an increase in cardiac demand for oxygen without an increase in supply, Black hypothesised, on the basis of his studies with the heart extract, that it might be possible to develop a new approach for the treatment of coronary artery disease through blockade of the action of adrenaline in the heart.

At that time Black does not appear to have been specific about the discovery of drugs for different types of coronary artery disease, e.g. acute myocardial infarction and angina pectoris. The signs and symptoms of coronary artery disease arise from an imbalance between oxygen supply and demand. Acute interruption of the oxygen supply gives rise to myocardial infarction and death from ventricular fibrillation whereas an imbalance during stress gives rise to reversible chest pain. It would appear that Black seemed to think that these two entities might be controlled at the same time.

Black came in contact with the Pharmaceuticals Division of Imperial Chemical Industries (ICI) in 1957. This Division had just moved into new purpose built facilities in pleasant surroundings in Alderley Edge, in rural Cheshire. The nature and circumstances which led Black to ICI are now confused. Black may have gone to ICI on a scientific visit, in response to an advertisement or ICI staff may have visited him in Glasgow in response to an application for funds. The link men at ICI were Dr. J.Y. Bogue (Research Director) and Dr. Garnet Davey who had been recently appointed to the post of Manager of the Biology Research Department.

Black appears to have described his novel ideas to ICI about a new type of drug for the treatment of coronary artery disease and they were sufficiently convinced to give him their backing and an opportunity to pursue his ideas when he joined in July 1958. These ideas are summarized in a *'Project Team Report'* from ICI in January 1959:

> 'There are two clearly differentiated sympathetic receptors $-\alpha$ receptors associated with excitatory effects on blood vessels and smooth muscle and β receptors associated with inhibitory effects on smooth muscle and possibly cardiac muscle. All the known adrenolytic agents are α receptor inhibitors. Presumably the unknown factor in heart muscle is a β receptor inhibitor and recently, the dichloro analogue of isoprenaline has been shown to be a powerful β receptor inhibitor. The question of whether this latter compound will effectively block the cardiac sympathetic responses remains to be satisfactorily answered.

> It seems clear that the search for compounds which will block cardiac sympathetic responses constitutes a clear-cut pharmacological problem and screening tests are being developed. In addition experiments are planned which will attempt to elucidate further the possible value of such compounds in coronary artery disease'.

1.6 Pronethalol

1.6.1 Discovery – studies in animals

Black established methods for the assessment of the activity of compounds in blocking beta adrenoceptors. He settled on 'heart rate' as the key measurement using a simple Langendorff preparation – isolated perfused spontaneously beating guinea pig heart (Black, 1967).

Black obtained a sample of DCI from Lilly in January 1959 – two months after Moran and Perkins published their paper. Within the next few months Black tested DCI on his Langendorff preparation and 'found it to be about as active as isoprenaline as a cardiac stimulant and rejected it as a suitable compound for antagonising the cardiac actions of catecholamines which had been our objective. Many months later we changed our technique and used rate-controlled guinea-pig papillary muscle preparations. When dichloroisoprenaline was retested it had practically no positive inotropic effects at doses which completely blocked the effects of catecholamines; as with the Langendorff preparations, however, the rate of contraction of isolated guinea-pig atria was also stimulated. Since the measurement of heart rate gave a simple means of assaying both beta-receptor blockade and the intrinsic activity of beta-receptor antagonists, the measurement of heart rate in the cat was used for further evaluations of potential antagonists (Black and Stephenson, 1962)' (Black, 1967).

By the end of 1959, Black had established a series of test preparations that demonstrated both the beta adrenoceptor blocking activity of DCI and its intrinsic sympathomimetic activity. During this time the testing of compounds continued but none was as active as DCI.

The important breakthrough came in January 1960, when John Stephenson – a medicinal chemist at ICI – conceived of replacing the two chlorine molecules in DCI by another phenyl ring to make a naphthalene. Stephenson synthesised this new compound (ICI 38174, pronethalol, 'Alderlin') in February, 1960, and it was tested by Black in March, 1960. For a short time this compound was called 'nethalide'. ICI 38174 was shown to block the positive inotropic and chronotropic effects of adrenaline on several isolated tissue preparations and the increases in heart rate produced by the intravenous injection of isoprenaline and by cardiac nerve stimulation in anaesthetised cats (*ICI Report,* June 1960). ICI 38174 had no intrinsic activity on isolated preparations and no effect on heart rate in anaesthetised cats. The drug was absorbed on oral administration and the LD_{50} values on IV and oral administration were 50 mg/kg and over 300 mg/kg, respectively. By June 1960 sufficient work had been completed to suggest that this compound possessed most of the properties that were postulated to be necessary in a compound to protect the heart from the effects of adrenaline (*ICI Project Team Report,* June 1960).

During the remainder of 1960, Black and his colleagues demonstrated that ICI 38174 blocked beta adrenoceptors in several species while producing few adverse physiological consequences. The only consistent change the animals developed was some degree of bradycardia which was attributed to blockade of cardiac sympathetic drive. A moderate lowering of blood pressure occurred in anaesthetised animals after intravenous injection of pronethalol, rapid injections reduced myocardial contractility and cardiac output. Intravenous injection in conscious and anaesthetised dogs produced a bright red flush of abdominal skin; Slater described a similar phenomenon with DCI which resulted in it being called the 'pinking compound'.

Black appears to have been concerned about the effect of pronethalol on cardiac contractility which at that time was difficult to assess in intact animals. One of Black's technicians, Brian Horsfall, made isometric strain gauge arches similar to those used by Moran (Shanks, 1966a). These were attached to the surface of the left ventricle in open chest anaesthetised dogs to assess the effects of pronethalol on cardiac contractile force and its effects on the inotropic responses to catecholamines and left cardiac sympathetic nerve stimulation. Pronethalol antagonised these responses. The rapid intravenous injection of pronethalol depressed cardiac contractions but slow intravenous infusion produced very small change. Black and Horsfall also constructed an acceleration ballisto-cardiograph to assess the cardiac actions of pronethalol. The drug produced effects opposite to those of adrenaline – slight prolongation of systole and decrease in the rate of development of change of tension (Black, 1967). The dog heart was shown to be capable of both adjusting its stroke volume to increased venous return and of maintaining its stroke volume with increased arterial pressure loading after treatment with pronethalol. There was no obvious evidence that pronethalol would cause cardiac failure in animals and no studies were made of the effects of the drug on cardiac work (Black, 1967).

Chronic toxicity studies were also started in rats during this period. Although some animals died during the first few days in the top dose (500 mg/kg/day) group, the study was completed satisfactorily when the dose was reduced to 250 mg/kg twice daily (*ICI Project Team Report*, February 1961). In further chronic toxicity studies in rats some animals died after becoming blue and wheezy within a short time of dose administration which was by an oesophageal catheter. Deaths occurred when the study had been in progress for several weeks. As a result it was decided to commence chronic toxicity tests in mice. Later it was suggested that the rats had died from ICI 38174 being administered into the pharynx and inhaled to produce death by drowning or from the rapid absorption of a large amount of drug.

The studies in animals were designed to demonstrate that pronethalol blocked beta adrenoceptors, from which Black predicted, on interpretation of the literature on angina pectoris, that beta adrenergic blockade would reduce the consumption of oxygen by the ischaemic myocardium and have the same net effect as increasing its oxygen supply (Black, 1967). Pronethalol was not tried in animals with experimentally induced pathological conditions before it was administered to man as Black believed 'that predictions based on the therapeutics of experimental disease are much less reliable than predictions based on pharmacological actions in normal animals' (Black, 1967).

Black and Stephenson described the properties of pronethalol in the *Lancet* of 18th August 1962. The concluding paragraph states:

> 'We are hoping that this compound will be sufficiently active to examine some pharmacological and clinical problems. For example, will conditions such as atrial fibrillation, and atrial and ventricular tachycardia, be helped by reducing the cardiac sympathomimetic responses to anxiety, emotion, and exercise? Again, will myocardial adrenergic blockade reduce the myocardial demand for oxygen, and, if so, will this be helpful to patients with angina? These are some of the problems we are currently investigating with compound 38174'.

1.6.2 Studies in man

Towards the end of 1961, Professor A.C. Dornhorst, of St. George's Hospital, London, visited Black at his laboratories to discuss investigation of the beta adrenoceptor blocking activity of pronethalol in man after we had published our abstract on DCI (Bharadwaj and Shanks, 1962). These studies were completed by the summer of 1962 and reported in the same issue of the *Lancet* in which Black and Stephenson described their findings (Dornhorst and Robinson, 1962). These investigators measured forearm blood flow, blood pressure and heart rate in normal subjects. The infusion of pronethalol into the brachial artery increased forearm blood flow and abolished the dilator response to the intra-arterial infusion of isoprenaline and adrenaline. In 6 subjects pronethalol (1–1.5 mg/kg) was infused intravenously over 6–10 minutes.

'Towards the end of the infusion, all the subjects developed a feeling of unsteadiness and some noted that objects appeared to move if the head was rotated suddenly while the gaze was fixed. These symptoms were never accompanied by nystagmus, but some subjects developed nausea and one had paraesthesiae. The disturbance of balance resulted in an uncertain gait on a wide base, but Romberg's sign was negative. Oral administration, either as a single dose of 200–300 mg, or as repeated doses of 100–200 mg three times a day, also produced unsteadiness, nausea and vomiting in some subjects; but the symptoms tended to subside with continued administration, and there was much variation in individual susceptibility. Other symptoms sometimes included sleeplessness and diarrhoea' (Dornhorst and Robinson, 1962).

In these subjects pronethalol had no consistent effect on resting heart rate or blood pressure; the increases in heart rate and forearm blood flow produced by the intravenous infusion of isoprenaline were abolished by pronethalol. In separate studies, the oral administration of pronethalol reduced resting heart rate in 10 normal subjects by 0–26% and in 14 patients with angina by 3 to 31%; exercise heart rate was reduced by 4 to 25% and by 10 to 31% in the two groups respectively. In 9 out of 10 patients with angina more work could be done before the development of anginal pain and in 5 out of 10 the electrocardiogram showed less abnormality than it had at comparable rates of work in the control run (Dornhorst and Robinson, 1962).

These observations clearly showed that on oral and intravenous administration pronethalol blocked cardiac beta adrenoceptors in man with no deleterious effects on the cardiovascular system although the authors indicated clearly that great caution may be required in patients with cardiac failure. The increase in exercise tolerance in patients with angina clearly indicated that the drug might be of value in the treatment of this condition through reducing cardiac work and myocardial oxygen requirements at any given level of exercise.

Clinical trials were established to assess the effectiveness of pronethalol in the treatment of angina pectoris at University College Hospital and St. George's Hospital London and in Stockport, Cheshire. In a double-blind comparison with placebo in 30 patients, these trials established that the active drug was effective in the relief of angina as shown by a reduction in the consumption of glyceryl trinitrate and in the number of anginal attacks and by an improvement in exercise tolerance (Alleyne et al., 1963). These studies probably commenced in the middle of 1962 and were published in the *British Medical Journal* in November 1963.

Mild side-effects occurred frequently in patients, but could be minimised by dosage reduction or by increasing the dose gradually. The side-effects were most commonly of central nervous origin consisting of paraesthesia, 'walking on air', visual disturbance, dreams, fatigue, dizziness, nausea and vomiting (Alleyne et al., 1963); mild side-effects were frequent (Fulton and Green, 1963).

Peter Stock, a cardiologist in Stoke-on-Trent, investigated Black's suggestion that pronethalol might be helpful in the management of atrial fibrillation and in ventricular and atrial tachycardias by reducing the cardiosympathomimetic responses to emotion and exercise (Stock and Dale, 1963). Pronethalol reduced the ventricular rate in undigitalized and digitalized patients with atrial fibrillation, and exercise rate in the latter group. Thirteen of 21 patients with atrial fibrillation claimed substantial symptomatic improvement when the heart rate was slowed by pronethalol. The drug had little effect in atrial flutter and paroxysmal tachycardia but abolished ventricular extrasystoles in 4 out of 6 patients. Pronethalol was most effective in abolishing the toxic rhythm in patients with digitalis intoxication. Stock concluded that pronethalol would be of value in combination with digitalis in patients with atrial fibrillation as together they prevented the excessive rise in ventricular rate on exercise which often occurs with digitalis alone.

Stock also reported that pronethalol precipitated cardiac failure in some patients and made it worse in patients already in failure. This was attributed to a weakening of cardiac contraction from removal of catecholamine drive and from a failure of stroke volume to increase to maintain cardiac output when ventricular rate is slowed (Stock and Dale, 1963). They recommended 'that the drug should be given with great caution in the presence of established or incipient heart failure'.

1.7 Propranolol

1.7.1 Discovery

Black was always of the opinion that although pronethalol fitted his concept of a beta adrenoceptor blocking drug and was a marked improvement on DCI, it was not ideal because of the occurrence of non-specific adverse effects in patients which would restrict its use. In a *Project Team Report* in January 1962 Black wrote 'that analogues of ICI 38174 (pronethalol) were being tested to find a compound which was longer acting, had greater resistance to catecholamine breakthrough and showed less penetration of the central nervous system'.

At I.C.I. many new compounds were synthesised and tested in anaesthetised cats for inhibition of the chronotropic and vasodilator actions of isoprenaline (Shanks, 1966a). These compounds were made for the completion of patents and on a speculative basis for increased beta adrenoceptor blocking activity. The first compound to show a marked increase in activity

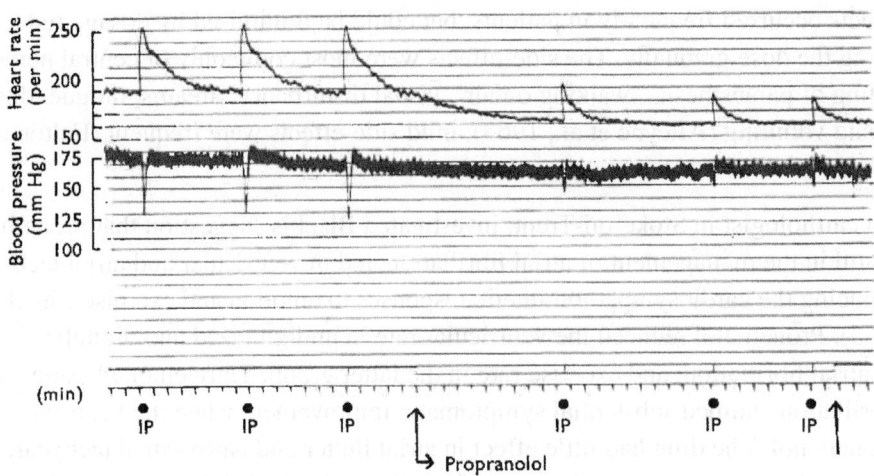

Cat, chloralose anaesthesia ; heart rate and femoral arterial pressure records. Responses to intravenous injections of isoprenaline (at IP ; 0.2 µg/kg) were obtained before and during the intravenous infusion of propranolol (between arrows ; 2.5 µg/kg/min).

Figure 1.3

Reproduced from the *British Journal of Pharmacology and Chemotherapy*, 1965, *25*, 581. By permission of the authors and editor.

over pronethalol was ICI 45520 (propranolol – 'Inderal'). This compound was conceived by A.F. Crowther and synthesised by L.H. Smith who were varying the distance of the CHOH group from the aromatic ring by the insertion of different groups; one of the groups selected was -OCH$_2$. This normally would have been done by a reaction involving β-naphthol but as α-naphthol was available Smith used this instead, and obtained ICI 45520; the compound made from β-naphthol is less active.

I joined I.C.I. in September 1962 to assist Black on the study of beta adrenoceptor blocking drugs. One of my first experiments was to administer ICI 45520 to a cat in November 1962. I found that it produced marked inhibition of the isoprenaline responses (Fig. 1.3); within a few days it was shown to be about 10 times more potent than pronethalol. In a few weeks it was found that the acute LD$_{50}$ values in mice for pronethalol and ICI 45520 were similar and that the intravenous dose required to produce neurological signs in conscious dogs was the same for the two compounds. As it was believed that these neurological signs in dogs correlated with the central side-effects in man, it was clear that ICI 45520 would have a greatly increased ratio between doses required to produce beta adrenoceptor blockade and adverse effects in patients.

By this time the stereoisomers of pronethalol had been synthesised at I.C.I. The laevo isomer was 40 times more potent than the dextroisomer in blocking beta adrenoceptors but the two isomers were equally effective in producing effects on the central nervous system and had the same acute LD_{50} in mice. These studies indicated that the adverse effects of pronethalol in patients might not arise from the beta blocking activity of the drug but from a non-specific action.

Propranolol

Pronethalol

Thus it was anticipated that ICI 45520 would block beta adrenoceptors in man with a reduced incidence of non-specific adverse effects.

Shortly after the discovery of propranolol, malignant tumours were found to occur with pronethalol in a chronic toxicity study in mice. These occurred first and most commonly in the thymus gland. As the study progressed generalised lymphosarcoma and reticulum-cell sarcomas of liver, spleen and genital tract developed (Paget, 1963). Repeat chronic toxicity studies confirmed the carcinogenic action of pronethalol (Alcock and Bond, 1964). Tumours did not occur in chronic toxicity studies in rats, guinea pigs, dogs or monkeys, although in the latter two studies these may have not continued sufficiently long to produce an effect (Alcock and Bond, 1964). The mechanism of this carcinogenic action of pronethalol has not been discovered.

These effects in mice were first reported in December 1962 when the clinical trials with pronethalol were almost complete. They were a major set-back to plans to market the drug which had to be delayed. Eventually the drug was marketed in the United Kingdom in November 1963 but with a restricted licence which would only permit its use in 'the treatment of conditions which themselves threaten life immediately or cause such morbidity that only short survival may be expected' (Paget, 1963).

This had been a difficult decision to reach although it was easier as propranolol had already been discovered and no tumours had developed in a chronic toxicity study in mice dosed at 200 mg/kg for 39 weeks. All effort was concentrated on the development of propranolol.

1.7.2 Studies in man

Early in 1964, studies with propranolol were started in man at ICI by J.W. Black, W.A.M. Duncan and myself. We showed that the oral administration of propranolol inhibited an isoprenaline tachycardia in 4 healthy subjects. In another 6 subjects an exercise tachycardia was reduced by 30 mg propranolol with the maximum effect occurring 1.5 hours after dosing but the tachycardia was still reduced after 6 hours (Shanks, 1966b) (Fig. 1.4). Resting heart rate was also reduced in the later study. Dornhorst confirmed the beta blocking activity of propranolol and that it did not produce light-headedness or incoordination (Black et al., 1964).

Pharmacological Studies with Propranolol (Inderal)

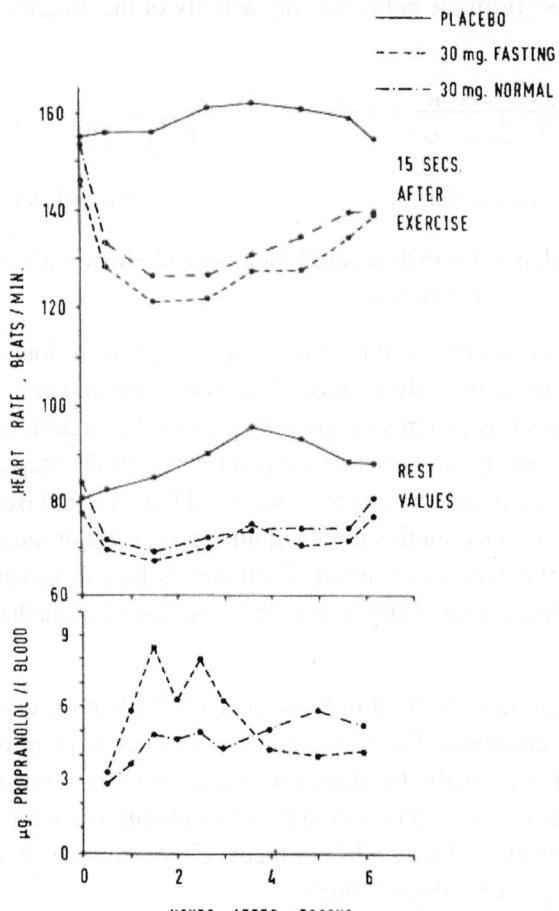

The effect of the oral administration of 30 mg placebo or propranolol on resting heart rate and the heart rate after 2 minutes of severe exercise in normal volunteers. These are the averaged results from groups of six. The concentration of propranolol in blood samples taken at regular intervals is also shown.

Figure 1.4
Reproduced from *Cardiologia Supplementum* 11, 1966, *49*, 15. By permission of the author and editor.

The properties of propranolol were described in a short paper published in the Lancet of 16th May 1964 (Black et al., 1964). The final paragraph reads: 'In conclusion, ICI 45520 is an adrenergic β-receptor antagonist which has a therapeutic ratio about ten times greater than that of pronethalol. It has not caused thymic tumours in mice, and in man does not produce the side-effects associated with pronethalol. The evidence suggests that ICI 45520 should have extended evaluation'.

Clinical studies commenced in the summer of 1964 and soon indicated that propranolol was a safe and effective drug for the treatment of angina pectoris and cardiac arrhythmias with a low incidence of adverse effects. Clinical evaluation progressed rapidly in the British Isles and in many other countries and confirmed the initial findings. Detailed studies were made on the effects of propranolol on many aspects of cardiac function in a variety of clinical conditions and it was used as a research tool to elucidate many aspects of cardiovascular function. The use of the drug in treatment was extended to hypertrophic obstructive cardiomyopathy, hypertension (see later), cardiac arrhythmias, tremor and hyperthyroidism. The main adverse effects could be attributed to the pharmacological effect of the drug inhibiting sympathetic drive to beta adrenoceptors. These effects included bronchospasm, bradycardia and cardiac failure. There was a low incidence of non-specific adverse effects (Stephen, 1966).

Within eighteen months sufficient experience had been obtained with propranolol to hold a major symposium entitled 'Beta adrenergic receptor blockade' in Buxton, England, on 10 and 11 November, 1965, at which thirty papers were given by investigators from different countries on the effects of propronalol in several conditions (Braunwald, 1966).

Sir Ian Hill stated in his closing remarks 'I think it has been established that propranolol is of both potential and established value' (Hill, 1966). I doubt if anyone at that meeting could have predicted the contribution of propranolol to many aspects of medical science. The literature on the drug is voluminous and continues to grow. Propranolol has become the standard reference beta adrenoceptor blocking drug.

It is interesting to note that at this meeting Dr. P.J.D. Snow from Bolton, England, described the results of the first secondary prevention study of a beta blocking drug in patients with acute myocardial infarction (Snow, 1966). Alternate patients admitted to hospital with a history of acute myocardial infarction within the preceding 24 hours were treated with propranolol; the remaining patients served as controls. In the control group of 55 patients, 16 (29%) died of cardiac causes and in the propranolol treated group of 52 patients 9 (13%) died. This difference between the two groups was highly significant. Although many aspects of this trial can be criticised, it is interesting that 17 years, many thousands of patients and many millions of dollars later, that it has been finally concluded that 'There is no doubt that late treatment with a beta-blocker reduces mortality in patients who have had a myocardial infarction' (Hampton, 1982).

Propranolol was first marketed in the United Kingdom in July 1965, two years and 8 months after the drug was first given to an animal. This was a remarkable achievement and was only obtained by a well organised research and development programme involving the Research, Development and Medical Departments at ICI. Excellent collaboration was provided by numerous clinicians. Pronethalol was withdrawn from the United Kingdom market in October 1965.

Unfortunately, J.W. Black left ICI in the middle of 1964 and was not present at the symposium in Buxton to see the fulfillment of his ideas. However, the research on beta adrenoceptor blocking drugs continued without interruption at ICI.

1.8 Ancillary properties of beta adrenoceptor antagonists

1.8.1 Intrinsic sympathomimetic activity (partial agonist activity)

As pronethalol, in contrast to DCI, produced little change in resting heart rate in animals, it was concluded that it was devoid of intrinsic sympathomimetic activity (Black and Stephenson, 1962). The administration of propranolol to anaesthetized or conscious animals always reduced resting heart rate (Black et al., 1965). Why was there this difference between pronethalol and propranolol? The answer was obtained when the effects were compared of the two drugs on heart rate in anaesthetized cats pretreated with syrosingopine – a derivative of reserpine – to deplete the cardiac stores of noradrenaline (Black et al., 1965; Shanks, 1966a). In these animals DCI produced a marked increase in heart rate, pronethalol a small increase (20–30 beats/min) and propranolol no change. It was concluded that propranolol had no intrinsic sympathomimetic activity and reduced heart rate in normal animals through blockade of tonic sympathetic drive to the sino-atrial node. Pronethalol had slight intrinsic sympathomimetic activity which balanced the blockade of sympathetic drive in normal animals and resulted in no change in heart rate.

Shortly after the discovery of propranolol, it was found that increasing the distance of the CHOH from the aromatic ring by the insertion of $-OCH_2$ enhanced the beta blocking activity of compounds when the aromatic moiety was phenyl or substituted phenyl. As it was not known if the 'naphthalene' part of pronethalol was responsible for its carcinogenic action, it was decided that a phenoxy derivative should also undergo carcinogenicity testing in mice along with propranolol. If propranolol was carcinogenic and the phenoxy compound was clear, the latter would have proceeded to clinical evaluation; but this did not occur as propranolol did not produce tumours. The compound chosen for testing was ICI 45763 which in animals was equipotent with propranolol in blocking beta adrenoceptors (Shanks, 1966a). Studies in mice showed that it was not carcinogenic. In laboratory animals ICI 45763 had intrinsic sympathomimetic activity. In man ICI 45763 had about one third the activity of propranolol in reducing an exercise tachycardia and had a shorter duration of effect (Shanks, 1966b). ICI 45763 was developed independently by Boehringer Ingelheim in West Germany and they eventually obtained a licence from ICI. This compound had pharmacological properties similar to alprenolol and oxprenolol.

When it was found that propranolol was not a carcinogen and was effective and well tolerated in patients, no further development work was undertaken by ICI with ICI 45763. Although we realised that it had intrinsic sympathomimetic activity, we were not sure of the importance of this in a beta adrenoceptor blocking drug. We were concerned that intrinsic sympathomimetic activity might increase myocardial oxygen consumption and thus be of little value in angina; we probably did not consider that intrinsic sympathomimetic activity might prevent some of the adverse effects (bradycardia, cardiac failure and bronchospasm) produced by propranolol.

Several beta adrenoceptor blocking drugs have been developed that possess intrinsic sympathomimetic activity including alprenolol, oxprenolol and pindolol. These are as effective as propranolol in the treatment of angina, cardiac arrhythmias and hypertension but there is no evidence that their use is associated with a lower incidence of adverse effects (Reale and Motolese, 1981; Shanks, 1981). Intrinsic sympathomimetic activity is now described as partial agonist activity.

1.8.2 Membrane stabilizing activity

In 1963 Vaughan Williams reported that pronethalol abolished and prevented ventricular arrhythmias produced by ouabain, a digitalis glycoside, in guinea pigs (Vaughan Williams and Sekiya, 1963), was more active than quinidine in conventional tests for anti-fibrillatory action (Sekiya and Vaughan Williams, 1963a, b) and was a powerful local anaesthetic (Gill and Vaughan Williams, 1964). This posed a most important question about the mode of action of pronethalol in patients. Was the anti-arrhythmic effect, especially on digitalis arrhythmias, due to a quinidine-like action and was the beneficial action in angina due to a local anaesthetic effect on the cardiac pain fibres? Although it was believed by the investigators at ICI that the effects of pronethalol in these two conditions resulted from blockade of beta adrenoceptors, it was some time before information accumulated to provide sufficient proof.

Resolution of pronethalol into its dextro and laevo optical isomers (Howe, 1963) was used to determine the contribution of the beta blocking effect and quinidine like effects to the anti-arrhythmic action of pronethalol (Lucchesi, 1965). As the dextro isomer, which had little beta blocking activity, and racemic pronethalol were equally effective in preventing cardiac arrhythmias produced by ouabain, and by methyl-chloroform and adrenaline, it appeared that the effects of pronethalol on digitalis arrhythmia in animals were not due to blockade of beta adrenoceptors but the clinical relevance of these findings was inclear.

Resolution of propranolol into its two optical isomers (laevo and dextro) confirmed the earlier observations with pronethalol. The laevo isomer was 60 to 100 times more potent than the dextro isomer in blocking beta adrenoceptors but the two isomers were equally effective in abolishing ouabain-induced arrhythmias in anaesthetised cats (Howe and Shanks, 1966). Further studies showed that the two isomers of propranolol were equi-potent as local anaesthetics (Shanks, 1969). Eventually clinical studies confirmed that the dextro isomer of propranolol was largely without effect in the clinical conditions responding to propranolol (Shanks, 1976). These studies clearly indicated that the therapeutic benefits of propranolol arose from blockade of beta adrenoceptors.

1.9 Practolol

1.9.1 Discovery

Another approach to this problem was opened up when scientists from the American Pharmaceutical Company, Mead Johnson, described the properties of a new compound MJ 1999 (sotalol) at the meeting of the Division of Medicinal Chemistry of the American Chemical Society, Philadelphia in April, 1964 (see later). In a variety of tests MJ 1999 was shown to be a beta adrenoceptor antagonist, devoid of partial agonist activity, with no local anaesthetic activity and low acute toxicity (Lish et al., 1965). The acute LD_{50} of sotalol appeared to be much greater than that of pronethalol. Sotalol had low central nervous system toxicity which was attributed to its low lipid solubility in contrast to the high lipid solubility of pronethalol. Although this paper was given to the meeting in April and the Abstract published in *Federation Proceedings,* we did not hear about sotalol at ICI until a few months later.

A.F. Crowther, who was leader of the synthetic chemical team on the beta adrenoceptor blocking drug project, attended a Gordon Research Conference in the summer of 1964 where he learned of the Mead Johnson compound. A cable was sent to ICI suggesting that a sulphonamide-substituted molecule be synthesised. At the meeting he also learned that sotalol had low lipid solubility and would be less likely to penetrate the central nervous system to produce adverse effects. In a short time Crowther's colleagues had synthesised sotalol, its phenoxy derivative (ICI 50232) and the acetamido derivative of ICI 50232. This latter compound (ICI 50172) was practolol ('Eraldin').

Within a short time we had confirmed that sotalol and ICI 50172 (practolol) and ICI 50232 were potent beta adrenoceptor blocking drugs with ICI 50232 being the most potent and comparable to propranolol; sotalol had about one eighth and practolol about one third of the activity of propranolol. Acute toxicity studies in mice showed that the LD_{50} for these three new compounds was much greater than for pronethalol and propranolol. Thus the therapeutic ratio for ICI 50232 was greater than that for propranolol while the ratios for sotalol and practolol were similar to that of propranolol.

As these three compounds were much less lipid soluble than pronethalol and propranolol, it was thought that they penetrated the central nervous system to a smaller extent and that this accounted for the increase in LD_{50}. It is interesting to note that 2 years earlier Black had suggested that the therapeutic ratio of pronethalol could be increased by reducing its lipid solubility.

As there was concern at ICI in the later part of 1964 about the possible adverse effects e.g. negative inotropic effect, that might result from the 'quinidine-like activity' of propranolol, it was decided to develop a compound for clinical study which was devoid of this property. Sotalol had been shown by Mead Johnson to have no local anaesthetic properties and within a short time we showed that ICI 50232 and practolol were also devoid of this property; it was assumed that local anaesthetic activity was a manifestation of the 'quinidine-like effect'.

Detailed pharmacological studies were carried out with ICI 50232 and practolol. The beta adrenoceptor blocking activity of both compounds was confirmed; they had no effect on ouabain induced arrhythmias and were not local anaesthetics. There was a difference in their effects on resting heart rate in conscious and anaesthetised animals; sotalol, propranolol and ICI 50232 reduced heart rate but practolol had no effect. Studies in syrosingopine treated rats showed that practolol increased heart rate due to intrinsic sympathomimetic activity (Dunlop and Shanks, 1968).

Practolol was chosen for comparison with the dextro isomer of propranolol in clinical studies to assess the role of the quinidine-like effect of propranolol in its therapeutic action. Initial plans had been to select a compound that was devoid of partial agonist activity, as the extent to which this influenced the therapeutic effect of beta blocking compounds was not known, but these were not implemented by the selection of practolol which may have been chosen as its structure was new, whereas ICI 50232 was closely related to sotalol. Studies with dextro propranolol were started in patients with cardiac arrhythmias in the first few months of 1966 but those with practolol were delayed by the submission to the Dunlop Committee. Only a few comparisons (Wilson et al., 1969) were made between practolol and the dextro isomer of propranolol to settle the question about the contribution of the quinidine-like effect to the therapeutic and adverse effects of propranolol as practolol was developed independently for its own unique property.

Confusion has persisted about the terminology used to describe this additional property of beta adrenoceptor blocking drugs. Pronethalol and propranolol were shown to be potent local anaesthetics and to have a 'quinidine-like effect' on the heart although this action was different to that of quinidine (Black and Prichard, 1973). For many years it has been accepted that these terms describe the same property of these molecules which results from an effect on the cell membranes. Thus the term 'membrane stabilizing activity' was introduced by Van Zwieten (1969) and by Fitzgerald (1969) to describe these effects of beta blocking drugs. As these drugs may have other effects on membranes, a re-definition of the term 'membrane stabilizing activity' may be required (Smith, 1982).

1.9.2 Discovery of cardioselectivity

During 1966 detailed pharmacological studies were continued with practolol and to a lesser extent ICI 50232. In April 1966 we observed in anaesthetized dogs that practolol antagonised the inotropic and chronotropic actions of isoprenaline but not the depressor response which results from a peripheral vasodilatation (Dunlop and Shanks, 1968) (Fig. 1.5). Further studies confirmed that practolol did not block the peripheral vasodilator action of isoprenaline in the

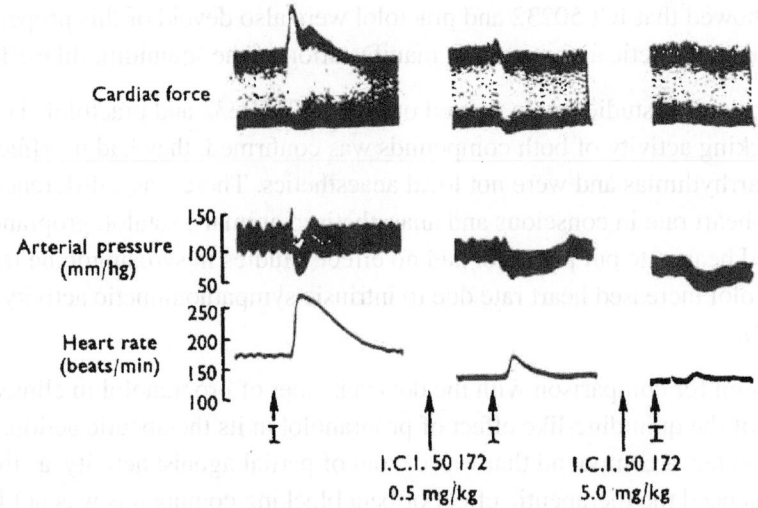

Cardiac force

Arterial pressure
(mm/hg)
1.50
100
50

Heart rate
(beats/min)
250
200
150
100

I.C.I. 50 172
0.5 mg/kg

I.C.I. 50 172
5.0 mg/kg

Dog anaesthetized with pentobarbitone. Records of cardiac contractile force (right ventricle), femoral arterial pressure and heart rate. Responses to the intravenous injection of isoprenaline (I) 0.4 µg/kg before and after the intravenous injection of I.C.I. 50172 (0.5 and 5.0 mg/kg).

Figure 1.5

Reproduced from *British Journal of Pharmacology and Chemotherapy*, 1968, *32*, 206. By permission of the authors and editor.

hind-limb of the dog (Dunlop and Shanks, 1968). Methods were then established to examine the effect of practolol on beta adrenoceptors in tracheal muscle. These showed that practolol had little effect in blocking the bronchodilator action of isoprenaline.

Almost by accident we had discovered that practolol had a new property that made it unique. Practolol blocked cardiac beta adrenoceptors but not those in bronchial muscle or in peripheral blood vessels. Practolol inhibited those beta adrenoceptors which were excitatory but not those that were involved in inhibitory responses (Dunlop and Shanks, 1968) and was described as being 'cardioselective'.

One of the main adverse effects of propranolol in some patients was wheezing due to bronchoconstriction induced by blockade of bronchial beta adrenoceptors (McNeill and Ingram, 1966). Theoretically this adverse effect should not occur in patients treated with practolol. ICI 50232 was also shown to be cardioselective. It was decided that practolol should be taken forward to clinical trial because it was cardioselective rather than a drug which was devoid of quinidine-like effect. Toxicity studies were completed by the end of 1966; practolol was not a carcinogenic agent in mice.

I left ICI in December 1966 to return to the Queen's University of Belfast to a post in the Department of Therapeutics and Pharmacology. Fortunately I was able to collaborate with my former colleaques in the Department of Physiology to examine the properties of practolol in man. By this time facilities had been introduced to enable heart rate and arterial pressure to be recorded in subjects and drugs were now given intravenously. In normal healthy subjects practolol reduced an exercise tachycardia but did not affect the peripheral vasodilator action of isoprenaline (Brick et al., 1968). These studies showed that practolol in doses which produced marked reduction in an exercise tachycardia had only a modest effect on an isoprenaline tachycardia. In contrast propranolol in doses which reduced an exercise tachycardia to the same extent as practolol produced much greater reductions in an isoprenaline tachycardia. The reason for the ineffectiveness of practolol, and other cardioselective drugs in inhibiting an isoprenaline tachycardia is still not known (McGibney et al., 1983).

In patients practolol was shown to block the chronotropic action of isoprenaline without reducing its bronchodilator action (Powles et al., 1969). Clinical studies confirmed the effectiveness of practolol in the treatment of angina, cardiac arrhythmias and hypertension while producing fewer side-effects of central nervous system origin and a lower incidence of bronchospasm. In patients practolol produced less cardiac depression than equi-active beta blocking doses of propranolol, especially in patients with impaired cardiac function (Jewitt and Croxson, 1971). It has not been discovered if this was due to partial agonist activity, cardioselectivity, a combination of both or to some novel feature of practolol.

Practolol was originally developed as a beta blocking drug devoid of local anaesthetic activity to be compared with the dextro isomer of propranolol to assess the importance of the quinidine-like activity. Few studies were completed (Wilson et al., 1969; Shanks, 1976).

Unfortunately practolol was withdrawn from general use in 1975, 5 years after its launch due to the development of the oculomuco-cutaneous reaction (Felix and Ive, 1974; Wright, 1974) which occurred on long term oral administration. Unlike the other beta adrenoceptor blocking drugs, practolol, causes little depression of cardiac function (Jewitt and Croxson, 1971) and is still available for intravenous administration.

As practolol was a less potent beta blocking drug and produced fewer adverse effects than propranolol (Wiseman, 1971) many doctors obtained confidence in beta adrenergic blockade by using practolol and although it had to be withdrawn it had served a most useful purpose. Other cardioselective beta adrenoceptor blocking drugs have been developed. The most widely used and studied are atenolol and metoprolol but they are probably less cardioselective than practolol and do not possess partial agonist activity and have not been a direct replacement of practolol.

When we discovered that practolol selectively inhibited cardiac beta adrenoceptors, practolol was described as a 'cardioselective' beta blocking drug (Dunlop and Shanks, 1968). During this period a number of compounds including isopropylmethoxamine, butoxamine and H35/25 were shown to produce selective blockade of vascular beta receptors in doses that produced no significant blockade of myocardial beta receptors (Levy and Wilkenfeld, 1969).

Independently from these studies Lands and his colleagues had compared the effect of a series of sympathomimetic amines on a number of organ systems. As a result they suggested that there were two types of beta adrenoceptor, β_1 mediating responses in the heart and β_2 mediating responses in bronchial smooth muscle and vascular smooth muscle (Lands et al., 1967). Although this paper was published before that on practolol (Dunlop and Shanks, 1968) the pharmacological classification of practolol had been completed before publication of the paper by Lands. Clearly practolol blocked those receptors which Lands had classified as β_1 and the methoxamine derivatives blocked β_2 receptors. However this terminology was not applied to the cardioselective drugs for some years and it has been difficult to determine when it was first used. No reference was made to it at a symposium on practolol in London in 1970 but metoprolol was introduced as a 'selective adrenergic β_1-receptor antagonist' in 1975 (Ablad et al., 1975).

1.10 Beta adrenoceptor blocking drugs in the treatment of hypertension

Black's original hypothesis had been that a drug which blocked beta adrenoceptors would be of value in the treatment of coronary artery disease, e.g. angina pectoris and acute myocardial infarction and in conditions characterised by an increase in activity of the sympathetic nervous system affecting beta adrenoceptors. It was not contemplated that these drugs would be of value in the treatment of hypertension in which there is an increase in peripheral resistance as a result of alpha adrenoceptor activity.

The acute intravenous injection of pronethalol reduced arterial pressure in anaesthetised and conscious animals and was accompanied by a peripheral vasodilatation (Black and Stevenson, 1962). The nature of the vasodilatation was not elucidated but, as it occurred with DCI, may have been a manifestation of partial agonist activity. The acute administration of pronethalol to man produced no change in heart rate or blood pressure (Dornhorst and Robinson, 1962).

We were surprised when Prichard (1964) reported that pronethalol had a hypotensive effect in 15 anginal patients who had been taking the drug for 3 months; 11 of the patients were hypertensive and 4 were normotensive being treated for angina pectoris. The mean fall in pressure in the supine position was 33/23 mmHg and in standing position 27/16 mmHg. He also reported small but significant falls in blood pressure in patients in a double blind trial of pronethalol in angina pectoris when patients were on active treatment. Later the same year Prichard described the effective use of propranolol in the treatment of hypertension (Prichard and Gillam, 1964).

The use of beta blocking drugs in the treatment of hypertension was only accepted slowly and it was not until 1972–1974 that these drugs began to be used widely as the drug of first choice or in combination with a diuretic in the control of raised arterial pressure even though their use had been shown to be associated with a low incidence of adverse effects and in particular the absence of postural hypotension (Prichard and Gillam, 1969). As the hypotensive effect was more often seen with larger doses (total daily dose of 400–1000 mg) than were used in angina and arrhythmias or were required to block an isoprenaline tachycardia, there was unjustified concern that adverse effects especially cardiac failure would develop.

Although several hypotheses have been advanced to explain the mechanism of the hypotensive effect of these drugs, none has yet been fully accepted and there may be several mechanisms, their contribution varying in different situations. Brian Prichard of University College Hospital London, has played a most important role in the development of beta blocking drugs in the treatment of hypertension; without his crusading zeal their use would probably be rather limited. He has recently published an excellent review article (Prichard, 1982).

1.11 Beta adrenoceptor antagonists – research in other pharmaceutical companies 1959–1964

Although most attention has been given to the contribution of scientists at the Pharmaceuticals Division of Imperial Chemical Industries to the development of beta adrenoceptor blocking drugs, many other pharmaceutical companies have been involved in the development of drugs of this type. While many of these only began research after the discovery of pronethalol and propranolol and were more involved in the synthesis of compounds not covered by ICI patents, at least three drug companies were already looking for beta adrenoceptor blocking drugs before the first publication on pronethalol appeared.

Research and development work began at AB Hassle in Göteborg in 1959 on cardiovascular drugs with the aim of obtaining a new anti-arrhythmic drug. In 1960 the object was 'to develop a drug, which should protect the diseased heart from too strong sympathetic stimulation caused by physical or emotional stress' (Östholm, 1982). In May 1961 Professor Arvid Carlsson became the pharmacological adviser to Hassle and on the basis of the reports on the properties of DCI suggested that the company develop a beta adrenoceptor blocking drug and begin by synthesizing compounds related to DCI. Many such compounds were made by a team led by Dr. Hans Corrodi and one of these, H29/50, was tested in man in 1963. At that time Dr. Bengt Ablad joined the company as a pharmacologist and became the leader of the project.

With the publication of the paper on pronethalol, Hassle discovered that ICI were working in the same field and were ahead of them. In 1963 and 1964 Hassle nearly stopped this research programme as there were many problems in finding compounds which had not already been patented. In 1963, Hassle began to synthesise compounds with an oxypropanolamine side chain as they could be made in a simple two step synthesis (this was before propranolol was described). In 1964 they found that the best compound was H56/28 – alprenolol (Ablad et al., 1967) which was shown to be an effective beta blocking drug in man.

It is interesting to note at this stage that at a research conference in 1961, one of the clinicians at Hassle said 'There may be a risk with the type of drug we are aiming at in this project. Due to a reduction of cardiac output, the drug may reduce blood pressure, which can be an undesirable effect'. After the publication of Prichard's paper on the hypotensive action of pronethalol (Prichard, 1964) these fears were forgotten and alprenolol was shown to reduce blood pressure in patients with hypertension (Bengtsson, 1972).

In 1963 Hassle developed a compound H35/25 which had less effect on beta adrenoceptors in the heart than on the receptors in the peripheral blood vessels and bronchi, thus indicating that beta receptors were probably not identical in all parts of the body; this drug was not taken into man (Levy and Wilkenfeld, 1969). In 1966 it was also discovered that para substituted alprenolol had a greater effect on beta receptors in the heart than on those in blood vessels and bronchi. A new objective was established which was to obtain a new cardioselective beta blocking drug as it would be expected to have less effect on the bronchi and peripheral circulation. This was before the description of practolol in the scientific literature. From the many compounds tested, two were taken to clinical trial – H87/07 which had partial agonist activity and H93/26 which had no such activity. As the latter compound was more potent in lowering blood pressure it was developed and marketed as metoprolol in 1975. It is interesting to note that H87/07 had essentially the same pharmacological properties as practolol.

The German pharmaceutical company Boehringer Ingelheim has a long history of innovation in medicinal chemistry. In June 1960, Dr. H. Köppe started to synthesise l-aryloxy-3-amino-2-propanols with the object of obtaining anorectic compounds without central stimulating effects. Single or multiple chlorine substitution was made with one of the first compounds synthesised being substituted with chlorine in the 2, 4 and 5 positions of the aromatic ring (Kö446). On account of the similarities in structure of DCI and these compounds, they were tested for anorectic activity but also for antagonism of the cardiac effects of isoprenaline. Kö446 was characterised by Dr. A. Engelhardt in May 1961 and was a highly effective beta adrenoceptor blocking drug. Later (May 1962) the phenoxy analogue of DCI was synthesised and shown to be a potent beta adrenoceptor blocking drug.

In July 1960, before ICI had synthesised pronethalol or propranolol, Dr. Köppe and his colleagues condensed α-naphthol with epichlorhydrine and then with isopropylamine to achieve a new series of substances related to those already described. Amongst the substances synthesised was '1-α-naphthoxy-3-isopropylamino-2-propanol (Lg 32)' which later became known as propranolol. Within a short time Dr. Engelhardt showed that Lg 32 was a potent beta adrenoceptor blocking drug. In August 1961, a new parent, meta-cresol, was used for the synthesis of new beta adrenoceptor blocking drugs and resulted in Kö592 which 18 months later was synthesised and tested independently as ICI 45763 at Imperial Chemical Industries. Dr. Engelhardt showed that Kö592 was a potent beta adrenoceptor blocking drug in April 1962.

Despite repeated proposals from the scientists (Köppe and Engelhardt) Boehringer Ingelheim did not envisage any commercial future for these compounds as there were no comparative sales figures and did not make a patent application for this class of drug until August 1963, by which time extensive patent applications had been made by ICI although the ICI patent application on ICI 45763 (Kö592) only preceded that by Boehringer by 8 months.

In the late 1950s the Mead Johnson Pharmaceutical Company, Evansville, Indiana, began testing new molecules for sympathomimetic properties using relaxation of intestinal, uterine and tracheal muscle (Lish et al., 1960). When Dr. A.A. Larsen joined Mead Johnson at this time, he had had considerable experience in the synthesis of sulphonamides. At Mead Johnson he proceeded to incorporate the alkylsulphonamide group into the benzene ring of phenethanolamines instead of a phenolic hydroxyl function. The second compound in the series had a methanesulphonamide group in the para position on the aromatic ring; this compound was MJ 1999 (sotalol) and was synthesised in October, 1960.

Initial studies showed that MJ 1999 had weak hypotensive activity in the anaesthetised dog but significantly blocked the tachycardia induced by adrenaline. As it was noted that MJ 1999 resembled DCI, tests were established to examine this activity further. On 22nd March, 1962, it was observed that MJ 1999 (0.01–0.1 μg/ml) blocked both the isoprenaline and adrenaline induced relaxation of the pitocin stimulated rat uterus in vitro (Larson and Lish, 1964). Dr. P.M. Lish, who was in charge of the programme commented on the test sheet that MJ 1999 (sotalol) was 'probably the first known and most potent drug capable of blocking beta stimulants in the uterus without simultaneously relaxing the uterus' (Stanton, 1982). Hence the beta blocking potency of sotalol without intrinsic sympathomimetic activity was discovered before the Black and Stephenson publication on pronethalol in the Lancet in August, 1962. A full scale pharmacological evaluation of sotalol confirmed that it was a beta adrenoceptor blocking compound without intrinsic sympathomimetic activity or local anaesthetic activity and had little or no effect on the central nervous system. Sotalol had low lipid solubility in contrast to the high lipid solubility of pronethalol (Lish et al., 1965). Lish and his colleagues had characterised the important differences between pronethalol and sotalol. Clinical studies commenced in July, 1965. We demonstrated that sotalol was a beta adrenoceptor blocking drug in man with a long duration of activity (Kofi Ekue et al., 1967). Sotalol unlike other beta adrenoceptor blocking drugs, prolongs the duration of the cardiac action potential – class III anti-arrhythmic activity (Singh and Vaughan Williams, 1970). The clinical significance of this finding is still speculative. Sotalol has been used for the treatment of angina pectoris, hypertension and cardiac arrhythmias in many countries but is not yet licensed in the United States. Sotalol would have been the ideal drug to compare with propranolol in elucidating the clinical importance of membrane stabilizing activity.

Alprenolol

Kö592 (ICI 45763)

Practolol

Metoprolol

Sotalol

1.12 Conclusions

Unknown to each other, five major pharmaceutical companies were involved in the late 1950s and early 1960s in studying the properties of novel compounds for blockade of beta adrenoceptors. The discovery at Lilly Laboratories of DCI provided a lead to two of the other companies, ICI and Hassle, to synthesise compounds of this type and to the other company, Boehringer, to test compounds they had already synthezised for beta adrenoceptor blocking activity.

The two companies which have benefited most from the discovery of these drugs have been ICI and Hassle (a subsidiary of Astra). Unlike the other two companies ICI and Hassle had already defined the type of drug for which they were searching when DCI was described and which they then used as a lead in obtaining a drug for clinical study. Both companies maintained their efforts to successfully market their new drug. In contrast Lilly and Boehringer had the active compounds but not the ideas to develop them into drugs for the treatment of disease.

Acknowledgements

I am deeply indebted to many people for the help they have given me in the preparation of this paper. Dr. H. Köppe, Dr. N.C. Moran, Dr. I. Ostholm, Dr. I. Slater and Dr. H. Stanton provided valuable information about developments in their own department or company. I also appreciated the help of Dr. J.D. Fitzgerald in reviewing my manuscript and making helpful suggestions and of Mrs. M. Scullion for typing the manuscript and preparing the references.

References

Ablad, B., Borg, K.O., Carlsson, E., Ek, L., Johnsson, G., Malmfors, T., Regardh, C.G., 1975. Acta Pharmacol. Toxicol. 36 (suppl. V), 7–23.

Ablad, B., Brogard, M., Ek, L., 1967. Acta Pharmacol. Toxicol. 25 (Suppl. 2), 9–40.

Ahlquist, R.P., 1948. Am. J. Physiol. 153, 586–600.

Ahlquist, R.P., 1980. J. Auton. Pharmacol. 1, 101–106.

Alcock, S.J., Bond, P.A., 1964. Proc. Eur. Soc. Stud. Drug Tox. 4, 30–39.

Allen, W.J., Barcroft, H., Edholm, O.G., 1946. J. Physiol. 105, 255–267.

Alleyne, G.A.O., Dickinson, C.J., Dornhorst, A.C., Fulton, R.M., Green, K.G., Hill, I.D., Hurst, P., Laurence, D.R., Pilkington, T., Prichard, B.N.C., Robinson, B., Rosenheim, M.L., 1963. Br. Med. J. ii, 1226–1229.

Apthorp, G.H., Chamberlain, D.A., Hayward, G.W., 1964. Br. Heart J. 26, 218–226.

Apthorp, G.H., Wedgwood, J., Hayward, G.W., 1960. Proc. Third European Congress of Cardiology, Rome 1960. Altera, A, Pars, p. 51.

Beck, C.S., 1957. Annal. Surg. 145, 439–460.

Bengtsson, C., 1972. Acta Med. Scand. 191, 433–439.

Bharadwaj, U.R., Shanks, R.G., 1962. J. Physiol. 160, 5P.

Black, J.W., 1960. J. Pharm. Pharmacol. 12, 87–94.

Black, J.W., 1967. Drug Responses in Man. CIBA Foundation Symposium, pp. 111–117.

Black, J.W., Crowther, A.F., Shanks, R.G., Smith, L.H., Dornhorst, A.C., 1964. Lancet i, 1080–1081.

Black, J.W., Duncan, W.A.M., Shanks, R.G., 1965. Br. J. Pharmacol. 25, 577–591.

Black, J.W., Prichard, B.N.C., 1973. Br. Med. Bull. 29, 163–167.

Black, J.W., Stephenson, J.S., 1962. Lancet 2, 311–314.

Braunwald, E., 1966. Am. J. Cardiol. 18, 303–307.

Brick, I., Hutchison, K.J., McDevitt, D.G., Roddie, I.C., Shanks, R.G., 1968. Br. J. Pharmacol. 34, 127–140.

Chamberlain, D.A., 1966. Am. J Cardiol. 18, 321–325.

Cotton, M., Moran, N.C., Stopp, P.E., 1957. J. Pharm. Exp. Ther. 121, 183–190.

De La Lande, I.S., Whelan, R.F., 1959. J. Physiol. 148, 548–553.

Dornhorst, A.C., Robinson, B.F., 1962. Lancet ii, 314.

Dresel, P.E., 1960. Can. J. Biochem. 38, 375–381.

Duff, R.S., Swan, H.J.C., 1951. J. Physiol. 114, 41–55.

Dunlop, D., Shanks, R.G., 1968. Br. J. Pharmacol. 32, 201–218.

Felix, R., Ive, F.A., 1974. Br. med. J. 2, 333.

Fitzgerald, J.D., 1969. Clin. Pharmacol. Ther. 10, 292–306.

Fulton, R.M., Green, K.G., 1963. Brit. Med. J. ii, 1226–1229.

Furchgott, R.F., 1959. Pharmacol. Rev. 11, 429–441.

Gill, E., Vaughan Williams, E.M., 1964. Nature 201, 199.

Glover, W.E., Greenfield, A.D.M., Shanks, R.G., 1962. Br. J. Pharm. Chemother. 19, 235–244.

Hampton, J.R., 1982. Brit. Med. J. 285, 33–36.

Hill, I., 1966. Am. J. Cardiol. 18, 185–187.

Howe, R., 1963. Biochem. Pharmacol. 12 (suppl), 85.

Howe, R., Shanks, R.G., 1966. Nature 210, 1336–1338.

Jewitt, D., Croxson, R., 1971. Postgrad. Med. J. Suppl. 47, 25–29.

Kofi Ekue, J.M., Lowe, D.C., Shanks, R.G., 1970. Br. J. Pharmacol. 38, 546–553.

Lands, A.M., Arnold, A., McAuliff, J.P., Ludena, F.P., Brown, T.G., 1967. Nature 214, 597–598.

Larson, A.A., Lish, P.M., 1964. Nature 203, 1283–1284.

Levy, B., Wilkenfeld, B.E., 1969. Eur. J. Pharmacol. 5, 227–234.

Lish, P.M., Dungan, K.W., Peters, E.L., 1960. J. Pharmacol. Exp. Ther. 129, 191–199.

Lish, P.M., Weikel, J.H., Dungan, K.W., 1965. J. Pharmacol. Exp. Ther. 149, 161–173.

Lucchesi, B.R., 1965. J. Pharmacol. Exp. Ther. 148, 94–99.

Moran, H.C. (1982) Personal communication.

Moran, H.C., Perkins, M.E., 1958. J. Pharmacol. Exp. Ther. 124, 223–237.

Moran, H.C., Perkins, M.E., 1961. J. Pharmacol. Exp. Ther. 133, 192–201.

McGibney, D., Singleton, W., Silke, B., Taylor, S.H., 1983. Br. J. Clin. Pharmacol. 15, 15–19.

McNeill, R.S., Ingram, C.G., 1966. Am. J. Cardiol. 18, 473–475.

Nickerson, M., 1949. Pharmacol. Rev. 27–101.

Ostholm, I., 1982. Personal communication.

Paget, G.E., 1963. Br. Med. J. ii, 1266–1267.

Powell, C.E., Slater, I.H., 1958. J. Pharmacol. Exp. Ther. 122, 470–488.

Powles, R., Shinebourne, E., Hamer, J., 1969. Thorax 24, 616–618.

Prichard, B.N.C., 1964. Br. Med. J. 1, 1227.

Prichard, B.N.C., 1982. Br. J. Clin. Pharmacol. 13, 51–60.

Prichard, B.N.C., Gillam, P.M.S., 1964. Br. Med. J. 2, 725–727.

Prichard, B.N.C., Gillam, P.M.S., 1969. Br. Med. J. 1, 7–16.

Reale, A., Motolese, M., 1981. Eur. Heart J. 2, 245–251.

Riddell, D.H., Schull, L.G., First, T.F., Baker, T.D., 1963. Annal. Surg. 157, 980–988.

Sekiya, A., Vaughan Williams, E.M., 1963a. Br. J. Pharmacol. 21, 462–472.

Sekiya, A., Vaughan Williams, E.M., 1963b. Br. J. Pharmacol. 21, 473–481.

Shanks, R.G., 1966a. Methods in Drug Evaluation, 1965. North Holland Publishing Company, Amsterdam, pp. 183–198.

Shanks, R.G., 1966b. Cardiologia Supplementum II 49, 1–16.

Shanks, R.G., 1969. Irish J. Med. Sci. 2, 351–367.

Shanks, R.G., 1976. Postgrad. Med. J. 52 ((Suppl) 4), 14–20.

Shanks, R.G., 1981. Eur. Heart J. 2, 253–255.

Singh, B.N., Vaughan Williams, E.M., 1970. Br. J. Pharmacol. 39, 675–687.

Slater, I.H. (1982) Personal communication.

Slater, I.H., Powell, C.E., 1957. Fed. Proc. 16, 336.

Smith, H.J., 1982. J. Mol. Cell. Cardiol. 14, 495–500.

Smith, G., Lawson, D.A., 1958. Scot. Med. J. 3, 346–350.

Snow, P.J.D., 1966. Am. J. Cardiol. 18, 458–462.

Stanton, H.C. (1982) Personal communication.

Stephen, S.A., 1966. Am. J. Cardiol. 18, 463–468.

Stock, J.P., Dale, N., 1963. Br. Med. J. ii, 1230–1233.

Van Zwieten, P.A., 1969. Br. J. Pharmacol. 35, 103–111.

Vaughan Williams, E.M., Sekiya, A, 1963. Lancet i 420–421.

Von Euler, U.S., 1946. Noradrenaline. Charles C. Thomas, Springfield.

White, J.C., 1943. Res. Publ. Assoc. Neurol. Ment. Dis. 23, 373–390.

Wilson, A.G., Brooke, O.G., Lloyd, H.J., Robinson, B.F., 1969. Br. Med. J. 4, 399–401.

Wiseman, R.A., 1971. Postgrad. Med. J. suppl. 47, 68–71.

Woodbury, R.A., Abreu, B.E., 1944. Am. J. Obst, Gynecol. 48, 706–708.

Wright, P., 1974. Br. Med. J. 2, 560.

Can drugs be devised to lower elevated blood pressure by blocking sympathetic autonomic traffic? Commentary on Ganglion and adrenergic neurone-blocking agents by Alan L.A. Boura and Alan F. Green

John Christie McGrath

Autonomic Physiology Unit, School of Cardiovascular & Metabolic Health, University of Glasgow, Glasgow, Scotland

In this article from 1984, A.L.A. Boura and A.F. Green discuss the development of ganglion-blockers and adrenergic neurone blockers as anti-hypertensive drugs in the period of the 1950s and early 1960s. It was known that high blood pressure was undesirable since it led to further morbidity and mortality. There was no understanding of the cause of hypertension nor drugs that could reliably and safely lower blood pressure. Several drugs were known that could lower blood pressure in experimental animals by interrupting the activity of the sympathetic nervous system, though there was little evidence that elevated activity was responsible for a blood pressure that was higher than normal or that lowering activity would normalize it. Nevertheless, blocking sympathetic activity was considered a logical target and the technology was available to monitor the cardiovascular system and other examples of sympathetic nervous transmission in anesthetized and conscious animals. Synthetic chemistry was available that could produce novel compounds based on known toxins, drugs, or physiologically active molecules. So, there was an experimental basis for inventing drugs that could reduce sympathetically mediated physiological responses.

Discoveries in Pharmacology, Volume 3, Hemodynamics and Immune Defense.
DOI: https://doi.org/10.1016/B978-0-443-18442-0.00010-0

Options for blockade of sympathetic autonomic traffic

The sites considered useful for blocking sympathetic nerve activity were the two junctions in the autonomic pathway outside the central nervous system (CNS): the sympathetic ganglia and the junction between the sympathetic post-ganglionic nerve and the relevant target organs, i.e., the smooth muscle of the vascular wall and the cardiac muscle. Each had complications in devising selectivity.

The ganglia of the parasympathetic and sympathetic systems, often mediating opposing end-organ effects, had the same transmitter, acetylcholine, and the archetypal blocker of acetylcholine's action, nicotine, had a similar pharmacology at each. In the work described, many new antagonists of this transmission were found but no pharmacological selectivity between sympathetic and parasympathetic ganglia emerged. So, the blockade of the parasympathetic system remained a problem.

The pharmacology of the post-ganglionic transmission processes at the blood vessels and heart, both had the same transmitter, noradrenaline, but employed different receptors with different pharmacology, namely α-adrenoceptors and β-adrenoceptors, respectively. From long before the start of the 1950s, sympatholytic drugs, which were later known to be α-adrenoceptor antagonists, were available, but β-adrenoceptor antagonists were not invented until the mid-1960s, and it was considered essential to be able to attenuate both components to produce a stable lowering of blood pressure devoid of reflex compensation. So, if all of the cardiovascular effects of the post-ganglionic sympathetic system were to be reduced, some other pharmacological means were required.

In this scenario, Boura and Green document the development of drugs designed to lower blood pressure by targeting these two neuronal junctions. At this time, there was a symbiosis between drug invention and understanding the systems upon which the drugs worked so this adds historical interest.

Ganglion blockers: invention and aftermath

The intelligent, skillful, and effective development of ganglion blockers and their refinement to achieve properties suitable for therapeutic use is well described. In the end, the lack of discrimination between sympathetic and parasympathetic systems was fatal to their therapeutic usefulness. Also, from the start, an important issue was that the molecules were highly charged. This led to limited penetration from gut to bloodstream (a therapeutic disadvantage for the parenteral route desired for long-term anti-hypertensive treatment) and failure to pass through the blood–brain barrier (a therapeutic advantage when targeting peripheral synapses and avoiding the several CNS effects of the compounds). A balance had to be sought, which was not entirely resolved. However, in later repurposing of the drugs, having molecules with different permeabilities was useful. For example, when used in a surgical emergency targeted at the heart or blood pressure, a highly charged drug could be administered intravenously without CNS penetration, e.g., trimetaphan (Pubchem, 2022). Conversely, when the drugs were repurposed for CNS effects, such as interference with central effects of nicotine in suppression of addiction, then a less charged molecule could be administered parenterally and would cross the BBB, e.g., mecamylamine (Wonnacott et al., 1990; Lancaster et al., 2000).

Understanding of the chemistry of the nicotinic acetylcholine receptors (nACh) that were the target of ganglion blockers proceeded rapidly in the 1990s onwards as molecular biology developed. They were found to be transmitter-gated ion channels consisting of five subunits assembled in various combinations to make different receptors/channels at many sites including autonomic ganglia, somatic motor junctions, and many sites in the CNS (hence the early side effects). Ganglion blockers block the ganglion nACh and several more in the CNS (Gotti et al., 2021; Alexander et al., 2022); hence the early "side-effects" and later "repurposing."

Adrenergic neurone blockers: invention and aftermath

The development of adrenergic neurone blockers was an attempt to move the selectivity of the blockade to the sympathetic nervous system. The blockers were compounds that entered the neuronal noradrenaline storage/release sites by the same route as noradrenaline via transporters at the neuronal membrane and then at the intracellular storage vesicles. A molecular mechanism never fully resolved and likely different between agents, this led to reduced output of transmitter noradrenaline. This made them specific for blocking "noradrenergic" nerves. It was a theoretical improvement on the incomplete sympathetic blockade by α-adrenoceptors, which did not block the β-adrenoceptors of the heart. α-Blockers' relatively low effectiveness as anti-hypertensives was later an advantage when they were repurposed for alleviating symptoms of an enlarged prostate without lowering blood pressure. The successful development and refinement of adrenergic neurone blockers is another story well told by Boura and Green. The wider family of adrenergic neurone blockers was extensively used as experimental tools for understanding sympathetic neurotransmission, first for understanding noradrenaline's uptake and release processes. Later they helped establish the concept of co-transmission; adrenergic neurone blockers were specific for the noradrenaline-containing nerves, but their action was on the release process *per se*, so they also blocked transmission by other transmitters released by these nerves, such as ATP (Adenosine Triphosphate) and NPY (Neuropeptide Y). However, the therapeutic success of adrenergic neurone blockers was short-lived. In practice, blocking the sympathetic nervous system alone could not produce a sustained lowering of peripheral resistance due to countervailing compensatory mechanisms. Bretylium was later repurposed for its antiarrhythmic action (Leveque, 1965) in cardiac resuscitation of ventricular tachycardia/ventricular fibrillation (Somberg et al., 2020) by a mechanism thought to be due to the inhibition of Na, K-ATPase (Helms et al., 2004). In this case, its original employment to reduce blood pressure by adrenergic neurone blockade is a dangerous side effect.

Anti-hypertensive drugs after ganglion blockers and adrenergic neurone blockers

From the mid-1960s, other anti-hypertensive strategies came along which were safer and more effective than ganglion blockers and adrenergic neurone blockers.

They were developed from knowledge of mechanisms discovered in vascular physiology, pharmacology, and toxicology, which had not necessarily been targeted at hypertension but turned out to be highly effective anti-hypertensives.

β-adrenoceptor antagonists (β-blockers) were invented by JW Black and colleagues to prove that sympathetic transmission to the heart could be selectively blocked. The objective was to spare the failing heart from over-stimulation in cardiac insufficiency (Black, 1989; McGrath and Bond, 2021). However, in the clinic, they turned out unexpectedly to be effective in lowering the blood pressure in hypertension (Prichard et al., 2000; Wiysonge et al., 2017) and became hugely successful clinically and financially. JW Black was awarded the 1988 Nobel Prize in Physiology or Medicine for his method of rational drug design, including inventing β-blockers by modifying the structure of natural hormones or neurotransmitters, in this case noradrenaline/adrenaline.

Calcium channel blockers disrupt the movement of Ca^{2+} through calcium channels into many cell types including muscle, a key stage in activating many cellular processes. Selective block-ade of appropriate channels reduces muscle contraction, for example, causing vasodilation and lowering blood pressure. Developed mostly in the late 1960s and 1970s in cardiac and smooth muscle research (Godfraind, 2017), they came into use as antihypertensives in the 1980s (Zhu et al., 2022).

The renin-angiotensin system was researched in the late 1960s through the 1970s and be-came an antihypertensive target in the early 1980s. The initial target was the inhibition of the angiotensin-converting enzyme inhibitors (ACEI) to reduce levels of angiotensin II, a power-ful vasoconstrictor. Later, blockers were developed of the receptor through which angiotensin II caused vasoconstriction (angiotensin receptor inhibitors) to avoid side effects from elevated levels of bradykinin and angiotensin I through ACEI. Renin-inhibitors were also developed to interrupt the system at an earlier stage. On balance, ACEI was preferred for antihypertensive treatment (Chen et al., 2018).

Thiazide diuretics had been known to be antihypertensive from the early 1950s at doses lower than that which produced their main diuretic effect and by further mechanisms. They are effective as monotherapy and, importantly, augment the efficacy of other classes of antihyper-tensives when used in combination. So, their most effective use grew as other therapies were developed (Wright et al., 2018).

At the time of writing this commentary, the recommendations of national agencies for antihypertensive treatment vary somewhat but generally are based on statistical evaluation of large clinical trials, comparing the various options against one another. There is broad agreement on a scientific level that combinations of thiazide diuretics with one or more of the other options, namely ACEI, β-blockers, and/or Ca antagonists are the most efficacious strategy (Davis et al., 1996, 2004). Since the drugs are all out of patent, it is also the most economical.

References

Alexander, S.P., Mathie, A., Peters, J.A., Veale, E.L., Striessnig, J., Kelly, E., et al., 2021. The concise guide to pharmacology 2021/22: ion channels. Br. J. Pharmacol. 178, S157–S245.

Black, J., 1989. Drugs from emasculated hormones: the principle of syntopic antagonism. Science 245 (4917), 486–493. https://doi.org/10.1126/science.2569237.

Chen, Y.J., Li, L.J., Tang, W.L., Song, J.Y., Qiu, R., Li, Q., Xue, H., Wright, J.M., 2018. First-line drugs inhibiting the renin angiotensin system versus other first-line antihypertensive drug classes for hypertension. Cochrane Database Syst. Rev. 11 (11), CD008170. https://doi.org/10.1002/14651858.CD008170.pub3.

Davis B.R., Cutler J.A., Gordon D.J., Furberg C.D., Wright J.T. Jr, Cushman W.C., Grimm R.H., LaRosa J., Whelton P.K., Perry H.M., Alderman M.H., Ford C.E., Oparil S., Francis C., Proschan M., Pressel S., Black H.R., Hawkins C.M. Rationale and design for the antihypertensive and lipid lowering treatment to prevent heart attack trial (ALLHAT). Am. J. Hypertens. 9(4):342–60. https://doi.org/10.1016/0895-7061(96)00037-4.

Davis, B.R., Furberg, C.D., Jr, W.J.T., Cutler, J.A., Whelton, P.A. Collaborative Research Group, 2004. ALLHAT: setting the record straight. Ann. Intern. Med. 141 (1), 39–46. https://doi.org/10.7326/0003-4819-141-1-200407060-00013.

Godfraind, T., 2017. Discovery and development of calcium channel blockers. Front. Pharmacol. 8, 286. https://doi.org/10.3389/fphar.2017.00286.

Gotti C., Marks M.J., Millar N.S., Wonnacott S., 2021. Nicotinic acetylcholine receptors (nACh) in GtoPdb v.2021.3. IUPHAR/BPS Guide to Pharmacology CITE. 2021 (3). https://doi.org/10.2218/gtopdb/F76/2021.3.

Helms, J.B., Arnett, K.L., Gatto, C., Milanick, M.A., 2004. Bretylium, an organic quaternary amine, inhibits the Na,K-ATPase by binding to the extracellular K-site. Blood Cells Mol. Dis. 32 (3), 394–400. https://doi.org/10.1016/j.bcmd.2004.01.013.

Lancaster, T., Stead, L.F., 2000. Mecamylamine (a nicotine antagonist) for smoking cessation. Cochrane Database Syst. Rev. 1998 (2), CD001009. https://doi.org/10.1002/14651858.CD001009.

Leveque, P.E., 1965. Antiarrhythmic action of bretylium. Nature 207, 203–204.

McGrath, J.C., Bond, R.A., 2021. Sir James Whyte Black OM. 14 June 1924—22 March 2010. Biogr. Mem. Fellows. R. Soc. 70, 23–40.

National Center for Biotechnology Information, 2022. PubChem compound summary for CID 23576, Trimethaphan. https://pubchem.ncbi.nlm.nih.gov/compound/Trimethaphan. (Accessed 26 January 2022).

Prichard, B.N., Graham, B.R., Cruickshank, J.M., 2000. New approaches to the uses of beta blocking drugs in hypertension. J. Hum. Hypertens. 14, S63–S68. https://doi.org/10.1038/sj.jhh.1000989.

Somberg, J., Molnar, J., 2020. What is new in pharmacologic therapy for cardiac resuscitation? Cardiol. Res. 11 (3), 141–144. https://doi.org/10.14740/cr1058.

Wiysonge, C.S., Bradley, H.A., Volmink, J., Mayosi, B.M., Opie, L.H., 2017. Beta-blockers for hypertension. Cochrane Database Syst. Rev. 1 (1), CD002003. https://doi.org/10.1002/14651858.CD002003.pub5.

Wonnacott, S., Drasdo, A., Sanderson, E., Rowell, P., 1990. Presynaptic nicotinic receptors and the modulation of transmitter release. Ciba Found Symp. 152, 87–101. https://doi.org/10.1002/9780470513965.ch6.

Wright, J.M., Musini, V.M., Gill, R., 2018. First-line drugs for hypertension. Cochrane Database Syst. Rev. 4 (4), CD001841. https://doi.org/10.1002/14651858.CD001841.pub3.

Zhu, J., Chen, N., Zhou, M., Guo, J., Zhu, C., Zhou, J., Ma, M., He, L., 2022. Calcium channel blockers versus other classes of drugs for hypertension. Cochrane Database Syst. Rev. 1 (1), CD003654. https://doi.org/10.1002/14651858.CD003654.pub6.

Peripheral anti-hypertensives: Ganglion and adrenergic neurone-blocking agents

Alan L.A. Boura and Alan F. Green

Contents

2.1 Introduction

Pharmacologists carrying out research into medicinal chemistry are particularly fortunate people. The intellectual stimulation, resulting from encouragement to unleash their inquisitive natures and satisfy their curiosities regarding the nature of physiological mechanisms and the action of drugs, ensures a high level of personal satisfaction. An added bonus is the continuous stimulus of innovatory ideas from close collaboration and argument with able and indispensable colleagues of many different disciplines. The consequence is a high level of

---

Disclaimer: The original text that follows is reproduced from the first edition and carries errors and omissions from it. The editors and publisher agreed to retain them and honor the original authors and challenges they had to deal with in publishing back in those times.

Discoveries in Pharmacology, Volume 3, Hemodynamics and Immune Defense.

DOI: https://doi.org/10.1016/B978-0-443-18442-0.00062-8

enthusiasm and team work which hopefully leads to finding new drugs – though serendipity at one stage or another is likely to be a factor in discovering agents with entirely novel properties. A marketed drug may represent one step in a succession of small improvements on existing therapy, and the discovery of a new drug class, providing the possibility of a major exciting advance, is relatively uncommon. When this occurs, an inevitable sequel is an opportunity for acquisition of new knowledge of the physiological systems and diseases affected by the drugs.

The most successful drug companies have been those who have followed this philosophy by providing time and encouragement to laboratory workers to pursue research programmes and incidental chance observations which excite them. So, from the beginning, has it been in the discovery of new drugs that affect peripheral autonomic mechanisms.

In 1904 Mr. (later Sir Henry) Wellcome, then the sole proprietor of Burroughs Wellcome & Co., mentioned to his recently appointed research physiologist, Dr. H.H. Dale, that it would give him special satisfaction if an attempt was made to clarify the confusion which then existed regarding the pharmacology of ergot (see chapt. 1), providing it did not interfere with Dale's own plans for research. Dale (also later Sir Henry) was not at all anxious to enter 'the ergot morass' (Dale, 1953), but, when he did, a mixture of serendipity and astute observation led him to a wealth of pharmacological and physiological discoveries, which probably will never be equalled. Terms such as adrenaline reversal, sympathomimetic, adrenergic and cholinergic are among the many he first coined (see *Discoveries in Pharmacology,* Vol. 1, chapt. 2).

$$MeCO_2.CH_2.CH_2.N^+Me_3 \quad MeO.CH_2.CH_2.N^+Me_3 \quad ON.O.CH_2.CH_2.N^+Me_3$$

(1) Acetylcholine   (2)   (3)

One of the many constituents of ergot extract which excited Dale was that which caused intense bradycardia when injected into anaesthetised cats and which he and A.J. Ewins later identified as acetylcholine (compound 1). Thus stimulated, Dale embarked on an investigation of the pharmacological effects of esters and ethers of choline together with compounds (2) and (3) (Dale, 1914) following up the earlier work of Crum Brown and Fraser (1869) and Hunt and Taveau (1911) who had already shown that quaternary ammonium salts caused powerful circulatory effects. Extension of this work might have led him to the discovery of adrenergic neurone blocking agents as happened when others pursued this line some forty years later (see Section 2.3.1). In that event the discovery of such substances could have preceded that of specific ganglion blocking agents. But Dale's interests turned to the further investigation of other bases including tetraethylammonium which was identified as a selective ganglion blocking agent (Burn and Dale, 1915) and to another constituent of ergot, namely histamine (Dale and Richards, 1918), with far reaching consequences in terms of new physiological knowledge and later of drug discovery in the shape of histamine H_1 and H_2 antagonists.

2.2 Ganglion blocking agents

2.2.1 Tetraethylammonium (TEA)

As already mentioned, the discovery of the ganglion blocking action of tetraethylammonium (4) was made by Burn and Dale in 1915, who found that whereas tetramethylammonium caused first stimulation followed by depression of ganglion cells, effects known to be caused by nicotine (Langley and Dickinson, 1889), its tetraethyl analogue (TEA) displayed only the depressant property. It was some thirty years later before a thorough pharmacological study was made of TEA, as a result of which a rational basis was found for the use of ganglion blockade to lower arterial blood pressure in hypertension and the effectiveness of TEA in this condition was demonstrated (Acheson and Moe, 1946; Acheson and Pereira, 1946; Hoobler et al., cit. Moe and Freyburger, 1950). The short persistence of TEA by injection and its ineffectiveness by mouth ruled it out for general use as a hypotensive agent.

Whereas TEA was the first ganglion blocking agent shown to be effective in hypertension, the discovery of pentamethonium (5, $n = 5$) and hexamethonium (5, $n = 6$) (Section 2.2.2) was essentially independent of it. Nevertheless knowledge that TEA lowered arterial blood pressure in hypertensive subjects must have accentuated the desire to evaluate pentamethonium and hexamethonium when their ganglion blocking properties were found. On the other hand, it seems that both the discovery and exploitation of trimetaphan were inspired by TEA (Section 2.2.5). TEA is perhaps now best known for its ability to block potassium currents in the nerve membrane, an effect considered a likely cause of the paraesthesias it produces (Paton, 1982).

$$N^+Et_4 \qquad\qquad Me_3N^+ \cdot [CH_2]_n \cdot N^+Me_3 \qquad \left[\begin{array}{c} N^+ \cdot [CH_2]_5 \cdot N^+ \\ Me \qquad\qquad Me \end{array}\right]$$

(4) Tetraethylammonium   (5)   (6)

(TEA)

2.2.2 Hexamethonium and other symmetrical bisquaternary compounds

The fascinating chain of events that led to the synthesis and evaluation of hexamethonium has been reviewed recently by Paton (1982). As a member of the Division of Biological Standards at the National Institute for Medical Research in Hampstead, England, W.D.M. Paton (now Sir William) joined F.C. MacIntosh in looking at the toxicity of licheniformin, an antibiotic isolated from cultures of *Bacillus licheniformis*. When this substance was injected intravenously into a cat under chloralose anaesthesia, it caused a precipitous fall in blood pressure, but the onset of the fall was delayed by some 20 seconds, in contrast to that caused by directly acting vasodilator substances. The delayed fall was subsequently shown to be due to endogenous histamine release (MacIntosh and Paton, 1949; Gray and Paton, 1949). The observation prompted examination of some other available chemicals and findings that many dibasic substances with the basic groups (amine, amidine, isothiourea, guanidine) separated by five or more methylene groups similarly released histamine to cause characteristically delayed depressor responses. This property was shown to be especially prominent in the basic polymer 48–80 (Paton, 1951a) whose powerful depressor action was hitherto unexplained.

Among the bases made available to Paton by Dr. Harold King, the senior chemist at the National Institute, was the C8 member of the methonium series, i.e. octamethonium (5, $n = 8$). It was to determine whether or not this compound released histamine that it was first injected into an anaesthetised cat. In fact it caused respiratory paralysis and a resulting asphyxial rise in blood pressure. The respiratory paralysis was soon shown to be attributable to the drug's powerful neuromuscular blocking properties.

Previously the essential structure of the neuromuscular blocking agent (+)-tubocurarine (curare) had been elucidated by King (1935) at The National Institute for Medical Research, providing the inspiration for the synthesis of the bisquaternary ammonium compound gallamine by Bovet et al. (1947). (Many years later Everett et al. (1970) demonstrated that only one of the amino groups of tubocurarine was quaternised rather than two as King had supposed.) Bovet's success, and continuing interest in the chemistry of neuromuscular blocking agents, led King to advise that Paton's finding of the powerful activity of octamethonium should be pursued by studying the complete methonium series. Their synthesis was undertaken by Zaimis (1950). Comparison of their neuromuscular blocking activities, after intravenous injection in anaesthetised cats, soon revealed that decamethonium (C10) was the most potent member and that as the methylene chain was reduced below C7 the curare-like activity faded out (Paton and Zaimis, 1948).

As Paton (1982) has pointed out, the methonium compounds are much more active after intravenous injection in cats than in tests in vitro using the rat isolated diaphragm; had only the latter been used the series would have appeared much less striking and perhaps might not have been studied so energetically. Tests using frog rectus abdominus muscle showed that whereas the longer chain compounds, C7 and upwards, resembled acetylcholine by causing contraction, in contrast tubocurarine acted as an antagonist of acetylcholine. Compounds with C6 or shorter chains lacked stimulant action on the rectus but, surprisingly resembled tubocurarine by antagonising contractions caused by the longer chain compounds, C5 and C6 being the most potent in this respect. As neuromuscular blockade by decamethonium, in contrast to that by tubocurarine, could not be readily antagonised by the anticholinesterase neostigmine, C5 and C6 became attractive candidates as potential clinical antagonists of the newly found methonium neuromuscular blocking agents.

Two other properties quickly revealed themselves in follow-up studies of C5 and C6. When injected intravenously into anaesthetised cats, they caused marked hypotension and during head-drop tests for neuromuscular blocking activity the ears of rabbits rapidly flushed bright red. The latter vividly reminded Paton of Claude Bernard's classical experiment which demonstrated the effects of section of the sympathetic trunk to the rabbit's ear. Assuming therefore that the effects of C5 and C6 were likely to be due to sympathetic ganglion blockade, experiments were done stimulating the pre- and post-ganglionic cervical sympathetic nerves to the nictating membranes of anaesthetised cats. It was soon demonstrated that this was indeed the site of action (Paton and Zaimis, 1949, 1951). Fortunately too, the availability at Hampstead of a technique allowing measurement of acetylcholine (ACh) release during preganglionic stimulation of the perfused superior cervical ganglion, provided opportunity for direct demonstration of lack of impairment of transmitter release. The actions of pentamethonium and hexamethonium were therefore attributable to antagonism of the effects of ACh on the postsynaptic neurones, an antagonism in keeping with their chemical structures for they, like ACh, are methylated quaternary ammonium compounds.

The potency of hexamethonium in blocking contractions of the preganglionic stimulated nictitating membranes of cats, after intravenous injection, was some seven times greater than that of TEA. Its action was also slower to reach a maximum and lasted considerably longer. Pentamethonium was somewhat less active.

Much of the further interest in the cardiovascular potential of these compounds followed from the knowledge that TEA was a hypotensive agent (Moe and Freyburger, 1950) and from the use of surgical sympathectomy as a therapeutic procedure. Once chronic toxicity tests had been completed (Paton and Zaimis, 1949) (these tests would be regarded as rudimentary by today's standards but they adequately covered all likely eventualities, especially for a highly ionised basic substance likely to remain essentially extracellular), exploration of the actions in man of hexamethonium and pentamethonium followed rapidly. Within a year of recognition of their ganglion blocking properties, reports on their clinical effects were beginning to appear. At first both drugs were given only parenterally but later hexamethonium was used by mouth despite knowledge that only some 5 -10% of the drug was absorbed and erratically at that. Arnold and Rosenheim reported an early study in patients in August 1949. This was followed by the finding in man of a marked and embarrassing hypotension after pentamethonium during a study of its ability to antagonise the neuromuscular paralysis caused by decamethonium which at the time was the action of prime interest. Then came reports of the use of hexamethonium for treating peptic ulcer (Kay and Smith, 1950) and of its effects on the peripheral circulation in peripheral vascular diseases (Arnold et al., 1949; Burt and Graham, 1950). Contemporarily, the technique was developed of reducing bleeding during surgery by making use of the marked postural hypotension that can be induced in the presence of pentamethonium (Enderby, 1950). Hexamethonium gradually took interest away from pentamethonium for ganglion blockade and its use expanded, despite a number of serious shortcomings attributable to widespread blockade of autonomic functions. The diversity of handicaps produced has been vividly portrayed by Paton (1954) in his description of 'hexamethonium man'. Manifestations of blockade of autonomic ganglia, included failure of salivation, loss of accommodation of the eye for near vision, failure of erection in men, a dry skin and constipation. Also, as the lowered blood pressure, being due to sympathetic block, was dependent upon the level of sympathetic nerve activity, patients often suffered severe hypotension and even syncope on standing and during exercise. Furthermore the actions of the substance were relatively short-lived so that frequent doses were required. A degree of tolerance to the drug also developed during its daily administration. This was not due to reduced absorption (Morrison and Paton, 1953). The explanation was advanced by Zaimis (1956) that tolerance was due to the cardiovascular system developing hypersensitivity to catecholamines released, in reduced quantity, from the postganglionic sympathetic nerve endings and from the adrenal medulla. Later the degree of hypersensitivity to catecholamines that developed during continuous ganglion blockade was shown to be similar to that following preganglionic nerve section (Emmelin, 1959; Boura and Green, 1962).

The discovery of hexamethonium and the clinical benefits that derived from it led inevitably to the synthesis and pharmacological study of a large number of other symmetrical bisquaternary compounds and the discovery of several with similar or greater potencies (Ing, 1956). Some of these were used in man the most successful being pentolinium (6), synthesised by Libman et al. (1952) and first described in the pharmacological literature by Mason and Wien (1955). This became a more popular therapeutic agent than hexamethonium because of lower dosage, less frequent dosing requirement and rather better absorption from the alimentary tract. Otherwise its use was attended by the same side effects.

2.2.3 Asymmetric bisquaternary derivatives: pentacynium and chlorisondamine

Whereas for several years symmetry and a chain length equivalent to that of five or six methylene groups between two quaternary ammonium groups was thought optimal for ganglion blocking activity, this turned out not to be so when asymmetric bisquaternary compounds were studied. Many such series were demonstrated to have very powerful ganglion blocking activity in studies reported by Adamson et al. (1956); Billinghurst (1956); Green (1956).

(7) BW229C48

(8) X = C(OH)CH$_2$ (11) X = C(CN)CH$_2$
(9) X = C:CH   (12) X = CH.O
(10) X = CH.CH$_2$ (13) X = CH.CO$_2$

(14) Pentacynium

During the period 1946–1951, Dr. D.W. Adamson and his colleagues at the Wellcome Research Laboratories in England, were examining derivatives of benzhydrylalkylamines in a programme that led to several marketed drugs including the histamine H$_1$ antagonist triprolidine, the anti-Parkinsonian agent procyclidine, and the analgesic diethylthiambutene. In 1948, as part of this study, the compound BW229C48 (7) was made and observed to cause powerful mydriatic effects in mice although it had no antimuscarinic action on the guinea pig isolated ileum. The possibility of any further work on BW229C48 was crowded out by exciting leads in the development of antihistamines, analgesics and anti-muscarinic agents. However, when these programme objectives were successfully achieved, attention was again focussed on this compound. Its actions were soon demonstrated to be attributable to ganglion blockade in which regard it was much more potent than hexamethonium and far more persistent. Activity was found not to depend on the piperazine moiety; powerful ganglion blocking properties were revealed in the diquaternary-amino-carbinols (8), -alkenes (9), -alkanes (10), -nitriles (11), -ethers (12) and -esters (13) where R1 and R2 are preferably phenyl or cyclohexyl or, less favourably, pyridyl or thienyl groups. N^1 and N^2 are fully substituted quaternary nitrogen atoms.

These compounds are, therefore, structurally related to the large group of tertiary and quaternary amines of the benzhydrylalkyl types which, as already mentioned, yielded a number of clinically useful drugs. Thus, compounds 8–10 are related to tricyclamol, procyclidine, triprolidine and the thiambutenes; while series 11, 12 and 13 are related to methadone, diphenhydramine and 'Trasentine' respectively. The introduction of the group consisting of two quaternary nitrogen atoms linked by a short polymethylene chain, in place of the tertiary or quaternary amino-group of the known compounds, conferred ganglion-blocking activity on all these classes of drugs and divested them of their previous types of activity.

In studies concentrated on the diphenyl compounds, activities were greatest when the substituents on N^1 and N^2 were no larger than ethyl, this also applying when N^1 performed part of a pyrrolidinium, piperidinium or morpholinium ring. The optimal value for *n* was 2 or 3 (in contrast to the methonium compounds) and as *m* was increased from 1 to 7 activity reached a maximum at 3 or 4 and then declined. Not only are several such compounds over a hundred times more active than hexamethonium subcutaneously in mice but their persistences are far greater (Adamson et al., 1956; Billinghurst, 1956). That most extensively examined was pentacynium (Green, 1956), (14). In a variety of tests of ganglion blocking activity its potency exceeded that of pentolinium some ten-fold, minimal effective parenteral dosages being 0.01 mg/kg or even less and its duration of action was far more persistent.

Pentacynium and several analogues examined were found effective by oral administration in experimental animals, principally mice, but the dosages required were about ten times those needed by subcutaneous injection. After carrying out subacute toxicity studies, selected compounds were examined by Dr. S. Locket for hypotensive action in patients with severe hypertension and found effective (Adamson et al., 1956; Locket, 1956). Pentacynium, the most potent, effectively lowered blood pressure for over 5 hours after a subcutaneous dose of 5 mg and for over 20 hours after 15 mg. Consistent results were obtained during repeated dosing over periods of up to 3 weeks.

During the pharmacological study of pentacynium and its forerunners there was an unexpected and perplexing variation in their mydriatic effects in mice, apparently depending upon the source of the mice, the day and the type of box in which the animals were housed (biscuit tins with holes punched in the lid or clear plastic containers). An explanation was provided when it was found that dilation of the mouse pupil by ganglion blockade was dependent upon light intensity (Green, 1956). When the mice were in boxes in which the only light source was from small holes in the lid, especially when the mice for some reason spent less time in peering through the holes or the day was dull, mydriasis was less. Also an occasion arose when paradoxically a dog which had received a threshold dose of pentacynium showed constricted pupils when kept in dim light and dilated pupils in bright light. Such findings well illustrated for the ciliary ganglia the conclusion of Paton (1951b, 1954) that, as a consequence of the diminishing release of acetylcholine from the preganglionic nerve endings in autonomic ganglia during continuous high rates of nerve traffic, the effects of ganglion blockade become more prominent. As the concentration of acetylcholine in the synapse becomes less the competitive blockade exerted by the ganglion blocking agent becomes greater. Another curiosity was the finding that the pupils of albino rats, in contrast with those of other species, failed to dilate when any ganglion blocking agent was administered, even though their responses to antimuscarinic drugs were in no way anomalous. An adequate explanation of this has still to be established.

(15)   (16)   (18)

(17)   (19)

High potency and long persistence of ganglion blocking activity was shown also by chlorisondamine at the Ciba Laboratories in the United States (Plummer et al., 1955; Green, 1956). Its discovery came about in the following circuitous manner (Dr. Charles Huebner, personal communication). In the late 1940s, lithium aluminium hydride, a revolutionary new reagent for reducing organic compounds was discovered by Dr. H.L. Brown (for which he was later awarded a Nobel Prize). It was reported that it reduced amides to amines. In 1952 Dr. Huebner and his colleagues wondered whether cyclic imides might similarly be reduced to cyclic imines and since the dimethylamino ethyl side chain is a common feature in many synthetic drugs this side chain was attached to the molecules under investigation. Thus compound (15) was converted to (16). The great facility of this reaction led to the preparation of congeners. The chemical precursor of (15) is phthalic anhydride and as tetrachlorophthalic anhydride is also readily available commercially, compound (17) was made. It was then realized that if the bifunctional tertiary amines were quaternised, the functional groups of ganglion blocking agents would be present. The products (e.g. 18, 19) showed this activity in abundance, and more especially (19) now known as chlorisondamine. For example chlorisondamine at dosages of 0.1–0.2 mg/kg i.v. or 2 mg/kg orally caused ganglion blockade over several hours in dogs (Plummer et al., 1955). Dr. A.J. Plummer (personal communication) recalls that he took a number of 50 mg tablets to Dr. Keith Grimson at Duke Medical School who became greatly excited by the initial tests: 'He had several resistant hypertensive patients on hand, and about 30 minutes after taking a tablet the leg skin temperature rose and the blood pressure fell. The effect lasted 12–18 hours and postural hypotension was a problem since the dose was too large. We split the tablets into quarters and got a good therapeutic effect'.

For a period chlorisondamine came to be used as a hypotensive agent to a fairly considerable extent, both by injection and orally, but it lost ground to the more fully absorbed drugs described in the next section and interest in it at Ciba waned after guanethidine was discovered.

Pentacynium was used in man to a much lesser extent and suffered an analogous fate at the hands of better absorbed ganglion blocking drugs and the arrival of bretylium the first clinically effective adrenergic neurone blocking agent (Section 2.3.2).

2.2.4 Secondary and tertiary amines: mecamylamine and pempidine

Mecamylamine (20) was the first discovered powerful and specific agent of this class. Being a secondary amine and therefore less highly ionised at physiological pH it has the major advantage over quaternary compounds of being well absorbed from the alimentary tract. However, an inevitable consequence of its more lipophilic character is that in contrast to quaternary compounds it has the attendant disadvantage of penetrating the blood-brain barrier into the central nervous system. Thereby its use in controlling hypertension can cause tremors, mental confusion, seizures, mania or depression. Nevertheless the balance of advantages can be judged from its more frequent use for treating hypertension and by the fact that it outlived any of the quaternary compounds for such a purpose.

The literature does not explain why chemists at Roche indulged in the chemistry that led to the synthesis of mecamylamine. However the first announcement of its synthesis and associated ganglion blocking properties (Stein et al., 1956) indicates at least an element of serendipity. The intermediate from which mecamylamine was prepared was an unexpected reaction product. A full account of the pharmacological properties of mecamylamine was presented by Stone et al. (1956).

(20) Mecamylamine   (21) Pempidine

A considerable stir was caused in circles of British medicinal chemistry and pharmacology in 1956 when contemporary but independent syntheses of pempidine (21) were announced by two British pharmaceutical companies together with their independent discoveries that this tertiary amine had ganglion blocking activity exceeding that of mecamylamine. The independent discoveries were those of Spinks and Young (1958) at the ICI Laboratories and Lee et al. (1958) of May and Baker. The pharmacologists of both groups, no doubt to their initial dismay, found themselves programmed to present results of their independent work at the same meeting of the British Pharmacological Society in Glasgow (July 1958) when hitherto each had supposed their findings to be unique. Overlap of chemistry was even greater. Quite independently of the two pharmaceutical groups and independently of one another two American laboratories, essentially unconnected with medicinal chemistry (one an academic department, and the other associated with textiles) had synthesised the same substance. (Leonard and Hauck, 1957; Hall, 1957). Quite understandably the latter publications were not concerned with any pharmacological potential of the many compounds they described. This is just one of many examples of chemists following fashions that depend on the availability of new routes of synthesis and often of fresh intermediates. However, there is no question but that the chemistry and attendant pharmacological studies conducted by the two British drug houses were inspired by knowledge of mecamylamine, which at that time was regarded as a therapeutic agent of great promise.

Pempidine is the more potent and shared with mecamylamine the advantage of good absorption from the alimentary tract and the disadvantages associated with penetration into the brain. It also shared in superseding the quaternary ganglion blocking drugs that were already in clinical use and encouraging the abandonment of other yet more powerful quaternaries, such as pentacynium and chlorisondamine, that were only just beginning to become known or had not reached the market. A further sequel was to encourage industrial researchers who had developed a keen interest in the sympathetic nervous system, while developing ganglion blocking agents, to focus their attention on better drugs for lowering blood pressure. To some extent, at least, this was subsequently reflected in the discoveries of adrenergic neurone blocking agents at the Wellcome Research Laboratories in England (bretylium and bethanidine) and at the Ciba Laboratories in the United States (guanethidine) which are described in Section 2.3.

2.2.5 Trimetaphan

Today the only therapeutically significant ganglion blocking agent still in clinical use, other than mecamylamine, is trimetaphan (22) (Randall et al., 1949). Its discovery was roughly contemporary with that of hexamethonium, inspired by the knowledge of the ganglion blocking properties of tetraethylammonium (TEA) and based on the anticipation that triethyl sulphonium salts might have analogous properties to quaternary ammonium salts. The paper of Randall et al. (1949) mentions that this particular sulphonium salt was available from the Roche synthesis of biotin giving insight into its choice. The pharmacological properties described show that its ganglion blocking potency is about thirty times that of TEA with a duration of action about twice as long in the cat, dog and monkey. By comparison with the ganglion blocking agents later discovered, this duration of action is short and ruled it out of consideration as a treatment of choice for the sustained medication of hypertensive subjects. On the other hand, the rapid onset and short duration of action of intravenous trimetaphan has led to its adoption and continuing use for the production of controlled hypotension during certain kinds of surgery. This can be used to minimise haemorrhage in the operative field especially during bone and vascular operations. Infusions of trimetaphan are also used in the management of autonomic hyperreflexia, a syndrome typically seen after injury of the upper spinal cord. In such patients the massive sympathetic discharge that occurs, for example during catheterisation, distension of the bladder or during cystoscopy, can be controlled by ganglion blockade; a use not envisaged at the time of the drug's inception. Intravenous infusions are also sometimes used in the emergency treatment of hypertensive crises.

(22) Trimetaphan   (23) Xylocholine (TM 10)

2.3 Adrenergic neurone blockade

The discovery of adrenergic neurone blocking drugs fully illustrates the exciting combination of serendipity and scientifically planned follow-up studies that has characterised so many successful searches for new and novel medicinal substances. The major compounds are described below in order of their discovery and attention is drawn to inter-relationships between them. The essential action of adrenergic neurone blocking agents is that they suppress the release of the transmitter noradrenaline from the terminals of peripheral sympathetic postganglionic nerves. Details of their pharmacological effects and studies concerning their mechanism of action are the subject of many reviews (Boura and Green, 1965; Maxwell and Wastila, 1977; Boura and Green, 1981, 1984; Green, 1982; Maxwell 1982).

2.3.1 Xylocholine (TM 10)

A masterly account of the complex series of events that led to the discovery of TM10 (23) at Leeds University, England was provided by Professor W.A. Bain in 1960 and recently an abridged version of this, containing some additional information, has been presented by

Fielden (1981) who was one of Bain's Ph.D. students in 1960. Bain and his colleagues established that TM10 had the hitherto unknown property of selectively suppressing the release of the adrenergic transmitter from peripheral adrenergic neurones. According to Fielden (1981), Bain referred to this action as adrenergic nerve blockade and the change to adrenergic neurone blockade was made at the suggestion of Sir Henry Dale. This is not in keeping with our recollection. Dale proposed the term antiadrenergic to define the similar action of bretylium and the change to adrenergic neurone blockade was made by the Editors of the *British Journal of Pharmacology* in 1959 (Boura and Green, 1959; Green 1982). This term received universal and rapid acceptance. The recent substitution of the historical 'adrenergic' by 'noradrenergic' by some workers and editors has been deprecated, but seems an inevitable consequence of the realisation that the major transmitter at peripheral sympathetic nerve endings is noradrenaline and that adrenaline is released by some central neurones which are therefore adrenergic.

The discovery of the unique action of TM10 was the culmination of a long sequence of chance observations. The circumstances were often fortuitous and whereas pharmacological interpretations were generally astute, they were often proved wrong by subsequent increased knowledge of adrenergic mechanisms. To understand this it needs to be appreciated that during the course of this work physiological knowledge concerning adrenergic neurones was rudimentary. For example, it had yet to be fully appreciated that the adrenergic transmitter was noradrenaline rather than adrenaline, and the means by which the transmitter became available for release and how its action was terminated were unknown. Subsequent knowledge of such matters owes much to the discovery of selective pharmacological tools, including the blocking agents discussed here. It also owes a lot to the development of new technology.

The story of TM10 may be considered to have started with work that led Bain and Dickinson (1938) to conclude that the raised arterial blood pressure in hypertensives might be due to delayed inactivation of adrenaline. The data and arguments are now not convincing and doubts were thrown on the hypothesis by Bain and his young Ph.D. student Jean Batty (now Dr. J.E. Olley) finding no correlation between raised blood pressure and the rate of noradrenaline inactivation by human liver slices (Bain and Batty, 1956). Nevertheless, Bain's interest in such matters continued. Synthetic organic chemistry in his department was being carried out by Dr. Peter Hey (1952) who was studying the relationship between chemical structure and nicotinic activity in a series of choline aryl ethers, in fact extending the early work of Dale referred to in Section 2.1. Among the compounds synthesised was choline-*p*-tolylether bromide (TM6) which, according to Hey's hypothesis, was expected to have only minimal nicotine-like activity. This was measured in terms of its pressor effects in spinal cats. Dr. Jean Olley (personal communication) recalls that the established practice, when testing newly synthesised compounds for the first time, was to use an animal which had already been used for the day's demands for the assay of noradrenaline from liver incubation experiments. It was into such an animal in the late evening of 12th April, 1951, that Jean Batty injected 10 mg of TM6, with Dr. Hey standing by expecting little change in arterial blood pressure. But an astonishingly large rise occurred. Hey displayed unshattered faith in his hypothesis on the structure-activity relationships, for among the explanations advanced was that the rise in blood pressure was not due to stimulation of nicotinic receptors but due to some other biological action. A suggested possibility was that TM6 might be an inhibitor of monoamine oxidase (MAO), and the rise in blood pressure therefore attributable to MAO inhibition blocking inactivation of noradrenaline retained in the cat following the repeated doses administered during the earlier assay. As an appropriate test system was to hand this possibility was readily tested. TM6 was found to be indeed a powerful inhibitor of MAO. Modern knowledge prompts us, like Fielden (1981), to doubt whether potentiation of the effects of residual injected noradrenaline by inactivation of MAO could provide a valid explanation of the pressor action of TM6. But fortunately this knowledge was not possessed.

The relationship of the MAO activity among choline aryl ethers was pursued by Brown and Hey (1952, 1956). One of the compounds Hey synthesised for this study was choline 2,6-xylylether bromide (TM10, xylocholine) (Hey and Willey, 1953, 1954). Willey enters the story because he, another research student, was examining the nicotine-like properties of the same newly synthesised compounds by injecting them intravenously into anaesthetised cats.

Again the unexpected happened. Following the first dose of TM10 (10 mg) there was a typical brief rise in blood pressure, not dissimilar from that of nicotine, but subsequent doses were ineffective. Willey then examined the effects of TM10 on contractions of the cat nictitating membrane caused by stimulation of the cervical sympathetic nerve. He found, even when stimulation was postganglionic, that TM10 abolished these responses without impairing, except briefly, responses to adrenaline. As later Bain (1960) put it: 'On the principle of explaining new actions by old ones, Hey and Willey (1953) tested TM10 for local anaesthetic activity, and it proved – unfortunately perhaps – to have a potent and exceptionally long-lasting action of this kind. It seemed logical to conclude that TM10 prevented the effects of nerve stimulation on the nictitating membrane by suppressing conduction in the postganglionic (adrenergic) nerves; but the means of testing this were not then available'. The matter became dormant while attention was focussed on the potentiality of TM10 and its analogues as local anaesthetics.

Arousal of interest in the systemic effects of TM10 began in May 1955 when Bain was seeking a longer acting local anaesthetic than lignocaine for use in status epilepticus. TM10 and related compounds were obvious candidates. As a first step to selecting a compound for this purpose, Dr. K.A. Exley was asked to compare the pharmacology of TM10 and that of its tertiary analogue. Whereas the tertiary compound was equally potent as a local anaesthetic, unlike TM10 it failed to produce comparable block of the sympathetic innervation of the nictitating membrane (Exley, 1957). The observation cast doubt on the validity of the earlier conclusion that TM10 acted by blocking conduction along sympathetic postganglionic nerves, as also did, in yet greater measure, his later electrophysiological experiments (Exley, 1957,

1960) which showed that the propagation of electrical impulses in such nerve trunks was unchanged. Later, Exley (1957) made a major contribution towards understanding how TM10 acted by showing that the drug blocked responses of a variety of tissues to adrenergic nerve stimulation without blocking responses to catecholamines. He also directly demonstrated that the drug acted by impairing transmitter release in the cat spleen. Unfortunately however, besides blocking adrenergic nerves, TM10 also caused powerful parasympathomimetic effects. Its muscarinic properties are very obvious in cats given sympathetic nerve blocking doses (Boura and Green, 1959; Fielden, 1981). The comment of Fielden (1981) suggests that nevertheless heroic procedures were undertaken to establish that the knowledge acquired from animal experiments was meaningful for man – 'The muscarinic properties of TM10 were much too unpleasant for TM10 to be used clinically (personal observation!).'

This fascinating story of accidents, chance and misinterpretation due to incomplete and inaccurate physiological knowledge might not have reached its exciting conclusion had it not been for yet another fortuitous occurrence. The only property of TM10 that attracted attention and led to its further examination was its pressor effect in the cat after a 10mg intravenous dose, that failed to be repeated following a second or subsequent doses in the same animal. This property was not due to TM10 itself but to the presence in the particular batch tested of about 1.25% of the o-tolyl analogue (Fielden, 1981). Had the original batch of TM10 been pure it seems likely that its adrenergic neurone blocking action would not have been found or that its discovery would have been delayed. Guanethidine would then have become the first blocking agent of this kind, its discovery, unlike that of bretylium, being independent of the finding of TM10.

2.3.2 Bretylium

The adrenergic neurone blocking and other properties of TM10 were reported by Professor Bain and his colleagues to a meeting of the British Pharmacological Society in Edinburgh in July 1956 (Fielden, 1981). One of us (A.F.G.) attended that meeting, at a time when enthusiasm for the powerful quaternary ammonium ganglion blocking agents developed at the Wellcome Research Laboratories was waning in consequence of the advent of the better absorbed secondary and tertiary amines (Section 2.2.4). TM10 seemed a likely lead to finding a new class of improved hypotensive agent, providing the muscarinic and nicotinic effects could be dissociated from depression of sympathetic nerve function. It seemed likely that such a drug would be comparably effective as an antihypertensive to the ganglion blocking agents, but would lack the troublesome side effects associated with parasympathetic ganglion blockade. Agents were already known which blocked the vasoconstrictor effects of sympathetic stimulation by inhibiting the actions of the released transmitter at what are now known as α-receptors, but these agents did not block cardiac responses to sympathetic activation mediated through the now-termed β-receptors. Consequently, when these so-called adrenolytic agents, such as phentolamine and phenoxybenzamine, were tried as hypotensives their vasodilator actions were accompanied by marked and often dangerous reflex tachycardia and increased myocardial contractility. Adrenergic neurone blockade was expected to act on the innervation to both blood vessels and heart so that such cardiac reflexes would be avoided. The failure of adrenergic neurone blocking agents, exemplified by TM10, to cause comparable block of the release of catecholamines from the adrenal medulla might limit their effectiveness by comparison with ganglion blockade, which fully blocks such release, but only time and clinical experience could demonstrate its significance.

This was the background that led to the setting up of a programme of research at the Wellcome Research Laboratories to find a compound with an action similar to that of TM10 on adrenergic nerves but devoid of the nicotinic and muscarinic properties that prohibited its clinical use. The programme got off the ground quickly for a number of reasons. Management at Wellcome at that time provided much freedom of action to its scientists and encouraged new enterprises at least at the exploratory stage. One of us (A.L.A.B.) had just joined the Company from University College London and was unentangled by other research commitments. The target was clearly defined and the probability of attaining it considered high. We, as pharmacologists, also had the good fortune of the co-operation of the chemist Dr. F.C. Copp who had already made many quaternary ammonium compounds, similar enough in structure to TM10 to be worth testing. As always he exhibited an insatiable desire to venture into new territories and make new compounds in rapid progression but with due regard to the pharmacological evaluation of each successive compound. He amply occupied the high throughput screens that we developed, to the extent that untested compounds rapidly accumulated when we took respites from screening to examine selected compounds in greater depth. It was during such a respite that one of our principal burdens of unease was lightened. In preliminary tests using anaesthetised cats, some of our best adrenergic neurone blocking agents not only failed to lower blood pressure but paradoxically caused marked rises in blood pressure. This worry was largely alleviated when the cats were tilted into a vertical position to encourage venous pooling and the arterial pressure dropped, as after ganglion blockade (e.g. Fig. 2.1).

Among the quaternary ammonium compounds that were our starting point were those made during the development of antihelminthics, such as bephenium (24) (Copp et al., 1958). When screening these compounds it gradually became clear that results from in vitro preparations such as that of Finkleman (1930) of rabbit ileum, which was favoured at Leeds (Bain, 1960), correlated badly with those obtained from in vivo tests. Compounds were often highly effective in vitro but poorly effective in intact animals. Moreover in vitro tests did not often reveal the high specificity of action sometimes found in vivo. Both kinds of discrepancy are attributable to the selective accumulation of the drugs in adrenergic neurones which is most prominent in vivo – see below. For the initial screen more reliable results were obtained by administering the test substance parenterally to conscious cats at one or two dose levels and then repeatedly measuring over the next 24 hours the degree of relaxation of the nictitating

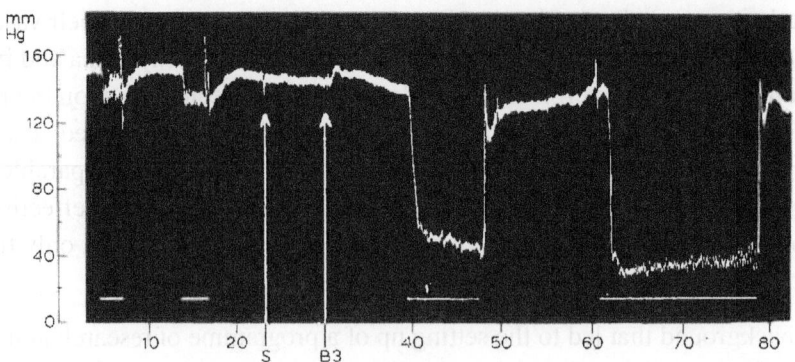

Figure 2.1

Postural hypotension after bretylium in a cat anaesthetized with chloralose. The cat was supine except when tilted through 75°, for the periods indicated by the horizontal white lines. Saline was injected intravenously at S and 3 mg/kg of bretylium at B3. The numerals 10 to 80 indicate the time in min. *Source: (After Boura and Green, 1959).*

membranes (Fig. 2.2). If the compound failed to relax the nictitating membrane after being injected subcutaneously at a dose level of 30 mg/kg it was rejected as inactive. Active compounds having unwanted properties were readily revealed, for example, ganglion blockade dilated the pupils and relaxed the nictitating membranes and muscarinic properties were indicated by salivation, lachrymation and diarrhoea. Effects on the central nervous system would have been indicated by behavioural changes but, because of the blood-brain barrier, these rarely occurred with the highly polar substances being investigated. The cats were used at weekly intervals for screening purposes and generally became increasingly friendly.

PhO.CH₂CH₂.N⁺Me₂.CH₂Ph   PhCH₂.N⁺Me₂.CH₂.CH₂OH

(24) Bephenium   (25) BW25C57   (26) Bretylium (BW373C57)

BW25C57 (25) was the first compound found to cause unequivocal blockade of sympathetic postganglionic nerve function. This was injected into a cat in the morning as was usual practice, at a dosage of 30 mg/kg subcutaneously. The nictitating membranes showed no signs of relaxing and thinking that the compound was probably inactive we went to lunch. On return, to the laboratory, we were gratified to find that the nictitating membranes were slightly relaxed. Moreover this effect developed still further as the afternoon progressed and persisted during the following day. To our delight, miosis, rather than mydriasis, was present indicating that the drug was not a ganglion blocking agent, and there were none of the parasympathomimetic effects associated with TM10. Later investigation using an anaesthetised cat demonstrated that the delay in apparent onset of the adrenergic neurone blockade was due to intervention of early sympathomimetic effects, manifested for example as contraction of

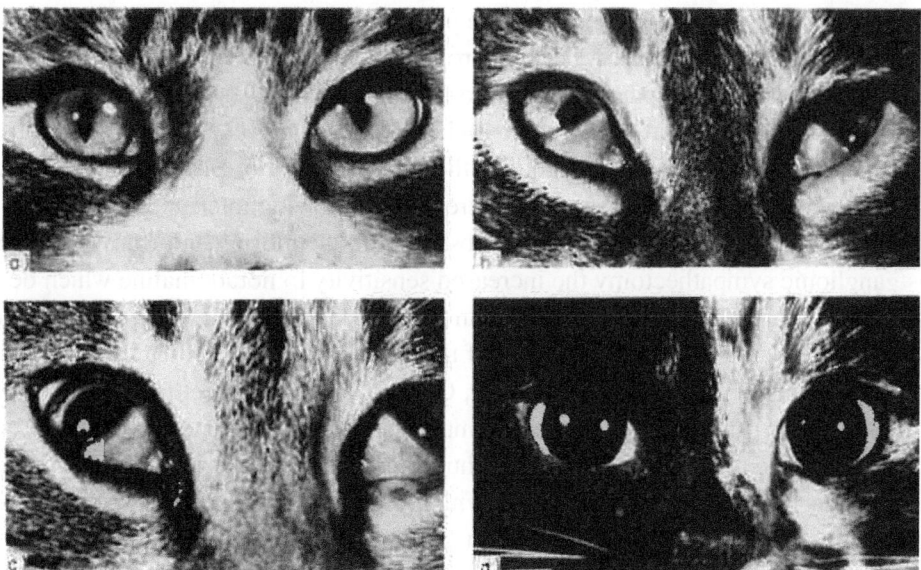

Figure 2.2
Effects of autonomic depressants on the eyes of cats. (a) Normal cat. (b) After adrenergic neurone blockade: the nictitating membranes are relaxed and the palpebral fissures narrowed. (c) After ganglion blockade: as after adrenergic neurone blockade, but the pupils are dilated. (d) After atropine: mydriasis only. *Source: (After Green and Boura 1964).*

the nictitating membranes, a rise of blood pressure and tachycardia. Such effects are now known to be common with adrenergic neurone blocking agents and are most prominent at elevated dosage. Relaxation of the nictitating membranes only occurs after this effect has worn off. Later in 1957 we found that BW373C57 (26) (bretylium) caused long lasting blockade of sympathetic post-ganglionic nerve function but less marked sympathomimetic effects than BW25C57. This led to our studying it in detail. The effects of bretylium on adrenergic mechanisms were shown to closely resemble those of TM10 but its muscarinic actions were minimal (Boura et al., 1959a; Boura and Green, 1959). Subacute toxicity studies revealed no contraindication to a study of the actions of bretylium in man which was arranged at University College Hospital Medical School following detailed discussions with Professor M.L. Rosenheim (later Lord Rosenheim) and Dr. (now Professor) D.R. Laurence. The effects of bretylium in volunteers confirmed the expectations from the animal studies. Trials in hypertensive patients therefore started and bretylium, at first, showed considerable promise (Boura et al., 1959b).

From data obtained from laboratory studies, we had forecast that tolerance to the antihypertensive action of bretylium might become a major problem in its clinical use. We had noticed (Boura et al., 1959b) that in cats, receiving daily substantial doses of the drug, the degree of relaxation of the nictitating membranes became progressively less. Concomitantly the smooth muscle of the nictitating membranes, became progressively more sensitive to the contractile effects of adrenaline and more particularly to noradrenaline (see also Green, 1960; Boura and Green, 1962). Development of hypersensitivity of smooth muscle during continuous adrenergic neurone blockade was analogous to the earlier finding of Bacq (1936) of increased sensitivity of the nictitating membrane to noradrenaline following interruption of transmitter release by nerve section. It also related to the observation of Bülbring and Burn (1949) that after postganglionic sympathectomy the increased sensitivity to noradrenaline which developed was approximately 5–10 times greater than that which developed to adrenaline. These findings were considered to be consequences of the phenomena exemplified in Cannon's Law of Denervation Supersensitivity (Cannon, 1939; Cannon and Rosenblueth, 1949). Hypersensitivity of the smooth muscle of the nictitating membrane, after either nerve section or during continuous adrenergic neurone blockade, was thus considered to be essentially due to reduced output of the transmitter noradrenaline at the sympathetic postganglionic nerve endings. (At the time it was not known that bretylium inhibited neuronal uptake of noradrenaline which contributes to the total hypersensitivity which develops.) Evidence in support of the conclusion that tolerance was a consequence of hypersensitivity was provided two weeks after cutting a preganglionic cervical sympathetic nerve of a cat. When the relaxation of the nictitating membrane on that side had ceased to be present, due to its hypersensitivity to circulating catecholamines, administration of bretylium did not affect the membrane on the operated side but relaxed the membrane which had not been decentralised. Our clinical colleagues concluded, in a joint paper with us, 'it seems likely that tolerance does occur in man but so far this has not been a serious problem' (Boura et al., 1959b). Nevertheless, as time elapsed it became increasingly evident that the degree of tolerance to bretylium which developed was a major handicap in its clinical use for lowering blood pressure. Bretylium was therefore rapidly superseded by guanethidine when this, the second adrenergic neurone blocking agent to be marketed, became available. Guanethidine is better absorbed than bretylium from the alimentary tract and tolerance to its action is far less.

A major step was taken towards an understanding of adrenergic neurone blockade when during studies of its distribution in the body we and our colleagues made the exciting observation that after subcutaneous administration to cats, [^{14}C]bretylium accumulated to surprisingly high concentrations in sympathetic postganglionic nerve trunks but not in cholinergic nerves (Fig. 2.3) (Boura et al., 1960b). Concentrations of bretylium found in sympathetic ganglia, their postganglionic nerves and tissues with dense sympathetic innervation were about thirty times greater than those found in blood at the same time. Obviously the drug was being selectively taken up by sympathetic postganglionic neurones against a concentration gradient, but it required much further work, largely in laboratories elsewhere, before it was appreciated that the concentrating mechanism was the same as that involved physiologically in re-uptake of noradrenaline – the process termed Uptake$_1$ by Iversen (1971). An early pointer that this

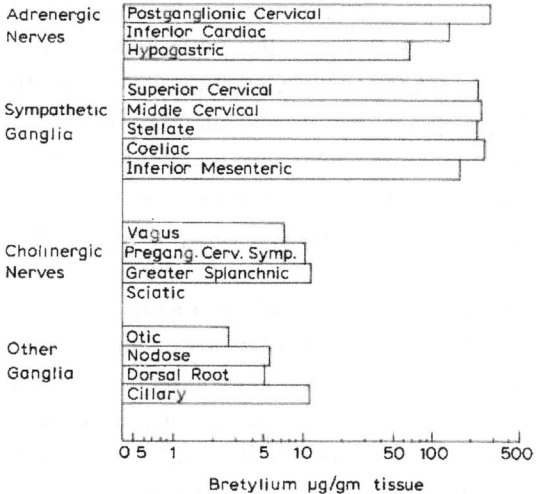

Figure 2.3

The concentration of ^{14}C-labelled bretylium in the peripheral nervous tissue of cats, at 12–18 hours after 10 mg/kg bretylium iodide subcutaneously. Bretylium: molecular weight = 243; 100 μg = 412 nmoles. *Source: (From findings of Boura et al., 1960b; after Green, 1962).*

was so had arisen however during studies of TM10. Cocaine, which blocks the re-uptake process, prevented the onset of TM10 induced adrenergic neurone blockade and partially restored transmitter release and function when given after the drug (Nasmyth and Andrews, 1959). Analogous observations were made during studies of bretylium in 1959 and later of bethanidine and guanethidine (reviewed by Boura and Green, 1965; Maxwell and Wastila, 1977). We also found that there was a temporal relationship between the concentration of bretylium in sympathetic postganglionic nerves and the degree of relaxation of the nictitating membranes (Boura et al., 1960b; Green, 1960). Later, similar observations of selective uptake into adrenergic nerves were made in studies of the blocking agents BW172C58 the 4-benzoyl derivative of TM10 (23) (Boura et al., 1960a; Boura et al., 1961b) and bethanidine (Boura et al., 1962) and analogous results were obtained for guanethidine and debrisoquin (see Maxwell and Wastila, 1977).

The very high concentrations of bretylium present in sympathetic postganglionic nerves led us to investigate whether they would be sufficient to impair axonal conduction. When applied topically they were sufficient to impair conduction in some but not all adrenergic nerve trunks, sensitivity varying substantially. It seemed more likely however that if block of conduction occurred it was at the nerve endings. The greater susceptibility of vasoconstrictor C nerve terminals than of their nerve trunks to depression of conduction was to be expected by analogy with their known susceptibilities to local anaesthetics. Moreover, the concentrations found in adrenergic nerves were fully adequate, when present in an organ bath, to suppress a variety of neuronally mediated end-organ responses not only to adrenergic but also to cholinergic nerve stimulation (Boura and Green, 1959; Boura et al., 1960b; Boyd et al., 1961). Also in 1960, similar observations were made using BW172C60 (Boura et al., 1960a, 1961b). Analogous observations using other blocking agents followed later. Exley (1957, 1960) showed that neither TM10 nor bretylium, which we found after intradermal injection also showed powerful and unusually persistent local anaesthetic properties (Boura and Green, 1959), blocked conduction in sympathetic postganglionic nerve trunks. However, his findings did not exclude the possibility that the depressant action of adrenergic neurone blockade might be explained in terms of an effect at adrenergic nerve terminals analogous to that of local anaesthetics. Much experimental work has led us for many years to conclude that on balance the evidence indicates that this is the mechanism of action and more recent observations using bretylium, guanethidine, bethanidine and other related substances, and in particular the electrophysiological studies of their effects on antidromic neuronal conduction carried out by Haeusler and his colleagues have provided strong support of this hypothesis (for recent reviews see Maxwell and Wastila, 1977; Boura and Green, 1981; Maxwell, 1982).

2.3.2.1 Other quaternary compounds

Whereas bretylium is the best known of the quaternary adrenergic neurone blocking agents, it is not the most active of the 450 compounds of this type that we examined in laboratory tests (for review of structure-activity relationships see Copp, 1964). The most outstanding of these, discovered in 1958, was the already mentioned para benzoyl analogue of TM10 (23), BW172C58 (Boura et al., 1960a). Studies using cats showed it to be 10–20 times more potent than TM10 and virtually devoid of parasympathomimetic properties. A particular asset of this compound, apart from its high activity and selectivity, is its rapid onset of action and relatively short persistence which makes it particularly useful as a pharmacological tool. Nevertheless, when tested in two hypertensive patients, it was found to be less potent than bretylium. BW172C58 exhibited species variation in another way too. Sympathomimetic manifestations after BW172C58 were minimal in cats but prominent in dogs. This only came to light when our colleague Dr. G.A. Stewart examined BW172C58 for effects on blood sugar of dogs and to our embarrassment observed a precipitous rise in blood pressure instead of the expected fall. Our investigation of further quaternary compounds was terminated following reports of the discovery of guanethidine.

2.3.3 Guanethidine

Dr. R.A. Maxwell has related how guanethidine had its pharmacological origin in experiments with the central nervous stimulant, methylphenidate (Maxwell and Wastila, 1977). This was discovered to block completely the pressor and cardiac effects of amphetamine in dogs (Maxwell et al., 1957). During the course of these experiments (carried out in the research laboratories of CIBA Pharmaceutical Products, Summit, NY, U.S.A.) it was the practice, for the purposes of economy, to utilize some dogs used previously for concluded unrelated studies. In this way it came about that cardiovascular experiments were conducted on anaesthetised dogs which previously had been given three or four new compounds at the rate of one a week to assess behavioural effects, a week elapsing between administration of the last compound and the cardiovascular experimentation. One of these dogs was given a large intravenous dose of amphetamine but responded by only a negligible increase in blood pressure. The blockade was as complete as if the animal had been given methylphenidate. This was a startling observation, bearing in mind that the last compound the dog had received had been administered seven days earlier. The cause was sought.

Each of the three or four compounds which the animal had received over the previous weeks was given singly to other dogs and a week allowed to elapse. After this time, the dogs were anaesthetised and challenged with amphetamine. In a most unlikely manner, it transpired that the compound which had been responsible for the blockade was the one which had been given three weeks earlier. This compound was hexahydro-1-azapinepropionamidoxime (Su-4029), (27) synthesised originally as part of an antitrypanosomal programme. Its pharmacology was subsequently examined (Maxwell et al., 1958) and led to Su-4029 being given a trial in man as an antihypertensive agent. This was unsuccessful because the drug caused fever, rash and headache. A systematic study was therefore undertaken of the capacity of congeners of Su-4029 to block the pressor effects of amphetamine given 24 h later. Compound Su-5864, (2-(octa-hydro-1-azocinyl)-ethyl)-guanidine sulphate (28), in addition to blocking pressor responses to amphetamine also relaxed the nictitating membranes of anaesthetised dogs, an action not shared by Su-4029. Relaxation of the nictitating membranes was indicative of reduced sympathetic tone. Su-5864, which was later to receive the generic name of guanethidine (28), received extensive examination and descriptions of its pharmacology appeared soon thereafter (Maxwell et al., 1959, 1960). Trial in man followed rapidly and guanethidine soon became, and has remained, an important drug for the control of hypertension.

$$[CH_2]_6 \; N-CH_2.CH_2.C \overset{\displaystyle NOH}{\underset{\displaystyle NH_2}{\diagup}} \qquad\qquad [CH_2]_7 \; N-CH_2.CH_2NH.C \overset{\displaystyle NH}{\underset{\displaystyle NH_2}{\diagup}}$$

(27) Su 4029   (28) Guanethidine

Largely because of the differences in species and experimental procedures used, it was uncertain at first as to whether the pharmacological properties orginally described for bretylium (Boura and Green, 1959; Green, 1960) and guanethidine (Maxwell et al., 1959, 1960) indicated a common mode of action, though it was noted that both were bases with some structural similarities. However, the biological similarity of the two latter compounds became increasingly clear as pharmacological investigations proceeded in their laboratories of origin and in a large number of academic institutions (for reviews see Green, 1962; Boura and Green, 1965; Maxwell and Wastila, 1977; Armstrong and Green, 1980; Boura and Green, 1981; Green, 1982; Maxwell 1982). Two major distinctions remain. The first is that guanethidine, in contrast to bretylium, causes a fairly rapid depletion of peripheral tissue noradrenaline content. Nevertheless it became clear in 1961, in acute studies of guanethidine, that depletion of tissue catecholamine levels followed the block of sympathetic postganglionic nerve function and was not the cause of it (Cass and Spriggs, 1961), as by this time had been accepted to be the case for reserpine. However, large doses of guanethidine can cause very substantial depletion of the adrenergic transmitter, especially when given daily, and this can sustain impairment of nerve function, particularly where the depletion is associated with neuronal damage (Maxwell, 1982; Boura and Green, 1984). The distinction between the two drugs is not absolute. Bretylium in high doses can also lower tissue catecholamine levels particularly after being given repeatedly. Thus a reduction in tissue catecholamines was found in the heart, spleen and sympathetic ganglia of cats given 14 large parenteral daily doses of 30 mg/kg bretylium (McCoubrey, 1962).

The second major distinction is the differing effects of the two drugs on the relationship between frequency of sympathetic nerve impulses and the response of the innervated tissue. This has considerable practical significance. In studies of the preganglionically stimulated nictitating membrane in anaesthetised cats, we found that bretylium depressed the slope of the curve relating the frequency of applied stimuli to the magnitude of the resultant contraction of the membrane (Boura and Green, 1959) (Fig. 2.4). Moreover when cats that had been dosed subcutaneously with 50 mg/kg bretylium each day for six months, in a chronic toxicity test, were examined their membranes showed small but definite responses to sympathetic nerve stimulation, whereas a single dose of 50 mg/kg was known to suppress fully contractions for over 24 hours (Green, 1960). The very small amounts of adrenergic transmitter that were still being released in the presence of the large dose of bretylium were apparently sufficient at that time to contract the membranes because of the high sensitivity to the transmitter which they had developed during prolonged exposure to the drug. As tolerance to bretylium in man was becoming increasingly troublesome, we examined this phenomenon in greater detail (Boura and Green, 1962). Maximum hypersensitivity to intravenous noradrenaline (approximately 30–100 fold, uncorrected for increased tone due to increased sensitivity to circulating cate-cholamines) occurred after daily subcutaneous doses in the range of 3–50 mg/kg bretylium had been administered for about 7 to 14 days. Its magnitude was comparable with that found 7 days after postganglionic sympathectomy in other cats. Moreover, situations were encoun-tered in which, following particular dosage regimes of bretylium, responses to low rates of nerve stimulation markedly exceeded those in control animals, even though responses to high frequencies were still diminished.

Tolerance was not a problem in the clinical use of guanethidine and when we examined its effects using the cat nictitating membrane model, some remarkable differences were found (Boura and Green, 1962). Guanethidine contrasted with bretylium by not depressing the slope of the curve relating nictitating membrane contraction to frequency of nerve traffic; instead it caused a parallel shift of the curve to the right (Fig. 2.4). The effects of daily administration

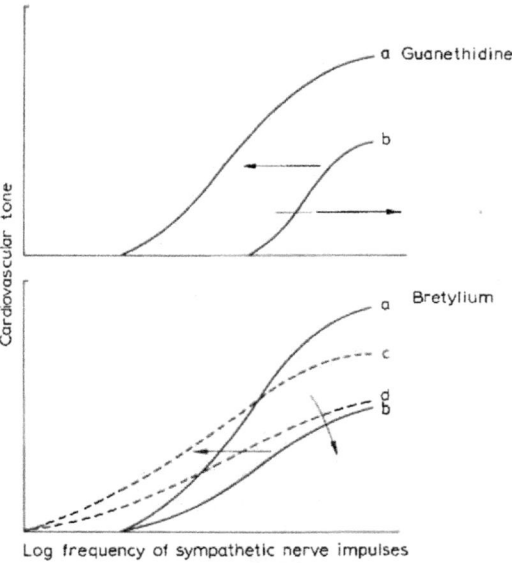

Figure 2.4

Theoretical curves illustrating a possible explanation for the finding that the incidence of tolerance to adrenergic neurone blockade may be higher with bretylium than with guanethidine. *Guanethidine*: the curve relating frequency of stimulation to effect produced in untreated animals (a) shifts to the right after giving the drug (b). The tendency for the curve (b) to shift to the left during the development of hypersensitivity to the adrenergic nerve transmitter that accompanies daily administration of the drug is apparently offset by the cumulative effect of the drug or can be overcome by increasing the dosage. *Bretylium*: the slope of the curve (a) is depressed after giving bretylium (b) to an extent dependent on dosage. When bretylium has been given daily the developed hypersensitivity to adrenergic transmitter may be expected to cause a parallel shift of the curve (b) to a position (c), so that responses to low rates of stimulation tend to exceed those before treatment (curve a). Increased dosage of bretylium is expected to depress the slope of the curve (c) to position (d), but, except when the dosage is large, responses to the lowest rates of stimulation may continue to exceed those before treatment. *Source: (After Boura and Green, 1962).*

of guanethidine were highly cumulative, tending to move the curve progressively to the right but the concomitant development of hypersensitivity to adrenergic transmitter (again comparable with that following postganglionic sympathectomy) had the opposing influence of pushing the curve to the left. The curve always remained roughly parallel with that in controls and exaggeration of responses to low rates of sympathetic nerve stimulation, such as was observed with bretylium, was never encountered. These findings provided a highly plausible explanation of the observed differences between the degrees of tolerance to bretylium and guanethidine which developed in man.

The different effects of bretylium and guanethidine on nerve impulse frequency curves were also thought likely to have relevance to their comparative hypotensive effects that depend

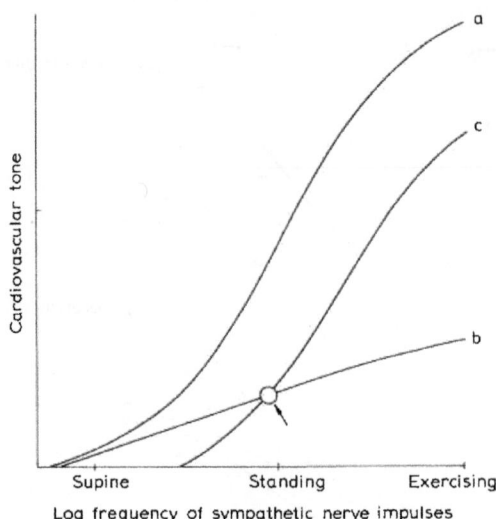

Figure 2.5

Expected relative effects of bretylium and guanethidine on cardiovascular tone in man depending on whether a subject is supine, standing or exercising. It is assumed that the frequency of sympathetic nerve impulses is least when the subject is supine and greatest during exercise and that the relation of this frequency to cardiovascular tone (control = a) is affected by bretylium (b) and guanethidine (c) in like manner to the nerve frequency-nictitating membrane response curves. The dose of bretylium or guanethidine usually given is that which causes the desired lowering of cardiovascular tone with the subject standing – this is represented by the circle at the intersection of the curves.
Source: (After Boura and Green, 1962).

on whether the subjects are supine, standing or exercising (Boura and Green, 1962). When dosage is chosen as that which causes the desired lowering of cardiovascular tone with the subject standing, (Fig. 2.5) bretylium would be expected to have the greatest hypotensive action when sympathetic traffic is high, for example, during exercise, whereas guanethidine, which in contrast preferentially abolishes responses to the lower frequencies of nerve traffic, would be expected to have a relatively greater effect on the blood pressure of supine subjects and be more liable to cause bradycardia. These expectations were paralleled by such clinical observations as were then available (Taylor and Donald, 1960; Dollery et al., 1960) and were supported by later clinical findings.

Although the initial studies on nerve frequency-end organ response relationships that led to the tentative proposal of the above hypotheses were carried out solely using cat nictitating membrane preparations, analogous differences between the effects of bretylium and guanethidine were later observed using a variety of other indirectly stimulated tissues (Green and Robson, 1964; Boura and Green, 1984). Similarly, hypersensitivity to noradrenaline and to adrenaline also develops in tissues other than the nictitating membranes, as following sympathectomy, but its magnitude varies substantially between tissues and in few reaches hypersensitivity levels comparable to that reached by the cat nictitating membrane (Green and Robson, 1965; Boura and Green, 1984). The extent of tolerance varies with the level of tissue hypersensitivity fortunately being less prominent for the cardiovascular system for example, than for the nictitating membranes.

These studies were of value not only for understanding the mechanism of action of bretylium and guanethidine and observed differences in their effects in clinical use, but also for setting criteria which could be used in the laboratory for selecting candidate adrenergic neurone blocking agents likely to show advantages over both bretylium and guanethidine. Thus it seemed that a preferred compound would not cause major depletion of the adrenergic transmitter. At this time guanethidine was considered by some clinicians to have an unduly prolonged duration of effect and there was reason sometimes to want more rapid recovery from its action during continuous therapy, for example to allow temporary recovery of ejaculatory function in males, or when the dose administered caused excessive hypotension. On the other hand, the nerve stimulation-frequency studies indicated that the effect of any new compound on the frequency-response curves should resemble that of guanethidine rather than that of bretylium. Studies in man provided two other opportunities of finding a better blocking agent than guanethidine. Whereas absorption of guanethidine from the alimentary tract was better than that of bretylium it was far from complete (Dollery et al., 1960). Additionally diarrhoea frequently developed and was often very severe with guanethidine, apparently more so than with bretylium. This action could have been simply a result of full unmasking of parasympathetic influences on the gut associated with complete suppression of responses to low rates of sympathetic traffic, but some observations of Cass and Spriggs (1961) had possible relevance. They found that guanethidine released endogenous 5-hydroxytryptamine in rats. This amine is well-known for increasing intestinal motility. Hence four possible ways of improving on guanethidine became known within a year or two of its introduction.

More recently it has been found that the high concentrations of guanethidine taken up into adrenergic neurones and responsible for their selective blockade can, when they have persisted over a prolonged period, result in neuronal damage (for review see Maxwell, 1982). Dr. Maxwell points out that it is not known if neuronal destruction is caused by guanethidine in man but the drug has been widely used over 20 years without effects attributable to irreversible sympathetic inhibition being reported. Nevertheless freedom from potential to cause irreversible neuronal damage would be advantageous in an alternative drug. Irreversible damage has been reported after guanacline (see below).

2.3.4 Bethanidine and other guanidines

At the time our chemist colleagues synthesised bethanidine and other benzyl and phenoxyethylguanidines (Boura et al., 1961a) the known differences between the pharmacological properties of bretylium and TM10 on the one hand and guanethidine on the other, which have already been mentioned above, raised doubt about whether they shared a common mode of action in blocking adrenergic neurones. Nevertheless it was argued that guanethidine could have a fundamentally similar action to that of the quaternary blocking agents and that the highly basic guanidine and quaternary ammonium groups, could have similar influences in governing pharmacological action. This prompted synthesis and our examination of the guanidine derivatives (29) to (32).

(29) R=H,Me,Cl,Br,NO$_2$;
R^1 and/or R^2= H,Me or Et

(30) R=H
(31) R=Me

(32)

(33) Debrisoquin

Among the most potent of these compounds was BW467C60 later called bethanidine (29, R = H: R1 = R2 = Me) and BW392C60 (29, R = Cl, R1 = R2 = Me). Both were more active than guanethidine when tested for their relaxant actions on the cat nictitating membranes and in contrast to guanethidine were approximately as effective orally as parenterally. In its effects on tissue noradrenaline and on responses to tyramine the effects of bethanidine were intermediate between those of bretylium and guanethidine, whereas the effects of BW392C60 mimicked those of bretylium. A particularly close analogy between the quaternary ammonium blocking agents and the related guanidine derivatives was found for the phenoxyethyl compounds. Adrenergic neurone blocking activity was attended by a strong muscarinic activity in compound (30) but not (31), just as it is in TM10 but not in its β-methyl derivative (Boura et al., 1961a).

Bethanidine and its ortho chloro derivative BW392C60 were subjected to more intensive pharmacological study (Boura and Green, 1963; Green and Robson, 1964, 1965) and were tested in man first by Montuschi and Pickens (1962), when toxicological evaluation had reached a suitably advanced stage. (Toxicological studies of bethanidine recently reported by Green and Weatherall, 1984, amply illustrate the fast escalation of standards of testing that was occurring by the early 1960s.) These and subsequent clinical reports on bethanidine, the preferred compound, were favourable (Johnston et al., 1962; Smirk, 1962, 1963) and bethanidine came to be accepted as an alternative and sometimes preferred therapy to guanethidine in the many countries in which it was introduced. Exceptionally, marketing did not take place in the United States, the submission, like many others on cardiovascular drugs, having been rejected by the F.D.A. despite the accumulated wealth of data showing its safety in animals and man (Green and Weatherall, 1984).

Bethanidine is a good but not an exact fit for our guiding specification of the ideal adrenergic neurone blocking agent, referred to in the previous section. It is well absorbed without change when given orally and rarely produces severe diarrhoea (Boura and Green, 1963; Boura and Green, 1984). Also it does not damage adrenergic neurones (Boura and Green, 1981) nor cause marked depletion of tissue noradrenaline (Costa et al., 1962; Boura and Green, 1963) and consequently its action can be more readily terminated than that of guanethidine by withholding treatment when desired. Less exact is the fit in relation to what are considered the wanted effects on the nerve-frequency and organ response curves. The effects of bethanidine in this respect are intermediate between those of guanethidine and bretylium. There is a right shift of the curves, showing a preferential suppression of the effects of low frequency traffic, but also some depression of the slope (Boura and Green, 1963; Green and Robson, 1964, 1965). Effects observed in man correspond well. The expectation of tolerance liability from the curves is that the dosage of bethanidine will more often require upward adjustment than is the case for guanethidine, but that run-away tolerance of the kind encountered with bretylium will not occur. This has been the situation during some twenty years use of bethanidine. Rather greater postural hypotension than with guanethidine is expected and was found (Prichard et al., 1968; Prichard and Waldren, 1979). Both the pharmacological and toxicological studies showed a high level of predictive accuracy (Green and Weatherall, 1984).

The question arises whether it might have been possible to have found an adrenergic neurone blocking agent that fulfilled all the desired criteria. This is questionable for as we have pointed out previously (Boura and Green, 1963, 1984) there seems to be a correlation among different compounds between ability to cause a parallel shift of the nerve frequency response curve and capacity to deplete tissue noradrenaline. Perhaps only a compromise on both properties can be realised, as in the case of bethanidine. An unequivocal answer to this question will probably never be obtained.

Many other companies also expended substantial resources in the search for improved guanidine derivatives following the discovery of guanethidine (see Maxwell and Wastila, 1977). The only one to stand the test of time in antihypertensive therapy is debrisoquin (33). It was discovered at the Roche Laboratories in the United States by Moe et al. (1964) and resembles bethanidine both chemically and pharmacologically. Some other long-acting guanidine derivatives such as guanacline have prominent irreversible damaging effects on adrenergic neurones (Burnstock et al., 1971) and cause persistent hypotension in patients after drug withdrawal (Dawborn et al., 1969).

The urge to seek better adrenergic neurone blocking agents passed when β-receptor antagonists were unexpectedly found to be effective antihypertensive agents. They together with the thiazide diuretics, α-methyldopa, clonidine and some recently discovered inhibitors of the angiotensin converting enzyme (captopril and enalapril) have the advantage of being able to control hypertension, without causing postural or exertional hypotension. Nevertheless adrenergic neurone blockade continues to be the treatment of choice for many severely hypertensive patients. The rate of progress in the discovery of new kinds of antihypertensive drugs since 1948 has been remarkable. It has been attended by stimulation and excitement for a large number of research workers in many disciplines, an enormous growth in knowledge of the physiology of peripheral autonomic mechanisms and, most importantly, a greatly prolonged and more agreeable life expectancy for a vast number of victims of hypertensive disease.

Acknowledgements

Our grateful thanks are due to Mrs. Rosemary Frigo, Mrs. Anne Grabinar and Mrs. Maureen Rose for skilful secretarial assistance and to Mr. Richard Crompton for photography.

References

Acheson, G.H., Moe, G.K., 1946. J. Pharmacol. Exp. Ther. 87, 220–236.
Acheson, G.H., Pereira, S.A., 1946. J. Pharmacol. Exp. Ther. 87, 273–280.
Adamson, D.W., Billinghurst, J.W., Green, A.F., Locket, S., 1956. Nature 177, 523–524.
Armstrong, J.M. and Green, A.F., (1980). In: Handbook of Experimental Pharmacology 54/1: (Szekeres, L., Ed.) pp. 135–221, Springer-Verlag, Berlin, Heidelberg, New York.
Arnold, P., Goetz, R.H., Rosenheim, M.L., 1949. Lancet ii, 408–410.
Arnold, P., Rosenheim, M.L., 1949. Lancet ii, 321–323.
Bacq, Z.M., 1936. Mem. Acad. R. Med. Belg. 25, 1–61.
Bain, W.A., (1960). In: Ciba Foundation Symposium on Adrenergic Mechanisms. (Wolstenholme, G.E.W. and O'Connor, M., Eds.), pp. 131–147, J. and A. Churchill, London.
Bain, W.A., Batty, J.E., 1956. Br. J. Pharmacol. 11, 52–57.
Bain, W.A., Dickinson, S., 1938. J. Physiol. 93, 54–55P.
Billinghurst, J.W., (1956). In: Hypotensive drugs (Harrington, M., Ed.), pp. 35–39, Pergamon, New York.
Boura, A.L.A., Coker, G.G., Copp, F.C., Duncombe, W.G., Elphick, A.R., Green, A.F., McCoubrey, A., 1960a. Nature 185, 925–926.
Boura, A.L.A., Copp, F.C., Duncombe, W.G., Green, A.F., McCoubrey, A., 1960b. Br. J. Pharmacol. 15, 265–270.
Boura, A.L.A., Copp, F.C., Green, A.F., 1959a. Nature 184, 70–71 B.A.
Boura, A.L.A., Copp, F.C., Green, A.F., Hodson, H.R., Ruffell, G.K., Sim, M.F., Walton, E., Grivsky, E.M., 1961a. Nature 191, 1312–1313.
Boura, A.L.A., Duncombe, W.G., McCoubrey, A., 1961b. Br. J. Pharmacol. 17, 92–100.
Boura, A.L.A., Duncombe, W.G., Robson, R.D., McCoubery, A., 1962. J. Pharm. Pharmacol. 14, 722–726.
Boura, A.L.A., Green, A.F., 1959. Br. J. Pharmacol. 14, 536–548.
Boura, A.L.A., Green, A.F., 1962. Br. J. Pharmacol. 19, 13–41.
Boura, A.L.A., Green, A.F., 1963. Br. J. Pharmacol. 20, 36–55.
Boura, A.L.A., Green, A.F., 1965. Annu. Rev. Pharmacol. 5, 183–212.
Boura, A.L.A., Green, A.F., 1981. J. Auton. Pharmacol. 1, 255–267.
Boura, A.L.A. and Green, A.F., (1984). In: Handbook of Hypertension (van Zwieten, P.A., Ed.), vol. 3, 194–238, Elsevier, Amsterdam.

Boura, A.L.A., Green, A.F., McCoubrey, A., Laurence, D.R., Moulton, R., Rosenheim, M.L., 1959b. Lancet ii, 17–21.

Bovet, D., Courvoisier, S., Ducrot, R., Horclois, R., 1947. C.R. Acad. Sci. Paris 224, 1733–1734.

Boyd, H., Chang, V., Rand, M.J., 1961. Arch. Int. Pharmacodyn. 131, 10–23.

Brown, B.G., Hey, P., 1952. J. Physiol. 118, 15P.

Brown, B.G., Hey, P., 1956. Br. J. Pharmacol. 11, 58–65.

Bülbring, E., Burn, J.H., 1949. Br. J. Pharmacol. Chemother. 4, 202–208.

Burn, J.H., Dale, H.H., 1915. J. Pharmacol. Exp. Ther. VI (4), 417–438.

Burnstock, G., Doyle, A.E., Gannon, B.J., Gerkens, J.F., Iwayama, T., Mashford, M.L., 1971. Eur. J. Pharmacol. 13, 175–187.

Burt, C.C., Graham, A.J.P., 1950. Br. Med. J. 455–460.

Cannon, W.B., 1939. Am. J. Med. Sci. 198, 737–750.

Cannon, W.B., Rosenblueth, A., 1949. The supersensitivity of denervated structures. A Law of Denervation. Macmillan, New York.

Cass, R., Spriggs, T.L.B., 1961. Br. J. Pharmacol. 17, 442–450.

Copp, F.C., 1964. Adv. Drug Res. 1, 161–189.

Copp, F.C., Standen, O.D., Scarnell, J., Rawes, D.A., Burrows, R.B., 1958. Nature 181, 183.

Costa, E., Kuntzman, R., Gessa, G.L., Brodie, B.B., 1962. Life Sci 1, 75–80.

Crum Brown, A., Fraser, T.R., 1869. R. Soc. Edinburgh Proc. 6, 556–561.

Dale, H.H., 1914. J. Pharmacol. Exp. Ther. VI (2), 147–190.

Dale, H.H., 1953. Adventures in Physiology. Pergamon Press Ltd., London, p. 652.

Dale, H.H., Richards, A.N., 1918. J. Physiol. LII, 110–165.

Dawborn, J.K., Doyle, A.E., Ebringer, A., Howqua, J., Jerums, G., Johnston, C.I., Mashford, M.L., Parkin, J.D., 1969. Pharmacol. Clin. 2, 1–5.

Dollery, C.T., Emslie-Smith, D., Milne, M.D., 1960. Lancet ii, 381–387.

Emmelin, N., 1959. Br. J. Pharmacol. 15, 260–261.

Enderby, G.E.H., 1950. Lancet i, 1145–1147.

Everett, A.J., Lowe, L.A., Wilkinson, S.W., 1970. J. Chem. Soc. D. 16, 1020–1021.

Exley, K.A., 1957. Br. J. Pharmacol. 12, 297–305.

Exley, K.A., (1960). In: Ciba Foundation Symposium on Adrenergic Mechanisms (Vane, J.R., Wolstenholme, G.E.W. and O'Conor, M., Eds.), pp. 158–161, Churchill, London.

Fielden, R., 1981. J. Auton. Pharmacol. 1, 251–254.

Finkleman, B., 1930. J. Physiol. 70, 145–157.

Gray, J.A.B., Paton, W.D.M., 1949. J. Physiol. 110, 173–193.

Green, A.F., (1956). In: Hypotensive drugs (Harrington, M., Ed.), pp. 95–99, Pergamon, New York.

Green, A.F., (1960). In: Ciba Foundation Symposium on Adrenergic Mechanisms (Vane, J.R., Wolstenholme, G.E.W. and O'Connor, M., Eds.), March 28–31, London, pp. 148–157, Churchill, London.

Green, A.F., 1962. Adv. Pharmacol. 1, 161–225.

Green, A.F., 1982. Br. J. Clin. Pharmacol. 13, 25–34.

Green, A.F. and Boura, A.L.A., (1964). In: Evaluation of Drug Activities: Pharmacometrics, Vol. 1 (Laurence, D.R. and Bacharach, A.L., Eds.), pp. 369–430, Academic Press, London.

Green, A.F., Robson, R.D., 1964. Br. J. Pharmacol. 22, 349–355.

Green, A.F., Robson, R.D., 1965. Br. J. Pharmacol. 25, 497–506.

Green, A.F. and Weatherall, M., (1984). In: Safety Testing of New Drugs (Laurence, D.R., McLean, A.E.M. and Weatherall, M., Eds.), pp. 5–18, Academic Press, London.

Hall, H.K., 1957. J. Am. Chem. Soc. 79, 5444–5454.

Hey, P., 1952. Br. J. Pharmacol. 7, 117–129.

Hey, P., Willey, G.L., 1953. J. Physiol. 122, 75P–76P.

Hey, P., Willey, G.L., 1954. Br. J. Pharmacol. 9, 471–475.

Hunt, R., Taveau, R.de M., 1911. Bull. U.S. Hyg. Lab. 73, 11–136.

Ing, H.R., (1956). In: Hypotensive Drugs (Harrington, M., Ed.), pp. 7–27, Pergamon, New York.

Iversen, L.L., 1971. Br. J. Pharmacol. 4, 571–591.

Johnston, A.N., Prichard, B.N.C. and Rosenheim, M.L., (1962). Lancet *ii,* 996.

Kay, A.W., Smith, A.N., 1950. Br. Med. J. 1, 460–463.

King, H., 1935. J. Chem. Soc. 1381–1389.

Langley, J.N., Dickinson, W.L., 1889. Proc. R. Soc. 46, 423–431.

Lee, G.E., Wragg, S.J., Corne, S.J., Edge, N.D., Reading, H.W., 1958. Nature 181, 1717–1719.

Leonard, N.J., Hauck, F.P., 1957. J. Am. Chem. Soc. 79, 5279–5292.

Libman, D.D., Pain, D.L., Slack, L., 1952. J. Chem. Soc. 2305–2307.

Locket, S., (1956). In: Hypotensive Drugs (Harrington, M., Ed.), p. 142, Pergamon, New York.

Macintosh, F.C., Paton, W.D.M., 1949. J. Physiol. 109, 190–219.

Mason, D.F.K., Wien, R., 1955. Br. J. Pharmacol. 10, 124–132.

Maxwell, R.A., 1982. Br. J. Clin. Pharmacol. 13, 35–44.

Maxwell, R.A., Mull, R.P., Plummer, A.J., 1959. Experientia (Basel) 15, 267.

Maxwell, R.A., Plummer, A.J., Ross, S.D., Paytas, J.J., Dennis, A.D., 1957. Arch. Int. Pharmacodyn. 112, 26–35.

Maxwell, R.A., Plummer, A.J., Schneider, F., Povalski, H., Daniel, A.I., 1960. J. Pharmacol. Exp. Ther. 128, 22–29.

Maxwell, R.A., Ross, S.D., Plummer, A.J., 1958. J. Pharmacol. Exp. Ther. 123, 128–139.

Maxwell, R.A., Wastila, W.B., 1977. Handbook of Experimental Pharmacology. In: Gross, F. (Ed.), 39: Antihypertensive Agents. Springer-Verlag, Berlin, pp. 161–261.

McCoubrey, A., 1962. J. Pharm. Pharmacol. 14 772–734.

Moe, R.A., Bates, H.M., Palkoski, Z.M., Banziger, R., 1964. Curr. Ther. Res. 6, 299–318.

Moe, G.K., Freyburger, W.A., 1950. Pharmacol. Rev. 2, 61–95.

Montuschi, E., Pickens, P.T., 1962. Lancet 897–901.

Morrison, B., Paton, W.D.M., 1953. Br. Med. J. i, 1299–1305.

Nasmyth, P.A., Andrews, W.H.H., 1959. Br. J. Pharmacol. 14, 477–483.

Paton, W.D.M., 1951a. Br. J. Pharmacol. 6, 499–508.

Paton, W.D.M., 1951b. Br. Med. J. i, 773–778.

Paton, W.D.M., 1954. Lectures on the Scientific Basis of Medicine, II. University of London, Athlane Press, London, pp. 139–164.

Paton, W.D.M., 1982. Br. J. Clin. Pharmacol. 13, 7–14.

Paton, W.D.M., Zaimis, E.J., 1948. Nature 161, 718–719.

Paton, W.D.M., Zaimis, E.J., 1949. Br. J. Pharmacol. Chemother. 4, 381–400.

Paton, W.D.M., Zaimis, E.J., 1951. Br. J. Pharmacol. 6, 155–168.

Plummer, A.J., Trapold, J.H., Schneider, J.A., Maxwell, R.A., Earl, A.E., 1955. J. Pharmacol. Exp. Ther. 115, 172–184.

Prichard, B.N.C., Johnston, A.W., Hill, I.D., Rosenheim, M.L., 1968. Br. Med. J. 1, 135–144.

Prichard, B.N.C., Waldren, R.J., 1979. Pharmacol. Ther. 5, 55–59.

Randall, L.C., Peterson, W.G., Lehman, G., 1949. J. Pharmacol. Exp. Ther. 97, 48–57.

Smirk, F.H., 1962. N.Z. Med. J. 61, 608–609.

Smirk, H., 1963. Lancet i, 743–746.

Spinks, A., Young, E.H.P., 1958. Nature 181, 1397–1398.

Stein, G.A., Sletzinger, M., Arnold, M., Reinhold, D., Gaines, W., Pfister, K., 1956. J. Am. Chem. Soc. 78, 1514–1515.

Stone, C.A., Torchiana, M.L., Navarro, A., Beyer, K.H., 1956. J. Pharmacol. Exp. Ther. 117, 169–183.

Taylor, S.H., Donald, K.W., 1960. Lancet ii, 389–394.

Zaimis, E.J., 1950. Br. J. Pharmacol. 424–430.

Zaimis, E.J., (1956). In: Hypotensive Drugs (Harrington, M., Ed.), pp. 85–92, Pergamon, New York.

Commentary on The proliferation of non-steroidal anti-inflammatory drugs (NSAIDs) by T.Y. Shen

Kim D. Rainsford

Department of Biosciences and Chemistry, Sheffield Hallam University, Sheffield, United Kingdom

The large number of non-steroidal anti-inflammatory drugs (NSAIDs) that were discovered and developed in the period of 1955–70 has been aptly described by the author of this chapter as the "golden era of Edinsonian Empiricism" (Shen, 1985). The focus of this period was to develop drugs to control the pain and inflammation accompanying the development of rheumatoid arthritis, then considered the principal rheumatic disease in need of therapy. The drugs then available for treating these conditions included salicylates, aspirin, aminophenols (phenacetin), and pyrazalones that dated from the beginning of the 20th century. Phenylbutazone discovered at J.R. Geigy in the 1950s had been used to solubilize the analgesic aminopyrine but was accidentally discovered as an effective anti-inflammatory agent.

While phenylbutazone was a very effective drug, especially for ankylosing spondylitis it had concerns relating to the occurrence of agranulocytosis and other blood dyscrasias. Later, it was found that this was due to systemic drug accumulation. The corticosteroids discovered by Hench in the 1960s were heralded as magic drugs. But it was not long before their toxicity was proven of serious concern. We now know that this was a consequence of the use of excessively high doses. Now it is known that moderately low doses (e.g., 5–10 mg prednisolone daily) are very effective while having low and acceptable toxicity. Over the years, moderation in the use and dosage of many anti-inflammatory drugs has led to the recognition that potentially toxic agents can be relatively safe.

Since this review by Shen in 1984, the state of conditions that constitute rheumatic diseases as well as their therapies has changed dramatically (Whitehouse, 2005). Rheumatoid arthritis and psoriatic arthritis and other immunological conditions have been effectively reduced, especially in their severity by the application of synthetic disease-modifying antirheumatic drugs (DMARDs), among them low-dose methotrexate, sulphasalazine, minocycline, anti-cancer agents such as cyclophosphamide, cyclosporin A, and more recently by selective anti-cytokine biologics, e.g., anakinra, tocilizumab, anti-T-cell, and anti-B-cell antibodies which

Discoveries in Pharmacology, Volume 3, Hemodynamics and Immune Defense.
DOI: https://doi.org/10.1016/B978-0-443-18442-0.00003-3

have been applied in patients that have been less responsive to DMARDs. Each of these drug developments has resulted from extensive immunopathological and mechanistic investigations on rheumatic diseases. These research developments have been facilitated by major advances in cell and molecule biological techniques and technologies, most of which were hardly envisaged back in the time when Shen wrote his review. Likewise, advances in enzymology and molecular biology of the specific enzyme systems controlling the production of lipid mediators (prostaglandins, phospholipases, and leukotrienes), reactive oxygen species (ROS, e.g., nitric oxide, superoxide, and peroxynitrite), and modified proteins (e.g., oxyradicals). These advances have enabled specific targets to be identified for potential drugs. Furthermore, the involvement of these targets in the initiation and amplification of inflammatory processes has been quantified so enabling advances in therapeutic applications of new and established drugs.

Among the rheumatic conditions which have been investigated during the past century and found of great significance in human health, have been gout and hyperuricaemia. The biochemistry of gout was established by chemists and biochemists and biochemists around the late 19th century. With advances in the application of these techniques, gout, and hyperuricaemia are now recognized as being amongst the most prevalent arthritic conditions, having the most profound consequences, especially in aging populations. Among the most recently recognized comorbidities associated with gout and hyperuricemia have been the development of renal and cardiovascular complications. Drug treatments for gout include hyperuricaemic agents and potent anti-inflammatory analgesics for the relief of pain from tophic and leucocyte-mediated joint inflammation. The earliest therapies dating to Roman times were based on the application of extracts of salicylate-containing plants, colchicine (from *Colchicum autumnale*/or the autumn crocus), the latter still being employed extensively to this day. The salicylate-containing plants served as the basis for therapy not only of gout but also classically, other inflammatory conditions such as osteoarthritis. The post-World War II period saw the development of what are now termed non-steroidal anti-inflammatory drugs (NSAIDs) based on salicylates (and later aspirin) which include ibuprofen, naproxen, and diclofenac. While these developments relied on the classical structure-activity relationships among a whole range of acidic drugs, it was the isolation and characterization of two isoforms of the cyclo-oxygenase (COX-1 or the constitutive enzyme) and the inflammation-inducible COX-2) in 1994 that gave rise to an immense range and variety of new drugs (reviewed by Vane et al., 1996) as well as defining the COX-specificity of various established NSAIDs. Enormous efforts and commercialization of these inventions followed with some limited successes (Whitehouse, 2005) and in some cases untoward outcomes (Rainsford et al., 2016). Since the 1980s NSAIDs have been applied generically and are recognized as being safe in what are low-prescription level doses for use over short periods (3–10 days) in non-prescription or "over-the-counter" sales to the lay public. The focus on cyclo-oxygenase inhibitors exemplified by the development of the various NSAIDs has since been overtaken by elegant discoveries of drugs affecting the arachidonic acid cascade, microsomal PGE-2 synthase-1, phospholipase, leukotriene MAP kinase, II kappa/NF-kappa B inhibitors, cannabinoid antagonists, glucocorticoid receptor antagonists, and sphingolipid inhibitors (Levin and Laufer, 2012).

Recognition of the relative safety of these drugs and their safe application in a wide range of low-grade, mild inflammatory states has probably represented the most profound therapeutic advance in the past 3–4 decades. Moreover, the development of an immense number and type of oral or parenteral formulations of NSAIDs and paracetamol (acetaminophen) and other non-opioid analgesics (e.g., dipyrone or metamizole) has enabled these drugs to be applied for an immense range and type of inflammatory states. These advances have built upon the medicinal chemistry and biochemical pharmacology of drugs discussed by Shen from work carried out four or more decades ago, including the major contributions of Shen himself (Hannah et al., 1977; Shen, 1977; Hannah et al., 1978; Shen, 1985).

References

Hannah, J., Ruyle, W.V., Jones, H., Matzuk, A.R., Kelly, K.W., Witzel, B.E., Holtz, W.J., Houser, R.W., Shen, T.Y., Sarett, L.H., 1977. Discovery of diflunisal. Br. J. Clin. Pharmacol. 4 Suppl 1 (Suppl 1), 7S–13S.

Hannah, J., Ruyle, W.V., Jones, H., Matzuk, A.R., Kelly, K.W., Witzel, B.E., Holtz, W.J., Houser, R.A., Shen, T.Y., Sarett, L.H., 1978. Novel analgesic-antiinflammatory salicylates. J. Med. Chem. 21, 1093–1097.

Levin, J.I., Laufer, S. (Eds.), 2012. Anti-Inflammatory Drug Discovery, series 26. The Royal Society of Chemistry, Cambridge.

Rainsford, K.D., Kean, I.R.L., Kean, W.F., 2016. Gastro-intestinal complications of anti-rheumatic drugs. In: Font, J., Ramos-Casals, M., Rhodes, J. (Eds.). Handbook of Systemic Autoimmune Diseases, Vol. 8, second ed. Elsevier BV, Amsterdam.

Shen, T.Y., 1977. Expanding vistas of nonacidic antiarthritic agents. New anti-inflammatory and antarthritic drugs. In: Bertelli, A (Ed.), Drugs Under Experimental and Clinical Research, Vol. II. JR Prous Publisher, Barcelona, Spain, pp. 1–8.

Shen, T.Y., 1985. Indomethacin, sulindac, and their analogues. In: Anti-Inflammatory and Anti-Rheumatic Dugs. Volume 1: Inflammation Mechanisms and Actions of Traditional Drugs. CRC Press, Boca Raton Fl, pp. 149–159.

Vane, J., Botting, J., Botting, R. (Eds.), 1996. Improved Non-Steroid Anti-Inflammatory Drugs: COX-2 Enzyme Inhibitors. Kluwer Academic Publishers, Dordrecht and Lancaster, & William Harvey Press, Charterhouse Square, London.

Whitehouse, M.W., 2005. Drugs to treat inflammation: a historical introduction. Current Med. Chem. 12, 2931–2942.

The proliferation of non-steroidal anti-inflammatory drugs (NSAIDS)

T.Y. Shen

Contents

3.1 Introduction

NSAIDS are a new class of therapeutic agents largely developed in the past two decades for the treatment of inflammation and pain associated with arthritis and other inflammatory

---

Disclaimer: The original text that follows is reproduced from the first edition and carries errors and omissions from it. The editors and publisher agreed to retain them and honor the original authors and challenges they had to deal with in publishing back in those times.

Discoveries in Pharmacology, Volume 3, Hemodynamics and Immune Defense.
DOI: https://doi.org/10.1016/B978-0-443-18442-0.00063-X

Table 3.1: NSAIDS in clinical use.*

1. *Carboxylic acids*	R CO$_2$H	Pirprofen	
Aspirin		Carprofen	
Trilisate	(1978)	Benoxaprofen**	(1982)
Benorylate		Suprofen	
Diflunisal	(1982)	Tiaprofenic acid	
Fendosal		Indoprofen	
Mefenamic acid	(1967)		
Meclofenamate	(1980)		
			O
			‖
2. *Acetic acids*	R CH$_2$CO$_2$H	4. *Butyric acids*	R CCH$_2$CH$_2$CO$_2$H
Indomethacin	(1965)	Bucloxic acid	
Sulindac	(1978)	Fenbufen	
		Furobufen	
Diclofenac			
Fenclofenac		5. *Acidic enols*	R ⟍ ╱ OH
			C=C
Tolmetin	(1976)		
Zomepirac**	(1980)		
		Phenylbutazone	(1952)
		Oxyphenbutazone	(1960)
	CH$_3$	Piroxicam	(1982)
	|	Isoxicam	
3. *Propionic acids*	R CHCO$_2$H		
Ibuprofen	(1974)	6. *Nonacidic*	
Naproxen	(1976)	Proquazone	
Fenoprofen	(1976)	Ditazole	
Ketoprofen		Tiflamizole	
Flurbiprofen			

*Year of U.S. approval in parenthesis.
** Product withdrawn.

conditions. At the present time, there are approximately 60 NSAIDS widely used in the clinic or in various stages of development. (Some of these are listed in Table 3.1.) It has been estimated that approximately 7% of the total population worldwide are afflicted with various forms of arthritis. In arthritis therapy, the current world market of $2.5 billion per year is steadily growing and may reach $6 billion per year by 1991. Clearly, NSAIDS represent a major therapeutic class of drugs.

Aspirin
(1)

The usefulness of anti-inflammatory agents was recognized in early civilization. The discovery of salicylates and the development of aspirin (1) derivatives are described in the following chapter. While aspirin remains the first line of treatment for arthritic patients, the need for more effective and better tolerated agents was long felt but could not be addressed until some 30 years ago. The discovery of potent anti-inflammatory effects of corticosteroids in the clinic in the 1940s not only dramatically demonstrated the feasibility of finding more effective anti-inflammatory drugs but also facilitated the development of several animal models of acute and chronic inflammation suitable for drug testing. These models in turn encouraged the search for anti-inflammatory drugs of the non-steroidal type in the late 1950s, with the hope of dissociating some serious side effects of corticosteroids from their anti-inflammatory activities. In our laboratories an NSAID project was then initiated with the establishment of a pharmacological screening assay, using a cotton pellet granuloma assay which was devised previously for the investigation of a potent steroid, dexamethasone (Sarett et al., 1963). In this model, aspirin was still too weak to show a consistent and significant inhibition of the granuloma weight but phenylbutazone (41), which was originally used as a complexing agent to solubilize aminopyrine and serendipitously uncovered as an effective anti-inflammatory agent (Domenjoz, 1960), proved to be a more potent and useful reference standard. At the beginning of our pharmacological screening, concerns for toxicity or side effects of test samples were mainly focussed on body weight loss, which might give a false anti-inflammatory effect, and thymus involution, which is indicative of adrenal stimulation. Specific animal models for measuring gastrointestinal irritation and peripheral analgesic activity, two principal parameters in the development of newer NSAIDS later, were still not available. Nevertheless, such a simple start eventually led to the discovery of indomethacin (3) (Shen et al. 1963; Shen and Winter, 1977). Similar animal models of acute or subacute inflammatory responses were used subsequently by many laboratories to develop other NSAIDS. NSAIDS are generally characterized as antiinflammatory, antipyretic and peripheral analgesic agents for the symptomatic relief of inflammation and pain. However, recent studies indicate that several NSAIDS or their related compounds may possess modest effects on some immunopharmacological parameters or possibly even on some aspects of the disease process as well. Conceivably, further extension of the immunopharmacological potential of NSAIDS may broaden the activity profile of these widely used agents further.

In this chapter a brief overview of the proliferation of NSAIDS as a result of an extensive and fruitful anti-inflammatory search in many laboratories will be presented. An attempt will be made to illustrate some of the key concepts, strategic approaches, experimental findings and milestones in this field with a few specific examples. The selection of these examples is admittedly influenced by this author's personal experience. Other important contributions of many laboratories are to be found in several broad surveys published recently (Scherrer and Whitehouse, 1974; Vane and Ferreira, 1979; Shen, 1981). Following a description of the emergence of this class of drugs, the proliferation of NSAIDS will be discussed in terms of the proliferation of their chemical structures, biochemical actions, pharmacodynamic properties and rational clinical applications.

Table 3.2: The evolution of anti-inflammatory therapy.

Major research emphasis	Decade
1. Herbal plants *Salix, spiraea*	prior to 1760
2. Aspirin and salicylates	1900
3. Pyrazolones, phenylbutazone	1940
4. Corticosteroids	1950
5. Indomethacin, Ibuprofen, fenamates (NSAIDS)	1960
6. Proliferation of NSAIDS	1970
7. Immunopharmacological agents	1980

3.2 The emergence of NSAIDS

The evolution of anti-inflammatory therapy in the past several decades is summarized in Table 3.2. Prior to 1960 the limited research activities in studying this class of agents did not merit much attention on NSAIDS in most medicinal chemistry textbooks (e.g. *Burger's Medicinal Chemistry*). The emergence of a broad interest in developing NSAIDS was stimulated by the laboratory progress made in three independent studies, namely, the indole acetic acids, phenyl acetic acids, and *N*-phenylanthranilic acids (fenamates), and especially by the clinical acceptance and marketing success of the first two products, indomethacin and ibuprofen. The experimental approaches and some strategic issues encountered in the first decade of NSAIDS research are briefly discussed below.

In modern drug research, the period between 1955–1970 was sometimes considered as a 'golden era' of Edisonian empiricism. Large-scale pharmacological testing of thousands of compounds in numerous pharmaceutical laboratories uncovered many biologically active leads which were then chemically improved to yield most of the synthetic drugs in use today.

The discovery of NSAIDS followed the same empirical path. Indeed, given the limited understanding of the inflammation process in the mid-1950s, the experimental approach to find non-steroidal agents, hopefully with steroid-like anti-inflammatory actions but without hormonal side effects, had to rely much on serendipitous clinical observations or direct in vivo screening. Acute inflammatory models such as the U.V. erythema and the cotton pellet granuloma assays, previously used to characterize anti-inflammatory steroids, were adapted for the testing of non-steroidal compounds. In the cotton pellet assay phenylbutazone was active orally at 30–90 mg/kg to produce a 20–35% inhibition of the granuloma weight and provided a valuable reference compound. The early difficulties encountered in the laboratory were variability of in vivo responses, the shallow dose response curves and the low capacity of the assay. With emphasis on finding efficacy first, the potential gastro-intestinal (G.I.) side effects were not addressed during the initial development of the first three clinical candidates described below.

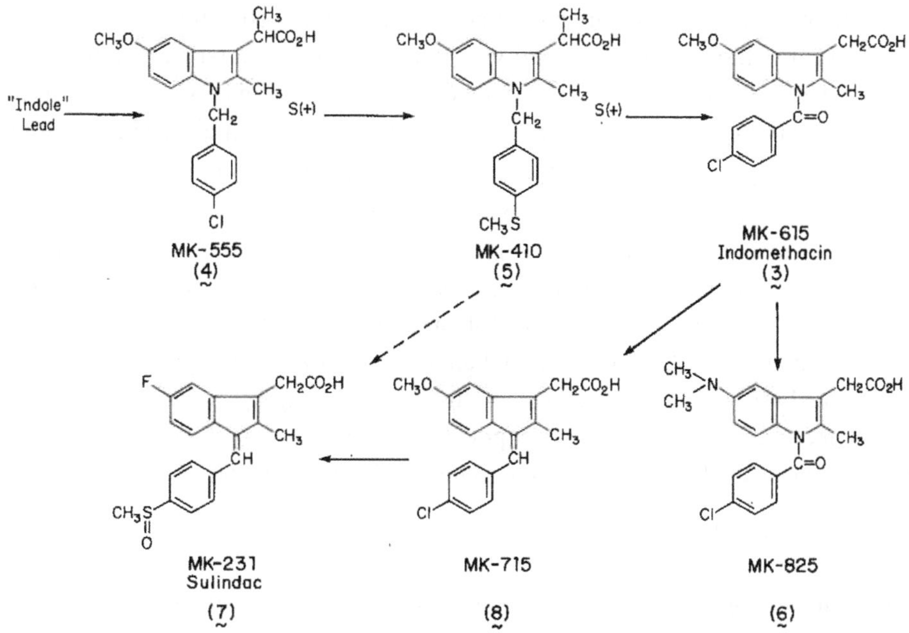

Figure 3.1
The development of indomethacin and sulindac.

3.2.1 The discovery of indomethacin (Shen and Winter, 1977)

The rationale of testing indoles at MSD was partly based on the hypothetical role of serotonin as a potent anti-inflammatory mediator in rodents. It was surmised that agents which could interfere with serotonin metabolism might have anti-inflammatory effects in our inflammatory models. Although the biochemical concept was simplistic, the interest in indole derivatives was further stimulated by the clinical observation of an abnormal tryptophan metabolism in rheumatoid arthritis patients. From an initial indole lead with a potency approximately ¼ that of phenylbutazone in the granuloma assay, a systematic structure-activity relationship study was able to identify the first clinical candidate (MK-555,4) (see Fig. 3.1) which has a

potency comparable to that of phenylbutazone. This compound enabled us to ask the critical question whether the activity of a non-steroidal compound in the cotton pellet granuloma assay would have any clinical significance in man. It was most gratifying to learn that, indeed, MK-555 was effective at 2–3 g/day in the treatment of arthritis although its G.I. side effects also soon became apparent. Further study of indole derivatives led to the selection of MK-410 (5) (which was 4 times more potent than MK-555 in our laboratory models). In an extended study MK-410 showed an improved clinical efficacy at 1–2 g/day and gave us further encouragement. The chemical structure of MK-410 also revealed two important medicinal chemical concepts (Shen, 1967). First, the chiral propionic acid side chain has a high degree of stereospecificity, the S-(+) optical enantiomer is much more active than the R-(−) isomer. Secondly, the methylthio group is an activity-enhancing substituent which can be metabolized to a sulphoxide with greatly increased aqueous solubility. This information was later used advantageously in the design of MK-231 (sulindac, 7) (Shen et al., 1972). Continued synthetic study eventually identified MK-615 (indomethacin) as the best compound among over 350 indole derivatives examined (Shen et al., 1963). The real breakthrough came when N-benzoyl indole acetic acid derivatives, contrary to the general notion regarding the chemical instability of N-acyl indoles, turned out to be adequately stable in vivo to give an increase in potency 30–40 fold over the corresponding N-benzyl indoles, MK-555 and MK-415. In fact, the unexpected potency of the first N-benzoyl analogue synthesized was almost overlooked when it was tested initially at the usual screening dose of 30 mg/kg and found to be toxic. In the clinic indomethacin was proven to be a potent and a novel anti-inflammatory agent for the treatment of arthritis. Its side-effects are mainly G.I. irritation and an idiosyncratic CNS symptom.

Since the CNS side-effect of indomethacin could not be measured in animals, a more polar 5-dimethylamino analogue of indomethacin, MK-825 (6), was investigated in the clinic. It was hoped that an altered metabolism and distribution of MK-825 in man might produce less CNS side effects. Disappointingly, MK-825 was found to be comparable to indomethacin in the clinic both in efficacy and in side effects and was, therefore, not pursued further. As described below, the CNS side-effect (and to some extent the gastrointestinal irritation) of indomethacin was eventually circumvented by the development of an indene isostere sulindac (7).

As indicated in Fig. 3.5, a large number of indomethacin analogues and derivatives were investigated by many laboratories later. Several of them, tolmetin (21, Carson et al., 1971), zomepirac (22, Wong et al., 1973), acemetacin (23, Fisnerova et al., 1977) and proglumetacin (24, Vidal y Plana et al., 1979), have since been introduced to the clinic.

3.2.2 The development of ibuprofen

Meanwhile, independent studies at the Boots Laboratories in England led to the development of ibuprofen, another widely used NSAID (Buckler and Adams, 1968; Nicholson, 1982).

Their search for anti-inflammatory compounds more potent and better tolerated than aspirin was initiated with a newly modified ultraviolet erythema test (Adams and Cobb, 1958). In a random screening programme, a number of phenoxyalkanoic acids, originally synthesized as potential herbicides, showed encouraging activities. From more than 600 analogues evaluated, the most active 2-(4-phenylphenoxy) propionic acid was chosen for clinical trial and was

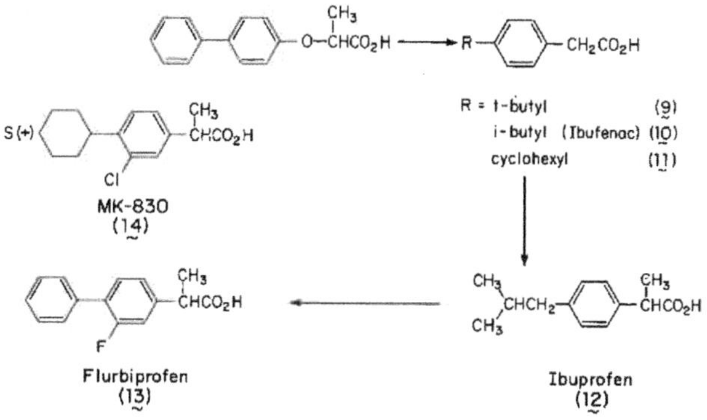

Figure 3.2
Development of ibuprofen and flurbiprofen.

found, disappointingly, ineffective in rheumatoid arthritis. Nevertheless, the corresponding phenylalkanoic acids were noted for their broader anti-inflammatory-analgesic-antipyretic profile and were pursued further in the laboratory. This extended effort culminated in the successful development of ibuprofen (12) and, later, flurbiprofen (13) (Fig. 3.2).

The development of ibuprofen revealed certain potential side-effects, in addition to the well-recognized G.I. irritation, likely to be encountered in the clinical study of new NSAIDS and illustrated the unpredictability of the structuretoxicity relationship. The first three phenyl acetic acids with 4-*t*-butyl (9), isobutyl (ibufenac) (10) and cyclohexyl (11) substituent, respectively, produced successively skin rash, hepatotoxicity and skin rash in patients. Through perseverance, the α-methyl homologue of ibufenac, ibuprofen (12), with antiinflammatory, analgesic and antipyretic activities 16–32 times those of aspirin in animal screens was eventually found to be clinically effective and well tolerated at 1.2–2.4 g daily. Both the (+) and (–) optical isomers of (12) were comparatively active in the U.V.-erythema test, so a racemic mixture was developed as ibuprofen. Interestingly, the two principal urinary metabolites in man are both dextrorotatory isomers. Since the same chiral metabolites were obtained from the administration of the *R*-(–) enantiomer to man (Mills et al., 1973), an inversion of the *R*-(–)-ibuprofen in vivo probably accounts for the isolation of the dextrorotatory metabolites.

The phenylacetic (or propionic) acid lead turned out to be a broad and highly rewarding one. Extension of MSD's study of indolyl and aryl acetic acids independently revealed the activities of 4-phenyl and 4-cyclohexyl phenylacetic acids and the activity-enhancing effects of halo substituents (Cl, F) at the meta position of the phenyl ring. MK-830 (14) was reported to be a most potent compound, being 10–20 times more active than indomethacin (Shen, 1972), and inspired various structure modifications to reduce its G.I. side effects. As shown in Fig. 3.6, a large family of NSAIDS today are related to this class of chemical structure.

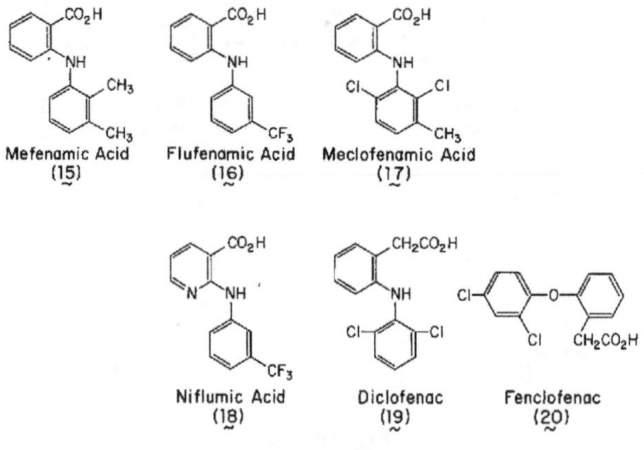

Figure 3.3
Fenamates and analogues.

3.2.3 The investigation of fenamates

At the same time the Parke-Davis Laboratories were interested in the study of a series of *N*-phenyl anthranilic acids (Winder et al., 1962; Scherrer, 1974).

The fenamates, *N*-aryl anthranilic acids, represent another major class of NSAIDS, with some notable differences in their biochemical and pharmacological actions as compared to aryl alkanoic acids. The three products derived from this series are mefenamic acid (15), flufenamic acid (16) and meclofenamic acid (17) (Fig. 3.3). As a group, the fenamates are more effective in inhibiting the U.V. erythema in the guinea pig than the carrageenan-induced paw oedema in the rat. All three compounds are potent cyclooxygenase inhibitors (see Section 3.2) but differ significantly in various anti-inflammatory and analgesic assays. Flufenamic acid was also reported to have a modest prostaglandin antagonistic activity. As a result, mefenamic acid was introduced as a short-term analgesic agent whereas flufenamic acid and meclofenamic acid were developed as anti-inflammatory drugs. Although the laboratory investigation of fenamates was also initiated in the mid 1950s along with the indomethacin and ibuprofen studies, the completion of their clinical development was somewhat delayed.

The heterocyclic analogues of fenamates were also studied. A pyridyl analogue, niflumic acid (18) was developed early in 1970 (Boisser et al., 1970). Extending the carboxyl group in fenamates to an acetic acid side chain as in phenylacetic acids has afforded diclofenac (19) as a potent NSAID (Ku et al., 1975). Further replacement of the amino group in 19 by an oxygen atom yielded the basic structure for fenclofenac (20) (Atkinson and Leach, 1976).

In each of the above three NSAID series, several prototypes were studied in the clinic before the final drug candidate was chosen. Indomethacin was the third clinical candidate in the indole series and ibuprofen was the fourth candidate in the phenylalkanoic acid series which eventually became product. The perseverance of the research and medical management, especially in the face of some early discouraging side effects, clearly played an important role in the successful development of this class of therapeutic agents. The introduction of indomethacin and ibuprofen not only set standards for laboratory testing, regulatory guidelines and the clinical usage of NSAIDS, they also stimulated a broad interest in numerous laboratories worldwide to investigate other related structures.

3.3 The proliferation of isosteres and analogues

Following the introduction of indomethacin and ibuprofen, soon it became apparent that:

(1) There was a large reservoir of arthritic patients whose conditions would not justify the usage of corticosteroids and who were waiting to be treated with newer agents, more potent and less irritating than aspirin.

(2) The two forerunners of NSAIDS, indomethacin and ibuprofen, left room for further improvement in terms of potency, G.I. side effects and duration of action.

(3) The pharmacological models, though far from perfect, were adequate for the development of newer agents. The chemical structures of indomethacin and ibuprofen also suggested a variety of possible modifications.

With such a demonstration of technical feasibility and market potential, many laboratories embarked on the pharmacological search for new anti-inflammatory-analgesic agents. In the first few years alone, more than 300 chemical structure types were patented as potential anti-inflammatory agents. Most of them claimed anti-inflammatory activity based on the carrageenan-induced rat paw oedema assay (Winter et al., 1962) or the guinea pig U.V. erythema assay and showed similar pharmacological profiles. Their chemical structural types generally fall into several major categories (see Table 3.1). Most of these modifications were derived from a combination of pharmacological screening and structure-activity analysis. Some notable medicinal chemical considerations involved in the development of these newer agents are discussed below.

3.3.1 Structure-activity relationship analysis

The majority of NSAIDS are substituent aryl acidic substances. The aryl moiety is usually a phenyl with additional aryl, heterocyclic aryl or alkyl substituents to constitute a non-planar hydrophobic structure with certain stereochemical configurations. Cyclization of the two aryl rings or the α-propionic acid side-chain to the adjacent aromatic group provides the fused ring systems in some newer agents such as isoxepac (31) (Lassman, 1975), clidenac (40) (Sawa et al., 1976) or even etodolic acid (33) (Demerson et al., 1976). A preferred stereochemistry of NSAIDS was recognized early. Two hypothetical receptor contours were independently

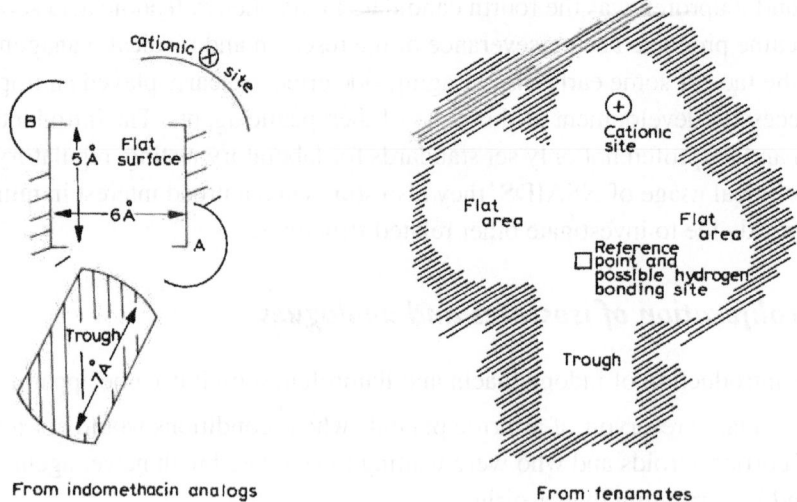

Figure 3.4
Two hypothetical receptor contours for NSAIDS.

proposed on the basis of some general structure-activity relationships of indomethacin (Shen, 1965) and fenamate analogues (Scherrer, 1974), even before any specific biochemical targets were identified (Fig. 3.4). These working models in turn facilitated the discovery of other active structures in many laboratories. The formal chemical lineage of many NSAIDS, though not necessarily the predominant reasoning in their development, is illustrated in Figs. 3.5 en 3.6.

The acidic group in NSAIDS can be a carboxyl, an acetic acid or an acidic enol group (as in phenylbutazone (41) and piroxicam, 49). The highly acidic tetrazole group was also investigated as a carboxyl substitute in a few studies (Juby and Hudyma, 1969). The contribution of the acidic function was highlighted by a correlation of their pKa value with serum half life and relative anti-inflammatory and uricosuric activities observed with phenylbutazone (41) and sulphinpyrazone (42) in the early 1950s. However, it became less critical in many recent series of anti-inflammatory compounds whose acidities are generally in the range of pKa. 4–6.5. A high degree of stereospecificity of the chiral propionic acid side chain in several series (Fig. 3.7) was also found to have a general application. For several potent agents, e.g. the α-methyl analogues of indomethacin (3) and sulindac (7), naproxen (26), flurbiprofen (13), MK-830 (14) and its cyclized analogue, clidenac (40), etc., the S-(+) enantiomers are much more potent than the R-(−) enantiomers in both in vivo anti-inflammatory-analgesic models and in vitro cyclooxygenase assays. However, for some others, e.g. ibuprofen (12), fenoprofen (27) and ketoprofen (28), while the S-(+) isomers are more active than the R-(−) isomers as

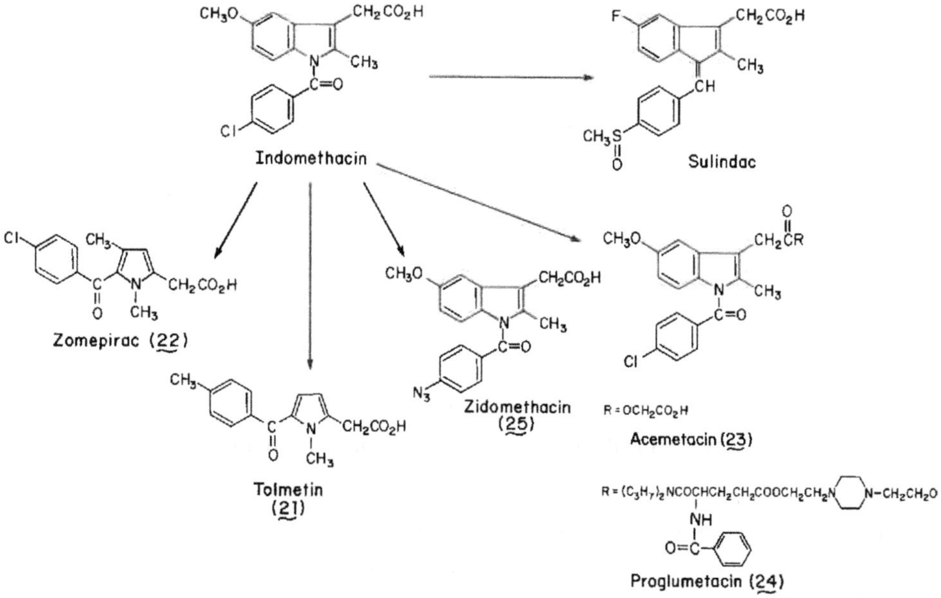

Figure 3.5
Indomethacin and analogues.

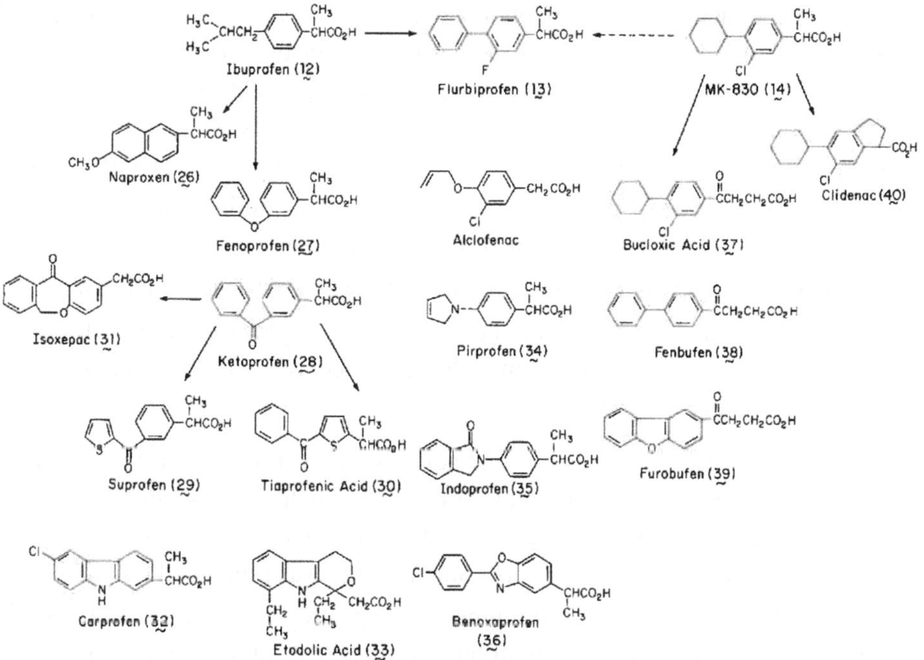

Figure 3.6
Structural relationship of substituted phenyl acetic acid analogues.

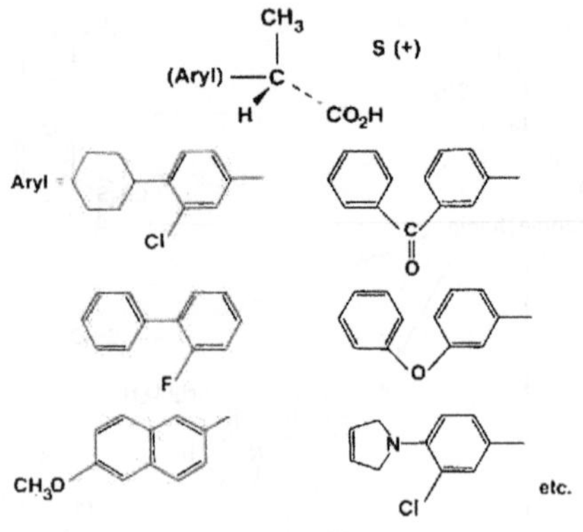

Figure 3.7
Stereospecificity of α-propionic acid side chain.

cyclooxygenase inhibitors in vitro, the potency differences between optical isomers are not always as much in vivo. Different modes of binding to cyclooxygenase by some of these isomers and the relative ease of in vivo racemization might account for this discrepancy. In practice, the racemic mixtures of these compounds are used in the clinic.

In addition to the simple ester and amides, complex carboxyl derivatives derived from various functionalized and chemically distinct alcohols or amines have also been used (Table 3.3). Possible advantages in terms of local G.I. irritation or pharmacokinetics were demonstrated in animal studies in some cases. Most of these are irreversible prodrugs acting through in vivo hydrolysis and liberation of the parent carboxylic acid. Interestingly, in the case of Proglumetacin (24) (Vidal y Plana et al., 1979), the derivative itself and some of the interme-diary metabolites are also active cyclooxygenase inhibitors and antiinflammatories in animal assays. Another nonacidic prodrug is nabumetone (56) which is oxidized in vivo to an active metabolite, 6-methoxy-2-naphthyl acetic acid, the acetic acid analogue of naproxen (26) and a potent cyclooxygenase inhibitor (Goudie et al., 1978; Boyle et al., 1982). The overall pharmacokinetics and the consequent pharmacological effect of such new analogues in man are obviously very complex.

It should be emphasized that the presence of an acidic group is not a general requirement for anti-inflammatory activity. Various non-acidic compounds such as shown in Fig. 3.9 were also found to be active compounds (Shen, 1974, 1977). The anti-inflammatory activity of indoxole (51) was detected early although its clinical usage was precluded by photosensitivity in patients (Szmuszkovicz et al., 1960). It represented a prototype of several highly potent diphenyl imidazoles studied later. A group of quinazolines (e.g. proquazone, 52) (Coombs et al., 1973) were also studied at an early stage. More recently several non-acidic agents, such as ditazole (54, Caprino et al., 1972) and the highly potent tiflamizole (55), which share the

Table 3.3: Prodrug modifications of NSAIDS.

general feature of a triaryl system as indicated in Fig. 3.9 were described. It is of interest to note that, biochemically, some of these aryl moieties can inhibit arachidonic acid cyclooxygenase in vitro at low concentrations equally well as the corresponding acidic derivatives.

NSAIDS in general possess a substituted aryl moiety with a molecular weight in the range of 250–400. The absence of hydrophilic substituents in active antiinflammatory compounds clearly indicate the importance of hydrophobicity and its associated protein-binding, membrane interaction, and tissue distribution properties. An attempted regressional analysis further pointed out the importance of the hydrophobicity of this class of compounds (Gund and Jensen, 1984). Regressional equations correlating the anti-inflammatory, analgesic activity and the buccal absorption of various series of structural analogues were examined but with limited predictability so far. The ulcerogenicity of NSAIDS has also been correlated with their lipophilicity (log P) (Rainsford, 1978). Sometimes the acidity (pKa) is also a contributing factor. A broader application of regressional analysis is hampered by the lack of quantitative data due to variability of in vivo testing, and by the difficulty to compare data, even on a few reference standards, generated from different laboratories. Further physicochemical studies

Table 3.4: Postulated and possible biochemical mechanisms of action of NSAIDS.

I. Earlier proposals (at drug concentration $\geq 10^{-4}$ M)
   1. Uncoupling of oxidative phosphorylation
   2. Inhibition of protein denaturation
   3. Stabilization of lysosomal and cellular membranes
   4. Inhibition of proteases
   5. Inhibition of complement activation
   6. Fibrinolytic activity
   7. Inhibition of protein kinase

II. Regulation of the arachidonic acid cascade (at $\leq 10^{-4}$ M)
   1. Inhibition of phospholipase A_2
   2. Inhibition of cyclooxygenase
   3. Inhibition of lipoxygenase
   4. Neutralization of oxygen radicals ($O_2^{-\cdot}$, $OH^{\cdot}$)

III. Regulation of leukocyte functions (at $\leq 10^{-4}$ M)
   1. Inhibition of receptor binding of f-Met-Leu-Phe
   2. Inhibition of chemotaxis
   3. Inhibition of phagocytosis
   4. Inhibition of degranulation and release of lysosomal hydrolases and mediators
   5. Inhibition of receptor binding of the platelet activating factor (PAF)

hopefully will continue to provide additional insight on factors influencing the interaction of NSAIDS with their active site and their pharmacokinetics in vivo.

3.3.2 Modulating biochemical mechanisms of action

Inflammation is a complex and dynamic process involving a myriad of cellular and humoral responses. Many of these can be suppressed by NSAIDS at mM concentration or higher, presumably due to their strong protein binding and membrane interaction properties. In fact, prior to recent studies of the biochemical mechanisms of NSAIDS, both protein denaturation (Mizushima, 1964, 1966) and membrane stabilization (Brown et al., 1967; Mizushima et al., 1970; Kalbhen et al., 1970), were investigated as possible primary in vitro screens for anti-inflammatory agents. Such non-specific or secondary actions are usually shown indiscriminately by both optical isomers of several aryl propionic acids, even though only the *S*-(+) isomers of these compounds are active in in vivo animal models. A list of these postulated biochemical mechanisms is shown in Table 3.4.

Of greater importance, the inhibition of cyclooxygenase (which generates prostaglandins from arachidonic acid) by aspirin and indomethacin, first reported by Vane and coworkers in 1971, has been established as a primary mechanism of action of many NSAIDS. The cyclooxygenase in the arachidonic acid cascade can be inhibited by NSAIDS at their physiological concentrations (μM range) with a structure-activity relationship and chiral specificity parallel to their in vivo anti-inflammatory actions. While aspirin exerts an irreversible enzyme inhibition,

Table 3.5: Relative potency of NSAIDS as cyclooxygenase inhibitors.

Drug	ID_{50} (μM), enzyme source*		
	SSV	*BSV*	*Human synovium*
Aspirin	72		
Diflunisal	28		
Indomethacin	0.4	0.6	0.003
Sulindac sulphide	2.2		
Ibuprofen	1.5	6	1
Flurbiprofen	0.7		0.01
Naproxen	6.1	0.8	
Diclofenac	0.3		
Mefenamic acid		0.7	
Meclofenamic acid		0.6	
Phenylbutazone	12.6	37	
Piroxicam			

* Enzyme source: SSV, sheep seminal vesicle enzyme (Ham et al., 1972).

                BSV, bovine seminal vesicle enzyme (Cushman and Cheung, 1976).

  Human synovium   (Kantrowitz et al., 1975).

by virtue of its reactive *O*-acetyl group which irreversibly acetylates the α-amino group of the N-terminal serine of the enzyme (Roth et al., 1975), most NSAIDS are substrate competitive reversible inhibitors. The relative potency of several NSAIDS are listed in Table 3.5. For some of them, e.g. flufenamic acid (16) and diflunisal (2), their ID_{50} are markedly influenced by the amount of phenolic cofactors present in the assay system. It should be pointed out that the relative potency of NSAIDS in cell-free in vitro systems may differ significantly from those obtained from the cellular (neutrophil or macrophage) systems or in vivo models. With many NSAIDS significant and intrinsic cyclooxygenase inhibitory activities are also obtained readily with their esters and amides derivatives and non-acidic analogues (alcohols, ketones, etc.) in vitro, but many of these are less effective in vivo. Variations of their cellular activities among different cells have also been noted. Some may possess superior pharmacokinetics or duration of action in animals, but their real therapeutic advantages must be demonstrated in clinical studies.

Recent studies have further established the important role of prostaglandins, thromboxanes, leukotriene B_4 and other arachidonic acid metabolites in inflammation and pain responses (Flower, 1974; Samuelsson and Paoletti, 1978; Vane and Ferreira, 1979; Smith et al., 1980; Samuelsson, 1982). A decrease of prostaglandin levels in the serum, joint fluid, urine and gastric juice of rheumatoid patients after administration of NSAIDS also correlated well with their anti-inflammatory activity and certain aspects of gastrointestinal irritation. From the medicinal chemical point of view, we can now consider cyclooxygenase as an important site of action for NSAIDS and model their possible mode of binding on the probable configuration of arachidonic acid at the enzyme site (Gund and Shen, 1977; Sankawa et al., 1982). While the validity of these models remains to be established by X-ray or other physicochemical studies with purified enzyme, they are still useful in the search for new active structures.

The involvement of reactive radical species derived from superoxide or hydrogen peroxide in various inflammatory and degenerative processes has received considerable attention in the past few years (Kuehl and Egan, 1980). Perhaps as a secondary action, an oxygen radical scavenging effect has been shown by several NSAIDS which possess either a phenolic hydroxyl group as in phenylbutazone and MK-447 (58) (Kuehl et al., 1979; Payne et al., 1982), or a sulphide group as in the active sulphide metabolite of sulindac.

In recent years, the possible stabilization of lysosome membrane, the inhibition of cellular release of hydrolases and mediators (Brune et al., 1981; Bonney et al., 1983), and the blockade of chemotactic receptors (Abita, 1981; Perianin et al., 1982) by NSAIDS have also been investigated. As highly hydrophobic molecules, many NSAIDS interfere with the binding of hydrophobic mediators, such as f-Met-Leu-Phe, with their membrane receptors. In a comparative study, most of them are not inhibitors of the specific binding of a lipid mediator, platelet activating factor, with its receptor (Shen et al., 1983). Nevertheless, it is conceivable that some newer NSAIDS may possess a broader spectrum of activity blocking the action of multiple mediators.

Clearly continued biochemical studies may provide further insight to the antiinflammatory actions of NSAIDS, rationalize the improved patient tolerance in some cases and pave the way toward the discovery of superior agents.

3.3.2.1 Characterization of diflunisal

Diflunisal (2) is a new analogue of salicylic acid with improved potency, tolerance and duration of action (Winter et al., 1981). Its inception was stimulated by an early suggestion from an authoritative rheumatologist, Dr. W. Bauer of Harvard Medical School in the U.S. (Sarett, 1977) but the technical feasibility was not available until our biological assays and chemical concepts were enriched by the experience in developing indomethacin and related NSAIDS. Consequently, it was discovered through an extensive synthetic and pharmacological effort which examined more than 500 salicylic acid derivatives (Hannah et al., 1977; Stone et al., 1977). Interestingly, the final selection of the diflunisal structure for clinical development was much influenced by the emerging knowledge of prostaglandin biochemistry (Shen, 1983). Chemically diflunisal differs from aspirin in two aspects, the addition of a 2,4-difluorophenyl group at the C_5 position and the absence of an *O*-acetyl group. The introduction of the hydrophobic difluorophenyl group was primarily based on an extensive structure-activity relationship study. It increases the protein-binding of the molecule and extends the duration of action (plasma $t_{1/2} = 8$–13 hours). The non-bonded interaction due to the ortho fluorine atom in the second phenyl ring forces the biphenyl group out of coplanarity and gives diflunisal a molecular conformation somewhat similar to other non-planar potent aryl acids. The absence

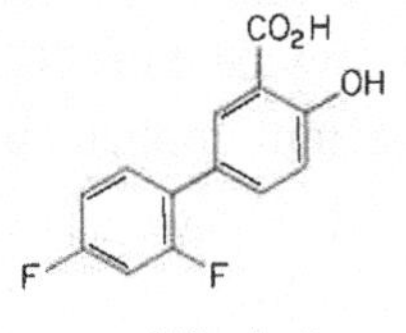

Diflunisal
(2)

of an *O*-acetyl group in diflunisal was a deliberate choice. As is well known, the *O*-acetyl group was first added to salicylic acid almost a century ago to reduce its gastrointestinal irritation and to improve its pharmacokinetics. Aspirin was also shown in recent years to be more potent than salicylic acid in anti-inflammatory and analgesic models in animals. Given the uncertainty of extrapolating the pharmacokinetics and tolerance of a new salicylate analogue from animals to man, there was a natural tendency to keep the *O*-acetyl group in any new aspirin derivative. Indeed, the clinical precursor of diflunisal, flufenisal (57), was the 5-(flurophenyl) analogue of aspirin, not of salicylic acid. Flufenisal was effective in the clinic but produced unsatisfactory gastrointestinal side-effects. At the time of selecting diflunisal several years later, the in vivo acetylation of membrane serum proteins by aspirin had raised some concern. The irreversible inactivation of platelet cyclooxygenase by aspirin through the reactivity of its *O*-acetyl group (transacetylation) was also under investigation. To circumvent these potential side effects, the *O*-acetyl group was purposely deleted from the difluoro analogue of flufenisal. Fortunately, in this case, the free phenolic compound, diflunisal, was fully active and well tolerated in various animal models, so there was no compelling reason to retain the *O*-acetyl group further.

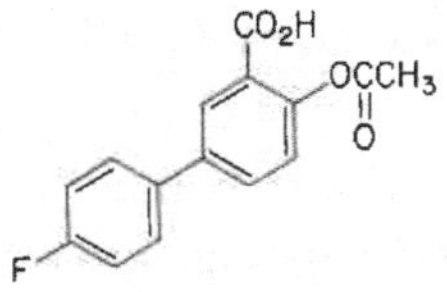

Flufenisal
(57)

The pharmacological profile of diflunisal indicates that it is 5–10 times more potent than aspirin as an anti-inflammatory-analgesic agent but only 1.5 times as an antipyretic agent. In vitro diflunisal is a moderately active inhibitor of cyclooxygenase (IC_{50} 28 μM), with a dependence of phenolic cofactor(s) in the medium, presumably related to the level of cyclooxygenase activating lipid peroxide. The relatively weak antipyretic and G.I. irritating properties of diflunisal may be attributed to its pharmacokinetic properties. The level of diflunisal in the CNS system was shown to be relatively low. In contrast to several potent NSAIDS, autoradiographic examination showed that diflunisal does not accumulate in the gastric mucosal tissue (Brune et al., 1977). Clinical studies also showed that the concentration of prostaglandin E_2 in gastric fluid was not significantly reduced after oral administration of diflunisal at the therapeutic level of 0.5–1 g twice daily (Cohen et al., 1980). As a secondary biochemical mechanism, diflunisal, like acetaminophen and the phenolic MK-447 (58), is capable of inactivating the reactive oxygen radicals generated as by-products in the arachidonic acid cascade. However, the possible in vivo significance of this secondary property remains to be demonstrated (Payne et al., 1982).

MK-447
(58)

3.3.2.2 Lipoxygenase inhibition

Following the elucidation of the lipoxygenase pathway (generating leukotrienes from arachidonic acid), a general concept that compounds capable of inhibiting both cyclooxygenase and lipoxygenase may possess greater antiinflammatory activity attracted much interest. As LTB_4 is a potent chemoat-tractant for leukocytes, such secondary action may decrease leukocyte infiltration (Snyderman and Goetzl, 1981). Such dual actions would result in the blockade of the entire arachidonic acid cascade analogous to the action of lipomodulin induced by corticosteroids (see Chapt. 10, Part 2). An experimental agent BW 755C (Higgs et al., 1979) was found to inhibit both lipoxygenase and cyclooxygenase. Although BW 755C was precluded from clinical investigation by its toxicity, it has been used widely to illustrate the biological effects of a dual inhibitor. Most cyclooxygenase-inhibitory NSAIDS are not lipoxygenase inhibitors, despite the fact that the first step in cyclooxygenase action is formally hydroperoxidation of arachidonic acid at the 11-position, equivalent to 11-lipoxygenase action, and that the stereoconfiguration of many NSAIDS have shown certain similarities with that of arachidonic acid (Gund and Shen, 1977). Nevertheless, several NSAIDS were reported to inhibit 5-lipoxygenase either in the cell-free system or in intact macrophage (sulindac sulphide) or neutrophils (benoxaprofen). The non-acidic timegadine (53) is another dual enzyme inhibitor with moderate potency (Ahnfelt-Rønne and Arrigoni-Martelli, 1982). In general the concentrations required for lipoxygenase inhibition by these compounds are much higher than their cyclooxygenase inhibitory concentrations, but are still within the range of their plasma or demonstrated cellular concentrations. It was also noted that the inhibitory effect varies according to cellular types and other factors. Nevertheless, the preliminary impressions of the antiarthritic effects of benoxaprofen and timegadine, while remaining to be verified, further stimulate the continued search for dual enzyme inhibitors with greater potency and safety profiles.

3.3.3 Changing pharmacodynamics

An increased duration of action is often the objective for developing second generation drugs. A growing interest in longer-acting NSAIDS, to be used on a twice daily (b.i.d.) or once daily (q.d.) regimen, for better patient compliance and convenience has also been developed in recent years. Some NSAIDS, by virtue of their chemical structure and fortuitous pharmacokinetics, were found to have relatively long plasma half-lives, and presumed sustaining tissue level, in man (Hucker et al., 1980). The enolic phenylbutazone was first noted for its long plasma half-life (72 hours in man), although it is usually administered on a three times daily (t.i.d.) schedule. More recent aryl alkanoic acids such as naproxen ($t_{1/2} = 13$ hours in man), benoxaprofen ($t_{1/2} = 38$ hours) and fenclofenac ($t_{1/2} = 12$ hours) required b.i.d. or even q.d. dosing only. Unfortunately, such clinical findings were largely empirical. As species differences in drug metabolism are still unpredictable, even multi-species laboratory studies could not provide much guidance except for closely related analogues. Nevertheless, several potential approaches to prolong the duration of action can be illustrated by the laboratory considerations and pharmacodynamic data of three recently developed long-acting NSAIDS, sulindac, fenbufen and piroxicam.

3.3.3.1 Sulindac –A reversible prodrug

The importance of pharmacodynamics to both the selectivity and the duration of drug action was recognized in recent years. An early attempt to use such an approach to improve patient tolerance was the study of an indomethacin analogue, MK-825 (6). In order to circumvent the CNS side effect of indomethacin, the mechanism of which is still unclear and animal models are still unavailable today, an active analogue with a 5-dimethylamino substituent and with an altered tissue distribution and metabolism was investigated. The efficacy of MK-825 was comparable to that of indomethacin in the clinic, but so was its CNS side effect. Nevertheless, these findings encouraged the further study of other isosteres. Soon afterwards an indene analogue of indomethacin, MK-715 (8), was found to be nearly half as potent as indomethacin in animals and in man. Interestingly, it was less irritating to the G.I. tract and devoid of any significant CNS side effect. Since MK-715 is a relatively insoluble compound, other more soluble analogues were sought. Among various solubilizing functional groups, the methylthio-methylsulphoxide system, which was studied earlier in the case of MK-410, was of special interest. Such a system offered the advantages of: (1) compatibility with potent biological activities in the indomethacin series; (2) the methylsulphoxide group increased both the aqueous solubility and the distribution coefficient of the parent compound very significantly; (3) the dynamic and complex metabolism of this system would lead to the formation of multiple metabolites and thus reduce the probability of accumulating any single metabolite beyond its solubility in biological fluids.

The result of such a study was the development of sulindac (Shen et al., 1972; Van Arman et al., 1972). The pharmacodynamics of sulindac in animals and man were subsequently delineated by extensive metabolism and clinical pharmacology studies (Duggan et al., 1977) (Fig. 3.10). As a new type of reversible prodrug, based on in vivo redox systems, the prodrug sulindac is interconvertible with its active sulphide metabolite in different tissues and cells to sustain therapeutic levels of the active metabolite for a long duration. A b.i.d. or even q.d. dosing schedule was amply supported by detailed pharmacodynamic data. As a consequence of the local redox enzyme activity, differential membrane permeability and cellular distribution of the more hydrophilic sulindac vs. the more hydrophobic sulphide metabolite, a certain degree of selective prostaglandin inhibition in the gastrointestinal tract and kidney (Ciabattoni et al., 1980; Bunning and Barth, 1982) was also fortuitously achieved.

3.3.3.2 Fenbufen –an irreversible prodrug

An extension of the (α-methyl) acetic acid side-chain in biphenyl acetic acids to various metabolizable precursors was found by several laboratories to yield moderately active NSAIDS, some with reduced gastrointestinal side effects. Among a hundred or so side-chain modifications, the α-ketobutyric acid derivative, was first used in bucloxic acid (37) as an analogue of MK-830 (14) (Navarro et al., 1974). Recently, fenbufen (38), was found to have interesting pharmacodynamic properties in man (Cuisinaud et al., 1979). The metabolism of fenbufen varies significantly among species and yields more than 10 metabolites (Chiccarelli et al., 1980). The formation of the most active metabolite, biphenylacetic acid (BPAA), was found to be 27, 3.1, 8.1, 37.2, 53.6 and 10% in the mouse, rat, guinea pig, dog, monkey and man, respectively. Clearly, any extrapolation of pharmacodynamic data from laboratory animals to man would incur much uncertainty. Fortuitously, in man, the plasma concentration of BPAA could be sustained at a steady level ($10\mu g/ml$) on a 800 mg b.i.d. schedule and thus provide an effective and long duration of action. The oral administration of the prodrug fenbufen, like sulindac, reduces local mucosal irritation and the inhibition of prostaglandin synthesis in the gastric tissue and thus improved its G.I. tolerance to some extent.

3.3.3.3 Piroxicam –an enolic NSAID

The development of piroxicam (Lombardino et al., 1973; Wiseman et al., 1981) culminated an extensive study of aryl compounds containing an acidic enol, instead of a carboxylic acid, following the example of phenylbutazone. As metabolic conjugation of the acidic enol in these molecules is generally less facile than the glucuronide formation of carboxylic acids, a longer serum half-life and duration of action might be expected. 'Starting from a group of 2-aryl-l,3-indandiones (44, pKa 5.4), after investigations of various 2-arylbenzo(b)thiophenone-1,1-dioxide (45, pKa 5) and 1,3-dioxoiso quinoline-4-carboxanilides (46), the N-heteroaryl carboxamides of 4-hydroxy-2-methyl-2H-1,2-benzothiazine-1,1-dioxides (47) were found to be highly potent antiinflammatory agents (Fig. 3.8). The plasma half-lives of these com-

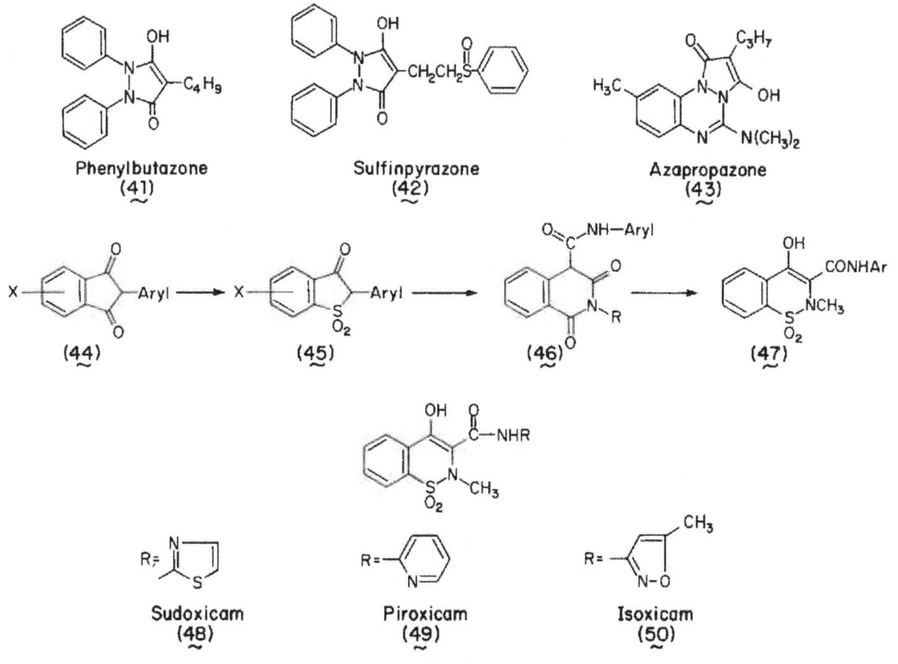

Figure 3.8
Enolic NSAIDS.

pounds vary considerably in different species. In general, the half-lives are only several hours in the rat, rabbit and monkey, but 12–60 hours in the dog. In man, the two clinical candidates, sudoxicam (48) and piroxicam (48) have plasma half-lives ranging from 24–96 and 38–45 hours, respectively. The first clinical candidate, sudoxicam, is three times more potent than indomethacin in the rat carrageenan paw oedema assay. Its plasma concentrations accumulated steadily upon repeated dosing and decayed slowly (1–2 weeks) after drug withdrawal. One of the metabolites of sudoxicam was identified as a thiourea derivative (Lombardino and Wiseman, 1982) which might account for some hepatotoxicity in early clinical trials. The second candidate piroxicam, with an amino pyridyl instead of the aminothiazole group, was further developed as a long-acting new NSAID active at 20–40 mg once per day.

The success of piroxicam in reducing the daily dose level to 1/10 that of most NSAIDS demonstrated the importance of pharmacokinetics as an integral part in drug design. A close analogue, isoxicam (50) (DePasquale et al., 1975), has displayed similar activities.

In summary, as shown in Table 3.6 there are at least four approaches to achieve a longer duration of drug action. The intrinsic properties of the chemical structures (e.g. naproxen and benoxaprofen), a retarded metabolism (piroxicam) and prodrugs with a reversible activation (sulindac), or irreversible activation (fenbufen) have all been used successfully in developing long-acting NSAIDS.

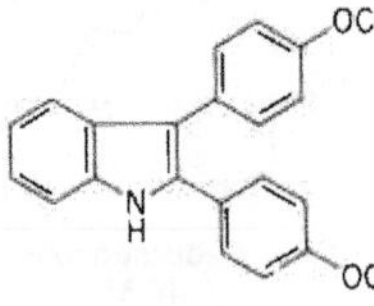

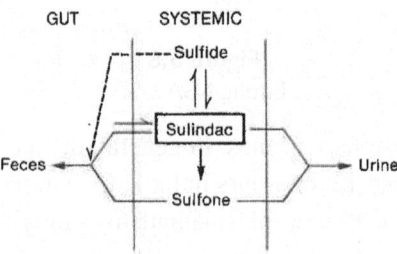

Indoxole
(51)

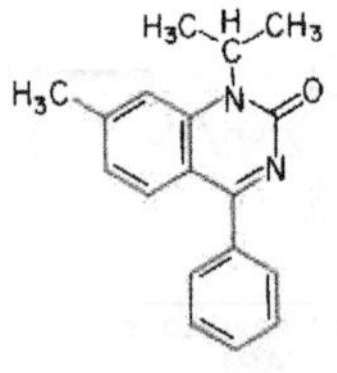

Proquazone
(52)

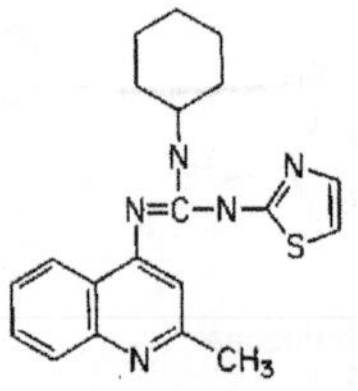

Timegadine
(53)

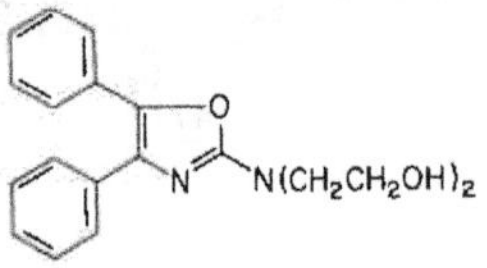

Ditazole
(54)

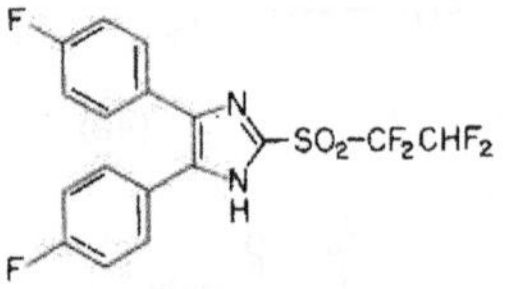

Tiflamizole
(55)

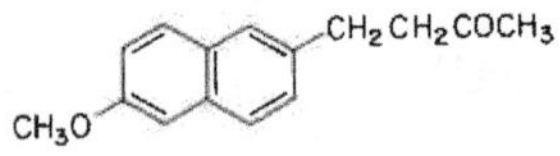

Nabumetone
(56)

Figure 3.9
Non-acidic NSAIDS.

Figure 3.10
Pharmacodynamics of sulindac.

3.4 Unexpected clinical observations

NSAIDS were developed mainly for the treatment of the chronic degenerative arthritic disorders. The laboratory models currently available are still oversimplified versions of the complex disease process, mostly reflecting the acute responses involving cellular dynamics, inflammatory mediators, etc. Species difference in drug metabolism complicates the selection of drugs with desired pharmacokinetics. The wide range of side-effects observed in chronic therapy, G.I. symptoms, renal, hepatic or CNS disorders, also lack convenient and predicative assays. The withdrawal of two major new NSAIDS, benoxaprofen and zomepirac, in the past year after extensive clinical usage and marketing development dramatically underscores the uncertainty of long-term drug safety. The fatal hepatotoxicity of benoxaprofen may be related to the slow excretion and continued drug accumulation as indicated by its steadily increasing

Table 3.6: Approaches to long duration of drug action.

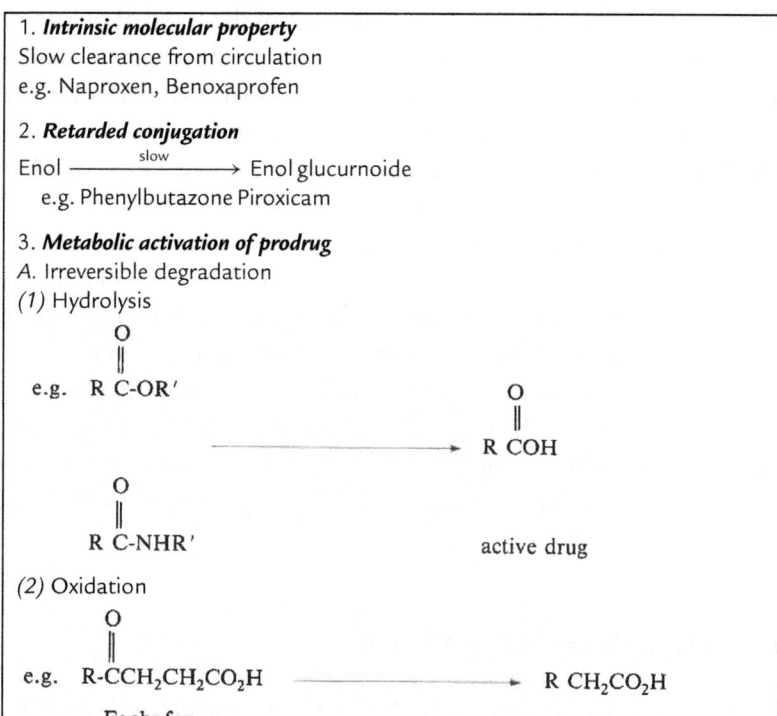

1. *Intrinsic molecular property*
Slow clearance from circulation
e.g. Naproxen, Benoxaprofen

2. *Retarded conjugation*

Enol $\xrightarrow{\text{slow}}$ Enol glucurnoide
   e.g. Phenylbutazone Piroxicam

3. *Metabolic activation of prodrug*
A. Irreversible degradation
(1) Hydrolysis

e.g. $\underset{\text{}}{R\,\overset{O}{\overset{\|}{C}}\text{-OR}'}$

$\longrightarrow\; R\,\overset{O}{\overset{\|}{C}}OH$

$R\,\overset{O}{\overset{\|}{C}}\text{-NHR}'$ active drug

(2) Oxidation

e.g. $R\text{-}\overset{O}{\overset{\|}{C}}CH_2CH_2CO_2H \longrightarrow R\,CH_2CO_2H$

    Fenbufen

B. Reversible oxidation-reduction

$R\text{-}\overset{O}{\overset{\|}{S}}CH_3 \rightleftharpoons R\text{-}SCH_3$

e.g. Sulindac

plasma level in certain patients. The anaphylactic allergic reaction to zomepirac observed at the rate of 11 000 per 15 million is obviously beyond any means of early detection. The unfortunate clinical problem was partly aggravated by the mistaken concept that zomepirac is an 'analgesic' agent like acetaminophen, etc. which could be used in salicylate-sensitive patients or in combination with other NSAIDS. On the positive side, it is gratifying to note that, over the years, the clinical trials of various experimental drugs have also uncovered unexpected results on efficacy, pharmacodynamics and tolerance which significantly influenced the course of NSAID research.

3.4.1 Analgesia of NSAIDS

It is well known that the antiarthritic effects of salicylates, gold preparations, antimalarials, corticosteroids, D-penicillamine and phenylbutazone were all discovered in the clinic by observant and ingenious rheumatologists. The analgesic effect of indomethacin was also first recognized in man. This observation led to the adaptation of the Randall-Selitto model of yeast-induced hyperaesthesia to measure the peripheral analgesic action of indomethacin and other NSAIDS. However, the acceptance of NSAIDS as effective analgesics in the treatment of more severe pains unrelated to arthritis was not realized until the last few years. The perception of the clinicians was favourably changed by the demonstration of a high degree of analgesia by zomepirac (Cooper, 1980), followed by diflunisal (Forbes et al., 1982), sodium naproxen and other NSAIDS, in several clinical pain models. As described above, zomepirac is a more potent analogue of tolmetin which was developed as an anti-inflammatory agent. In spite of their similar pharmacological profiles, the clinical investigation of zomepirac was focussed on its analgesic action first. Its efficacy in oral surgery patients compared favourably with narcotic analgesics. At a time when there was a general interest in finding non-narcotic substitutes for the much abused propoxyphene, this new recognition significantly broadened the usage of NSAIDS as analgesics. The incidence of zomepirac withdrawal further stimulated investigation of newer analgesics acting by somewhat different biochemical mechanisms.

3.4.2 'Disease modifying' potential of NSAIDS

The anti-inflammatory analgesic actions of NSAIDS, mainly mediated through their inhibition of the biosynthesis of prostaglandins, are generally considered to provide symptomatic relief only without affecting the disease process of arthritis. 'Disease modifying' properties are reserved for other slow-acting antirheumatic drugs such as D-penicillamine and anti-malarials. However, following the controversy of benoxaprofen, this general concept is being reexamined seriously at both the laboratory and clinical levels.

Benoxaprofen (36) is a heteroaryl analogue of phenylpropionic acids with a similar pharmacological profile. Reports from Lilly laboratories highlighted its effect to retard the joint erosion in adjuvant arthritic rats as shown in X-ray radiographs (Dawson, 1980) and its modest activity to inhibit leukocyte migration (Meacock and Kitchen, 1979). Several clinical reports suggested that it might have an antirheumatic effect more than those obtainable with other NSAIDS (Bluhm et al., 1982). However, independent comparative studies showed that the laboratory activities of benoxaprofen are apparently not unique. The pharmacological modulation of the actions of the chemotactic peptide f-Met-Leu-Phe and other inflammatory mediators on leukocytes, e.g. receptor binding, chemotaxis and release of lysosomal hydrolases etc. have been widely investigated (Smith and Iden, 1980; Ackerman et al., 1981). In newer cellular and enzymatic systems, the diversity of NSAID structures often produce inhibitors with varying degrees of activities. The correlation of these in vitro properties with 'disease-modifying' effect, if any, remains to be established. Although benoxaprofen was withdrawn shortly after its approval in the U.S. in 1982 because of unforeseen toxicity contributing to the death of patients, the controversial 'disease-modifying' potential of other NSAIDS, or new agents with greater inhibitory activities on leukocyte functions, lipoxygenase, etc. is being actively investigated. Aside from some ramifications produced by the brief history of benoxaprofen on clinical trials and drug regulation, a significant impact on current NSAID research is also evident.

3.4.3 Expansion of clinical utilities

A continued interest in developing newer NSAIDS is partly stimulated by the realization that, as potent cyclooxygenase inhibitors they may also be effective in the treatment of other clinical disorders mediated by the excessive production of cyclooxygenase metabolites, e.g. prostaglandins, thromboxanes or even oxidant radicals. The similarity between the pathogenesis mechanisms for rheumatoid arthritis and periodontitis was recognized early in the late 1960s. Other prostaglandin mediated clinical symptoms responsive to NSAID treatment are dysmenorrhea, patent ductus artereosis, Bartter's syndrome and Hodgkin's disease. As many of these are devoid of any satisfactory treatment, the availability of NSAIDS, in spite of their side effects offered a rational therapy. More recently, the usefulness of NSAIDS for alleviating general pain and certain types of headache further expanded the potential applications of this class of compounds. Topical formulations of NSAIDS have also been developed for dermatological and ocular inflammation without many systemic side effects.

As a broad chemical class with certain physicochemical characteristics, some NSAIDS and related structures may possess totally unexpected biological actions also. A case in point is the recent finding that sulindac turns out to be a potent inhibitor of aldose reductase in the lens (Sharma and Cotlier, 1982). Its potency ($ID_{50} \sim 10^{-7}$ M) is comparable to other specific inhibitors of this enzyme. Its sulphide and sulphone metabolites are approximately 10 times less active. This property of sulindac is clearly not associated with cyclooxygenase inhibitory activity. The possible role of lens aldose reductase, which reduces glucose to sorbitol, in the development of cataract and peripheral neuropathy in diabetic patients has received much attention in recent years. The advantage of combining analgesic-anti-inflammatory actions with aldose reductase inhibitory activity in treating these diabetic sequelae remains an intriguing possibility.

In conclusion, a highly productive and stimulating research on NSAIDS in the past two decades has provided a large number of antiarthritic drugs, which are commonly effective as anti-inflammatory-analgesic-antipyretic agents but differ in many specific aspects. Their biochemical properties, aside from cyclooxygenase inhibition, are far from understood and are continually being elucidated as new experimental systems on enzymes, mediators or receptors, become available. The availability of a variety of NSAIDS will undoubtedly foster more clinical explorations of their potential applications.

Acknowledgement

The author wishes to thank Ms. Betty Ann Mehl for her valuable assistance in the preparation of this manuscript.

References

Abita, J.P., 1981. Agents Actions 11, 610–612.

Ackerman, N.R., Jubb, S.N., Marlowe, S.L., 1981. Biochem. Pharmacol. 30 (15), 2147–2155.

Adams, S.S., Cobb, R., 1958. Nature 181, 773.

Ahnfelt-Rønne, I., Arrigoni-Martelli, E., 1982. Biochem. Pharmacol. 31 (16), 2619–2624.

Atkinson, D.C., Leach, E., 1976. Agents Actions 6, 657.

Bluhm, G.B., Smith, D.W., Mikulaschek, W.M., 1982. Eur. J. Rheumatol. Infl. 5, 186–197.

Boisser, J.R., Lwolf, J.M., Hertz, F., 1970. Therapie 25, 43.

Bonney, R.J., Wightman, P.D., Dahlgren, M.E., Sadowski, S.J., Davies, P., Jensen, N., Lanza, T., Humes, J.L., 1983. Biochem. Pharmacol. 32 (2), 361–366.

Boyle, E.A., Freeman, P.C., Mangan, F.R., Thomson, M.J., 1982. J. Pharm. Pharmacol. 34, 562–569.

Brown, J.H., Mackey, H.K., Riggilo, D.A., 1967. Proc. Soc. Exp. Biol. Med. 125, 837.

Brune, K., Graf, P., Rainsford, K.D., 1977. In: Rainsford, K.D., Brune, K., Whitehouse, M.W. (Eds.), Proceedings of the Symposium on Aspirin and Related Drugs: Their Actions and Uses, 1. Agents and Actions, Birkhaeuser Verlag, Basel, pp. 9–26.

Brune, K., Rainsford, K.D., Wagner, K., Peskar, B.A., 1981. Arch. Pharmacol. 315, 269–278.

Buckler, J.W., Adams, S.S., 1968. Med. Proc. 14, 574.

Bunning, R.D., Barth, W.F., 1982. J. Am. Med. Assoc. 248 (21), 2864–2867.

Caprino, L., Borrelli, F., Falchetti, R., 1973. Arzneim.-Forsch 23, 1972.

Carson, J.R., McKinstry, D.N., Wong, S., 1971. J. Med. Chem. 14, 646.

Chiccarelli, F.S., Eisner, H.J., Van Lear, G.E., 1980. Arzneim.-Forsch./Drug Res. 30 (1), 707–715 Nr. 4a.

Ciabattoni, G., Pugliese, F., Cinotti, G.A., Patrono, C., 1980. Eur. J. Rheumatol. Inflam. 3 (3), 210–221.

Cohen, M.M., Hughes, H., Cheung, G., Suedfeld, G., 1980. In: Beaver, W.T. (Ed.), Proceedings of the International Symposium on Diflunisal. Biomedical Information Corp., New York, N.Y, pp. 49–58.

Coombs, R.V., Danna, R.P., Denzer, M., Hardtmann, G.E., Huegi, B., Koletar, G., Koletar, J., Ott, H., Jukniewicz, E., Perrine, J.W., Takesue, E.I, Trapold, J.H., 1973. J. Med. Chem. 16, 1237.

Cooper, S.A., 1980. J. Clin. Pharmacol. 20, 230–242.

Cuisinaud, G., Legheand, J., Llorca, G., Belkahia, C., Lejeune, E., Sassard, J., 1979. Eur. J. Clin. Pharmacol. 16, 59–61.

Cushman, D.W., Cheung, H.S., 1976. Biochim. Biophys. Acta 424, 449–459.

Dawson, W., 1980. J. Rheumatol. 7 (suppl. 6), 5–11.

Demerson, C.A., Humber, L.G., Phillipp, A.H., 1976. J. Med. Chem. 19, 391.

DePasquale, G., Rassaert, C., Richter, R., Welaj, P., Gingold, J., Singer, R., 1975. Agents Actions 5, 256–263.

Domenjoz, R., 1960. Ann. N.Y. Acad. Sci. 86, 263.

Duggan, D.E., Hooke, K.F., Risley, E.A., Shen, T.Y., Van Arman, C.G., 1977. J. Pharmacol. Expt. Therap. 201, 9–13.

Fisnerova, L., Grimova, J., Rabek, V., Roubal, Z., 1977. Cesk. Farm. 26, 227; through (1978). Chem. Abstr. 88, 62247.

Flower, R.J., 1974. Pharmacol. Rev. 26, 33–67.

Forbes, J.A., Foor, V.M., Bowser, M.W., Calderazzo, J.P., Shackleford, R.W., Beaver, W.T., 1982. Pharmacotherapy 2, 43–49.

Goudie, A.C., Gaster, L.M., Lake, A.W., Rose, C.J., Freeman, P.C., Hughes, B.O., Miller, D, 1978. J. Med. Chem. 21 (12), 1260–1264.

Gund, P., Jensen, N.P. (1983) In: Quantitative Structure-Activity Relationships of Drugs (Topliss, J., Ed.), Academic Press, New York, NY, pp. 285.

Gund, P., Shen, T.Y., 1977. J. Med. Chem. 20, 1146–1152.

Ham, E.A., Cirillo, V.J., Zanetti, M., Shen, T.Y., Kuehl, F.A. (1972) In: Prostaglandins in Cellular Biology (Ramwell, P.W., Pharris, B.B., Eds.), pp. 345–352, Plenum Press, New York, NY.

Hannah, J., Ruyle, W.V., Jones, H., Matzuk, A.R., Kelly, K.W., Witzel, D.E., Holtz, W.J., Houser, R.W., Shen, T.Y., Sarett, L.H., 1977. Br. J. Clin. Pharmacol. 4, 75–135.

Higgs, G.A., Flower, R.J., Vane, J.R., 1979. Biochem. Pharmacol. 28, 1959–1961.

Hucker, H.B., Kwan, K.C., Duggan, D.E. (1980) In: Progress in Drug Metabolism (Bridges, J.W., Chasseaud, L.F., Eds.), Vol. 5, pp. 165–253, Wiley, New York, NY.

Hwang, S.B., Cheah, M.J., Lee, C.-S.C., Shen, T.Y. Eur. J. Pharmacol., in press.

Juby, P.F., Hudyma, T.W., 1969. J. Med. Chem. 12, 396.

Kalbhen, D.A., Gelderblom, P., Domenjoz, R., 1970. Pharmacology 3, 353–366.

Kantrowitz, F., Robinson, D.R., McCuire, M.B., Levine, L., 1975. Nature 258, 737–739.

Ku, E.C., Wasvary, J.M., Cash, W.D., 1975. Biochem. Pharmacol. 24, 641.

Kuehl, F.A., Egan, R.W., 1980. Science 210, 978–984.

Kuehl, F.A. Jr., Humes, J.L., Torchiana, M.L., Ham, E.A., Egan, R.W. (1979) In: Advances in Inflammation Research (Weissmann, G., Samuelsson, B., Paoletti, R., Eds.), Vol. 1, pp. 419–430, Raven Press, New York, NY.

Lassman, H.B., 1975. Pharmacologist 17, 226.

Lombardino, J.G., Wiseman, E.H., 1982. Med. Res. Rev. 2 (2), 127–152.

Lombardino, J.G., Wiseman, E.H., Chiani, J., 1973. J. Med. Chem. 16, 493–496.

Meacock, S.C.R., Kitchen, E.A., 1979. J. Pharm. Pharmacol. 31, 366–370.

Mills, R.F.N., Adams, S.S., Cliffe, E.E., Dickinson, W., Nicholson, J.S., 1973. Xenobiotica 3, 589.

Mizushima, Y., Sakai, S., Yamaura, Y., 1970. Biochem. Pharmacol. 19, 227–234.

Mizushima, Y., 1964. Arch. Int. Pharmacodyn. Ther. 149, 1–7.

Mizushima, Y., 1966. Lancet 2, 443.

Navarro, J., Stoliaroff, M., Savy, J.M., Berny, C., Brunaud, M., 1974. Arzneim. Forsch. 24, 1368.

Nicholson, J.S. (1982) In: Chronicles of Drug Discovery (Bindra, J.S., Lednicer, D., Eds.), Vol. 1, pp. 149–172, Wiley-Interscience, New York, NY.

Payne, T.G., Dewald, B., Siegl, H., Gubler, H.U., Ott, H., Baggiolini, M., 1982. Nature 296, 160–162.

Perianin, A., Labro, M.T., Hakim, J., 1982. Biochem. Pharmacol. 31 (19), 3071–3076.

Rainsford, K.D., 1978. Agents Actions 8, 587–605.

Roth, G.J., Stanford, N., Majerus, P.W., 1975. Proc. Nat. Acad. Sci. 72, 3073–3076.

Samuelsson, B., 1982. Agnew. Chem. Int. Ed. Engl. 21, 902–910.

Samuelsson, B., Paoletti, R., 1978. Advances in Prostaglandin and Thromboxane Research, 4. Raven Press, New York.

Sankawa, U., Shibuya, M., Ebizuka, Y., Noguchi, H., Kinoshita, T., Endo, A., Kitahara, N., 1982. Prostaglandins 24 (1), 21–34.

Sarett, L.H., 1977. Br. J. Clin. Pharmacol. 4 (Suppl. 1), 5S.

Sarett, L.H., Patchett, A.A., Steelman, S. (1963) In: Progress in Drug Research (Jucker, E., Ed.), Vol. 5, pp 11–153, Birkhauser Verlag, Basel.

Sawa, Y., Hattori, T., Kawakami, Y., Katsube, S., Goto, A., 1976. J. Pharmacol. Soc. Japan 96, 653.

Scherrer, R.A. (1974) In: Antiinflammatory Agents, Medicinal Chemistry Monographs, (Scherrer, R.A., Whitehouse, M.W., Eds.), Vol. 13–1, pp. 45–89. Academic Press, new York, NY.

Scherrer, R.A., Whitehouse, M.W., 1974. Antiinflammatory Agents. Medicinal Chemistry Monographs, 13–1. Academic Press, New York N.Y.

Sharma, Y.R., Cotlier, E., 1982. Exp. Eye Res. 35, 21–27.

Shen, T.Y., 1983. Pharmacotherapy 3 (2), 3S–8S Suppl. 1.

Shen, T.Y. (1981) In: Burger's Medicinal Chemistry (Wolff, M.E., Ed.), 4th edn., Part III, pp. 1205–1272, Wiley, New York, NY.

Shen, T.Y. (1977) New Antiinflammatory & Antirheumatic Drugs (Bertelli, A., Ed.), Vol. II, No. 1, pp. 1–8, J.R. Prous, Barcelona.

Shen, T.Y. (1974) In: Antiinflammatory Agents, Medicinal Chemistry Monographs (Scherrer, R.A., Whitehouse, M.W., Eds.), Vol. 13–1, pp. 180–207, Academic Press, New York, NY.

Shen, T.Y., 1972. Ang. Chem. 11, 460–742.

Shen, T.Y. (1967) In: Topics in Medicinal Chemistry (Rabinowitz, J.L., Myerson, R.M., Eds.), Vol. 1, pp. 29–78, Wiley-Interscience, New York, NY.

Shen, T.Y. (1965) In: Non-Steroidal Antiinflammatory Drugs (Garattini, S., Dukes, M.N.G., Eds.), pp. 13–20, Excerpta Medica Foundation, New York, NY.

Shen, T.Y., Winter, C.A. (1977) In: Advances in Drug Research (Harper, N.J., Simmonds, A.B., Eds.), Vol. 12, pp. 89–246, Academic Press, New York, NY.

Shen, T.Y., Windholz, T.B., Rosegay, A., Witzel, B.E., Wilson, A.N., Willet, J.D., Holtz, W.J., Ellis, R.L., Matzuk, A.R., Lucas, S., Stammer, C.H., Holly, F.W., Sarett, L.H., Risley, E.A., Nuss, G.W., Winter, C.A., 1963. J. Am. Chem. Soc. 55, 488–489.

Shen, T.Y., Witzel, B.E., Jones, H., Linn, B.O., McPherson, J., Greenwald, R., Fordice, M., Jacobs, A., 1972. Fed. Proc. 31, 577.

Shen, T.Y., Hwang, S.B., Cheah, M.J., Lee, C.S. (1983) In: Platelet Activating Factor, Inserm Symposium 23 (Benveniste, J., Arnoux, B., Eds.), pp. 167–176, Elsevier Science Publishers, New York, N.Y.

Smith, M.J.H., Ford-Hutchinson, A.W., Bray, M.A., 1980. J. Pharm. Pharmacol. 32, 517.

Smith, R.J., Iden, S.S., 1980. Biochem. Pharmacol. 29, 2389–2395.

Snyderman, R., Goetzl, E.J., 1981. Science 213, 830–837.

Stone, C.A., Van Arman, C.G., Lotti, V.J., Minsker, D.H., Risley, E.A., Bagdon, W.J., Bokelman, D.L., Jensen, R.D., Mendlowski, B., Tate, C.L., Peck, H.M., Zwickey, R.E., McKinney, S.E., 1977. Br. J. Clin. Pharmacol. 4, 19S–29S.

Szmuszkovicz, J., Glenn, E.M., Heinzelman, R.V., Hester Jr., J.B., Youngdale, G.A., 1966. J. Med. Chem. 9, 527.

Van Arman, C.G., Risley, E.A., Nuss, G.W., 1972. Fed. Proc. 31, 577.

Vane, J.R., 1971. Nature 231, 232–235.

Vane, J.R., Ferreira, S.H., 1979. Handbook of Experimental Pharmacology, 50/II. Springer-Verlag, Berlin.

Vidal y Plana, R.R., Makovec, F., Cifarelli, A., Bizzarri, D., Setnikar, I., Rovati, A.L., 1979. Arzneim. Forsch./Drug Res. 29 (11), 1122–1125.

Winder, C.V., Wax, J., Scherrer, R.A., Jones, E.M., Short, F.W., 1962. J. Pharmacol. Exp. Ther. 138, 1195.

Winter, C.A., Risley, E.A., Nuss, G.W., 1962. Proc. Soc. Exp. Biol. Med. 111, 544–547.

Winter, C.A., Shen, T.Y., Tocco, D.J., Robertson, R.T., Shackleford, R.W. (1981) In: Pharmacological and Biochemical Properties of Drug Substances (Goldberg, M.E., Ed.), Vol. 3, pp. 291–323, Am. Pharm. Assoc., Washington, D.C.

Wiseman, E.H., Lombardino, J.G., Holmes, C.L., Perraud, J. (1981) In: Pharmacological and Biochemical Properties of Drug Substances (Goldberg, M.E., Ed.), Vol. 3, pp. 324–346, Am. Pharm. Assoc., Washington, D.C.

Wong, S., Gardocki, J.F., Pruss, T.P., 1973. J. Pharmacol. Exp. Ther. 185, 127.

Harry Collier: Scientist and visionary. Commentary on The story of aspirin by Harry O.J. Collier

Roderick J. Flower

The William Harvey Research Institute, Queen Mary University of London, London, United Kingdom

Together with salicylic acid, chloral hydrate, and the "coal tar" analgesic/antipyretics, "Aspirin," was one of the first products of the emerging discipline of medicinal chemistry in the later part of the 19th century. These new types of synthetic medicines came to define our current concept of a "drug" as a single chemical entity of known composition and defined purity.

In his 1983 chapter, "*The History of Aspirin*," Harry Collier recounts significant landmarks in the story of this drug; its "herbal" origins in folk medicine, the identification, and synthesis in 1860, of the active principle, salicylate, and the subsequent search for a derivative by Bayer's CEO, Hermann Dreser, which culminated in the synthesis of a simple acetyl derivative in 1897. What was probably the first "me too" drug launched 2 years later in the hope that it would capture a part of the hugely lucrative salicylic acid market. It proved a runaway success, but from the start, it was clear that it was also something of an enigma.

In what was possibly another pharmaceutical "first," Dreser believed aspirin to be a "pro-drug" of salicylate but as it turned out, the two drugs had different therapeutic profiles. And then there was the puzzling connection between the apparently unrelated antiinflammatory, antipyretic, and analgesic actions and the seemingly inseparable side effects such as gastric irritation. What possible mechanism linked these seemingly disparate effects together?

A watershed discovery

Despite its ancient origins in herbal medicine and its 70-year commercial history as one of the most useful drugs ever developed, the world had to wait until 1971 when Vane and his

Discoveries in Pharmacology, Volume 3, Hemodynamics and Immune Defense.
DOI: https://doi.org/10.1016/B978-0-443-18442-0.00008-2

colleagues provided a solution to this conundrum, demonstrating aspirin's mechanism of action to be through the inhibition of the prostaglandin-forming cyclo-oxygenase (COX) enzyme. The other "aspirin-like" NSAIDs (non-steroidal anti-inflammatory drugs) were soon found to act through a similar mechanism. Not only did this solve the mechanism of action of one of the world's oldest synthetic drugs, but it neatly accounted for the apparently unrelated therapeutic and side effects of aspirin. The discovery also provided investigators with a useful set of tools with which to probe the physiological role of PGs *in vivo* and the *in vitro* cyclo-oxygenase assays developed to measure the inhibitory effect of NSAIDs also offered a cheap and practical method to screen for candidate anti-inflammatory drugs.

But few scientific discoveries are made in an intellectual vacuum. Of the many researchers who tackled the "aspirin problem" prior to 1971, Harry can confidently lay claim to have been the most influential and he cites many examples of his prescience in his chapter. In fact, it was a former colleague of his at Miles Laboratories, then working on one of his projects in Vane's lab, who turned out to make a key observation in the developing aspirin story (Piper and Vane, 1969).

COX isoforms

So much for the past: but how has the "aspirin" field changed since Harry wrote his chapter?

While other targets of NSAIDs have certainly been discovered (e.g., Wang et al., 2017), the intervening years have only served to substantiate and extend Vane's original concept. The COX enzyme was finally purified and cloned in 1988 (Merlie et al., 1988; Yokoyama and Tanabe, 1989). But perhaps the most significant advance in the field since 1983, was the discovery of another COX enzyme. As Harry notes in his chapter, hints that such an isoform may exist arose as early as 1972 (Flower and Vane, 1972), but it was not until 1991 that this long-held suspicion was unequivocally confirmed when what became known as the COX-2 isoform (the original was renamed COX-1) was cloned simultaneously by two groups, (Kujubu et al., 1991; Xie et al., 1991). Significantly, and unlike the "original" constitutive and widely distributed COX-1 enzyme, COX-2 was generally absent from cells except during inflammation. Even more importantly for pharmacologists, the two isoforms were differentially sensitive to the existing NSAIDs, a fact quickly seized upon by several groups (Kujubu et al., 1991; Xie et al., 1991; Mitchell et al., 1993).

Since it was by this time clear that prostaglandins, acting through a group of GPCR receptors (see, Narumiya et al., 1999), subserved a major homeostatic role as well as being inflammatory messengers, this discovery held a considerable promise for future drug development. "Selective" inhibitors of the COX-2 isoform ("Coxibs" as they were later called) would surely be expected to retain the therapeutic anti-inflammatory effects while producing less of the troublesome and unwanted effects on "physiological" prostaglandin production.

Space does not permit a detailed account of the subsequent race by pharma to produce the first truly selective coxib, but the rise of these drugs (and in some cases, their ignominious fall) has been extensively reviewed elsewhere (e.g., Flower, 2003; Smith, 2006). Sufficient to say that while these drugs have probably fallen short of their initial promise, some coxibs remain useful for the treatment of patients who are particularly susceptible to the gastric irritation produced by conventional NSAIDs. One problem noted with these drugs was an increased incidence of cardiovascular events and, oddly perhaps, an important unforeseen consequence of COX-1/COX-2 research was the surprising revelation that *all* NSAIDs caused hypertension when used chronically (Ray et al., 2009). It seems that even after all these years, the NSAIDs can still surprise us.

Unanswered questions

But despite all this progress, the enigmatic aspirin continued to pose some puzzling questions and, paradoxically, one of these concerns was salicylate itself. Dreser initially believed that aspirin owed its therapeutic activity to its conversion to salicylate in the body but as an inhibitor of COX *in vitro*, salicylate is distinctly feeble and much less active than aspirin. When administered to volunteers however, both drugs were equiactive in reducing the output of urinary prostaglandin metabolites (Hamberg, 1972). It seems therefore that aspirin is a "bifunctional" drug, with one effect dependent upon its ability to acetylate the cyclooxygenase in (for example) platelets, while the other is dependent upon its conversion to salicylic acid, although ironically, the exact mechanism of action of salicylate itself still remains unclear. Explanatory hypotheses abound, including suggestions that some metabolites have superior COX inhibitory potency (Flower, 1974; Hinz et al., 2000), that salicylate suppresses High Mobility Group Box 1 (HMGB1) protein action (Choi et al., 2015) or inhibits COX-2 induction (Xu et al., 1999) but none seem totally satisfactory.

Historically, the "coal tar" analgesics such as acetanilide (1886), phenacetin, and paracetamol (acetaminophen; 1887) antedated even aspirin. Paracetamol, like salicylate, has also proved to have an unexpectedly complex action as a drug. It is an excellent analgesic and anti-pyretic (and, interestingly, also has hypothermic activity) but lacks the systemic anti-inflammatory (and gastro-irritant) activity of the other NSAIDs.

It was an experiment with this drug that originally suggested that there could be isoforms of COX and many groups have investigated the basis of its apparently selective action on CNS COX. Several authors have advanced the concept that it is the unique redox environment of CNS tissue that is a key requirement for inhibition of the enzyme by paracetamol (e.g., Ouellet and Percival, 2001; Boutaud et al., 2002) but there are other suggestions too. A variant form of COX-1 (and later, two other partial transcripts of COX-1) was discovered in dog brains in 2002 (Chandrasekharan et al., 2002). Dubbed COX-3, this enzyme was reported to be more susceptible to paracetamol and some of the other "coal tar" analgesics. Supporting this idea was the later observation that there is a functional variant form of COX-1 in the CNS, and that paracetamol was observed to lack efficacy in COX-1 knockout mice (Ayoub and Flower, 2019). But this neat explanation for paracetamol's action was subsequently disputed when the variant could not be detected in other species, and the matter has not yet been settled to everyone's satisfaction (see Ayoub, 2021).

Other endogenous anti-inflammatory factors

It was interesting that Harry coined the term "anti-defensive drugs" for aspirin and its congeners because a very similar term was later applied to another group of anti-inflammatories, the glucocorticoids (Munck et al., 1984), and these drugs also crossed Harry's perceptive mental radar. He believed that there must be endogenous factors that controlled prostaglandin synthesis and in one of his papers (Saeed et al., 1977) he advanced the idea that these factors were present in mammalian serum and plasma and were increased by glucocorticoids thus providing a notional link between the anti-inflammatory effect of the two classes of drugs.

Once again, Harry's ideas were very much on target. Such a glucocorticoid-induced anti-inflammatory factor was later described, isolated, and cloned. Annexin (Anx) A1, as this factor is now known, has been shown by a variety of techniques to be a potent anti-inflammatory and a mediator of acute glucocorticoid actions through an effect on the FPR receptor family. A perusal of the methodology used by Harry's group suggests that Anx-A1 may have been present in some of their extracts, although it is probably not identical to the material described in his 1997 paper which apparently has a molecular weight in excess of the 37 kDa Anx-A1 molecule (see Sinniah et al., 2021).

Harry often visited the Vane lab during the "heroic" years of aspirin research. My personal recollection of him was that of a benign, bespectacled figure bustling around the lab, interested in everything and always happy to talk science with anyone. He was often observed ransacking the pockets of his tweed jacket for scraps of paper on which he had scribbled important questions that he wanted to ask or the timings of his next engagement.

When Harry died suddenly in 1983, one day after finishing the writing of his chapter, the "aspirin" story was just over 10 years old. His account of this episode of pharmaceutical history still makes for stimulating reading today, 50 years later, but since then the field has moved on a long way: new uses have been found for aspirin (e.g., Patrignani and Patrono, 2016) and the prostaglandin family itself has grown and, together with a profusion of other lipid mediators, now number >100 distinct species (Calder, 2020). Were Harry alive today then he would have had to greatly expand his chapter. He would have been fascinated by all the new science but, knowing Harry, probably not completely surprised.

References

Ayoub, S.S., 2021. Paracetamol (acetaminophen): a familiar drug with an unexplained mechanism of action. Temperature (Austin) 8 (4), 351–371.

Ayoub, S.S., Flower, R.J., 2019. Loss of hypothermic and anti-pyretic action of paracetamol in cyclooxygenase-1 knockout mice is indicative of inhibition of cyclooxygenase-1 variant enzymes. Eur. J. Pharmacol. 861, 172609.

Boutaud, O., et al., 2002. Determinants of the cellular specificity of acetaminophen as an inhibitor of prostaglandin $H_{(2)}$ synthases. Proc. Natl. Acad. Sci. U.S.A. 99 (10), 7130–7135.

Calder, P.C., 2020. Eicosanoids. Essays Biochem. 64 (3), 423–441.

Chandrasekharan, N.V., et al., 2002. COX-3, a cyclooxygenase-1 variant inhibited by acetaminophen and other analgesic/antipyretic drugs: cloning, structure, and expression. Proc. Natl. Acad. Sci. U.S.A. 99 (21), 13926–13931.

Choi, H.W., et al., 2015. Aspirin's active metabolite salicylic acid targets high mobility group box 1 to modulate inflammatory responses. Mol. Med. 21, 526–535.

Flower, R.J., 1974. Drugs which inhibit prostaglandin biosynthesis. Pharmacol. Rev. 26 (1), 33–67.

Flower, R.J., 2003. The development of COX_2 inhibitors. Nat. Rev. Drug Discov. 2 (3), 179–191.

Flower, R.J., Vane, J.R., 1972. Inhibition of prostaglandin synthetase in brain explains the anti-pyretic activity of paracetamol (4-acetamidophenol). Nature 240 (5381), 410–411.

Hamberg, M., 1972. Inhibition of prostaglandin synthesis in man. Biochem. Biophys. Res. Commun. 49 (3), 720–726.

Hinz, B., et al., 2000. Salicylate metabolites inhibit cyclooxygenase-2-dependent prostaglandin $E_{(2)}$ synthesis in murine macrophages. Biochem. Biophys. Res. Commun. 274 (1), 197–202.

Kujubu, D.A., et al., 1991. TIS10, a phorbol ester tumor promoter-inducible mRNA from Swiss $_3T_3$ cells, encodes a novel prostaglandin synthase/cyclooxygenase homologue. J. Biol. Chem. 266 (20), 12866–12872.

Merlie, J.P., et al., 1988. Isolation and characterization of the complementary DNA for sheep seminal vesicle prostaglandin endoperoxide synthase (cyclooxygenase). J. Biol. Chem. 263 (8), 3550–3553.

Mitchell, J.A., et al., 1993. Selectivity of nonsteroidal antinflammatory drugs as inhibitors of constitutive and inducible cyclooxygenase. Proc. Natl. Acad. Sci. U.S.A. 90 (24), 11693–11697.

Munck, A., Guyre, P.M., Holbrook, N.J., 1984. Physiological functions of glucocorticoids in stress and their relation to pharmacological actions. Endocr. Rev. 5 (1), 25–44.

Narumiya, S., Sugimoto, Y., Ushikubi, F., 1999. Prostanoid receptors: structures, properties, and functions. Physiol. Rev. 79 (4), 1193–1226.

Ouellet, M., Percival, M.D., 2001. Mechanism of acetaminophen inhibition of cyclooxygenase isoforms. Arch. Biochem. Biophys. 387 (2), 273–280.

Patrignani, P., Patrono, C., 2016. Aspirin and cancer. J. Am. Coll. Cardiol. 68 (9), 967–976.

Piper, P.J., Vane, J.R., 1969. Release of additional factors in anaphylaxis and its antagonism by anti-inflammatory drugs. Nature 223 (5201), 29–35.

Ray, W.A., et al., 2009. Cardiovascular risks of nonsteroidal antiinflammatory drugs in patients after hospitalization for serious coronary heart disease. Circ. Cardiovasc. Qual. Outcomes. 2 (3), 155–163.

Saeed, S.A., et al., 1977. Endogenous inhibitor of prostaglandin synthetase. Nature 270 (5632), 32–36.

Sinniah, A., Yazid, S., Flower, R.J., 2021. From NSAIDs to glucocorticoids and beyond. Cells 10 (12), 3524.

Smith, R., 2006. Lapses at the New England Journal of Medicine. J. R. Soc. Med. 99 (8), 380–382.

Wang, T., Cook, I., Leyh, T.S., 2017. The NSAID allosteric site of human cytosolic sulfotransferases. J. Biol. Chem. 292 (49), 20305–20312.

Xie, W.L., et al., 1991. Expression of a mitogen-responsive gene encoding prostaglandin synthase is regulated by mRNA splicing. Proc. Natl. Acad. Sci. U.S.A. 88 (7), 2692–2696.

Xu, X.M., et al., 1999. Suppression of inducible cyclooxygenase 2 gene transcription by aspirin and sodium salicylate. Proc. Natl. Acad. Sci. U.S.A. 96 (9), 5292–5297.

Yokoyama, C., Tanabe, T., 1989. Cloning of human gene encoding prostaglandin endoperoxide synthase and primary structure of the enzyme. Biochem. Biophys. Res. Commun. 165 (2), 888–894.

The story of aspirin

Harry O.J. Collier

Contents

Disclaimer: The original text that follows is reproduced from the first edition and carries errors and omissions from it. The editors and publisher agreed to retain them and honor the original authors and challenges they had to deal with in publishing back in those times.

Discoveries in Pharmacology, Volume 3, Hemodynamics and
Immune Defense.
DOI: https://doi.org/10.1016/B978-0-443-18442-0.00064-1

4.1 Introduction

For three reasons, aspirin (acetylsalicylic acid or acetylsalicylate) is an immensely important drug. First it is important because millions of people throughout the world can take it, without heavy expense or having to consult a physician, with no risk of addiction and little of serious toxicity, to combat several of the minor ills that flesh is heir to.

Second, acetylsalicylate is important because, as a result of these properties, it became for long the most widely used medicinal drug in the world. As such, it established the fortunes not only of the Rhineland firm of Bayer that introduced it to the world, but also of several other companies, which, for reasons of war, were able to take over part of its immense market.

Third, aspirin has proved of great importance to medical science, because an experimental analysis of its molecular mechanism of action has played a vital role in the discovery of a far-reaching system of bodily defences, based on the products of enzymes acting on arachidonic and related unsaturated fatty acids and their metabolites. We may call this the arachidonate defence system. It was for their outstanding contributions to unravelling the arachidonate and closely related systems of lipid local hormones that Sune Bergstrom, Bengt Samuelsson and John Vane were awarded the 1982 Nobel Prize for Physiology and Medicine.

The patho-physiological processes connected with the arachidonate defence system appear to be closely associated with some of the most important diseases of today – coronary infarction, stroke, rheumatism and allergy. This association in turn leads to the novel use or possible use of aspirin in controlling some aspects of these diseases.

The story of aspirin thus requires a book, rather than a chapter; but, since it must be compressed into a chapter, I have chosen to concentrate on the scientific elucidation of its molecular mechanism of action, which seems to me basic to the story.

In so doing, I may appear to the reader immodest, as I feel to myself embarrassed, to refer so often to the work of my colleagues and myself. This seems to be unavoidable because, during the 1960s, when several important steps were taken in elucidating the mechanism of action of acetylsalicylate, the group that I then headed was very active in this field. The work we did then was largely obscured and forgotten in the blaze of light and publicity that followed the discovery in 1971, by John Vane and his colleagues at the Royal College of Surgeons in London, that aspirin and like-acting drugs potently inhibit prostaglandin synthase. Nonetheless, our work brought the subject to the position from which Vane and his group could make that great step forward. And so it seems historically necessary to recall the forgotten groundwork, which we and other groups, such as that of Robert K. Lim, did during the 1960s. I must still beg the reader to forgive me, if he finds my account of the aspirin story during the 1960s too much of an 'ego-trip'.

As the story of aspirin unfolds, these reasons for its importance will take on a fuller meaning. As we shall see, the story illustrates the step-wise, zig-zag development of a scientific theme, resulting from the interlocking contributions of scientists of different nations or disciplines. It illustrates, too, the creative influence of the pharmaceutical industry on the development of pharmacology and, reciprocally, the effect of pharmacological discoveries on the growth of the industry; for, without the pharmaceutical industry, aspirin would not have been developed and, without aspirin, several pharmaceutical companies would not have reached their present stature. The story, like that of Man in Shakespeare's *'As You Like It',* may be divided into seven stages, although the last stage is not one of final deprivation, unlike Shakespeare's ('sans teeth, sans eyes, sans taste, sans everything'). Let us now turn to a brief outline (in Section 4.2 below) of the seven stages of the 'strange eventful history' of aspirin.

4.2 Seven stages of aspirin

4.2.1 Salicylate, a new, synthetic remedy

The first stage in its story occurred before aspirin existed. It was the discovery, by a cumulative process, during the 18th and 19th centuries, of the therapeutic value of salicylates and the establishment in the 1870s, that sodium salicylate was a new, synthetic remedy for rheumatic diseases.

4.2.2 Birth of Aspirin

The next stage was the birth of Aspirin. This occurred in 1897, when Felix Hoffmann, a chemist in the research laboratories of the German dyestuffs manufacturer, Friedrich Bayer, devised a way of preparing acetylsalicylic acid as the stable product of a manufacturing process (Fig. 4.1).

Acetylsalicylic acid was tested biologically by Hermann Dreser, Head of the new pharmacological laboratory at Bayer. Dreser concluded that acetylsalicylic acid was readily reconverted in the body to salicylic acid, which was the pharmacologically active form (Dreser, 1899). At the same time, aspirin was tested clinically, with favourable results.

Because the German Patent Office had refused a patent for acetylsalicylic acid, it was commercially important to introduce it quickly with a good tradename. For reasons given below (see Section 4.3), the name 'Aspirin' was chosen and, in 1899, Aspirin was introduced and marketed as a 'pro-drug' for salicylic acid.

Although Aspirin was patented in some countries, wars with Germany later removed its legal protection in the English-speaking world, where 'aspirin' was made by law a generic name for acetylsalicylic acid, as it remains in these countries to this day. In this chapter, a capital A will be used when the brand-name of the drug is intended, a lower case a indicates acetylsalicylic acid.

4.2.3 Aspirin acts in its own right

Sixty years were to elapse before the next major step in the history of aspirin. That step was the establishment that, at least in some actions, aspirin acts in its own right and not through being converted to salicylate, as Dreser had laid down.

To establish the distinct and independent identity of aspirin as a drug, it was necessary to find actions in which it was significantly more potent than sodium salicylate and therefore could not act by being converted to the less potent drug.

Three such actions came to light in the ten years between 1959 and 1968. In antinociceptive tests, in which a 'writhing' response of mice to intraperitoneal injection of a noxious substance was suppressed, aspirin was 4 to 7 times more potent than was sodium salicylate (Hendershot and Forsaith, 1959; Keith, 1960). In preventing the bronchoconstrictor response of the guinea-pig to intravenous injection of bradykinin or slow-reacting substance in anaphylaxis (SRS-A), aspirin was 32 times more potent than was sodium salicylate (Collier and Shorley, 1960; Berry and Collier, 1964). Lastly, in man, in preventing the aggregation of platelets in shed blood in response to certain agents, a small oral dose of aspirin was remarkably effective, whereas a large oral dose of sodium salicylate was without effect (O'Brien, 1968a, b).

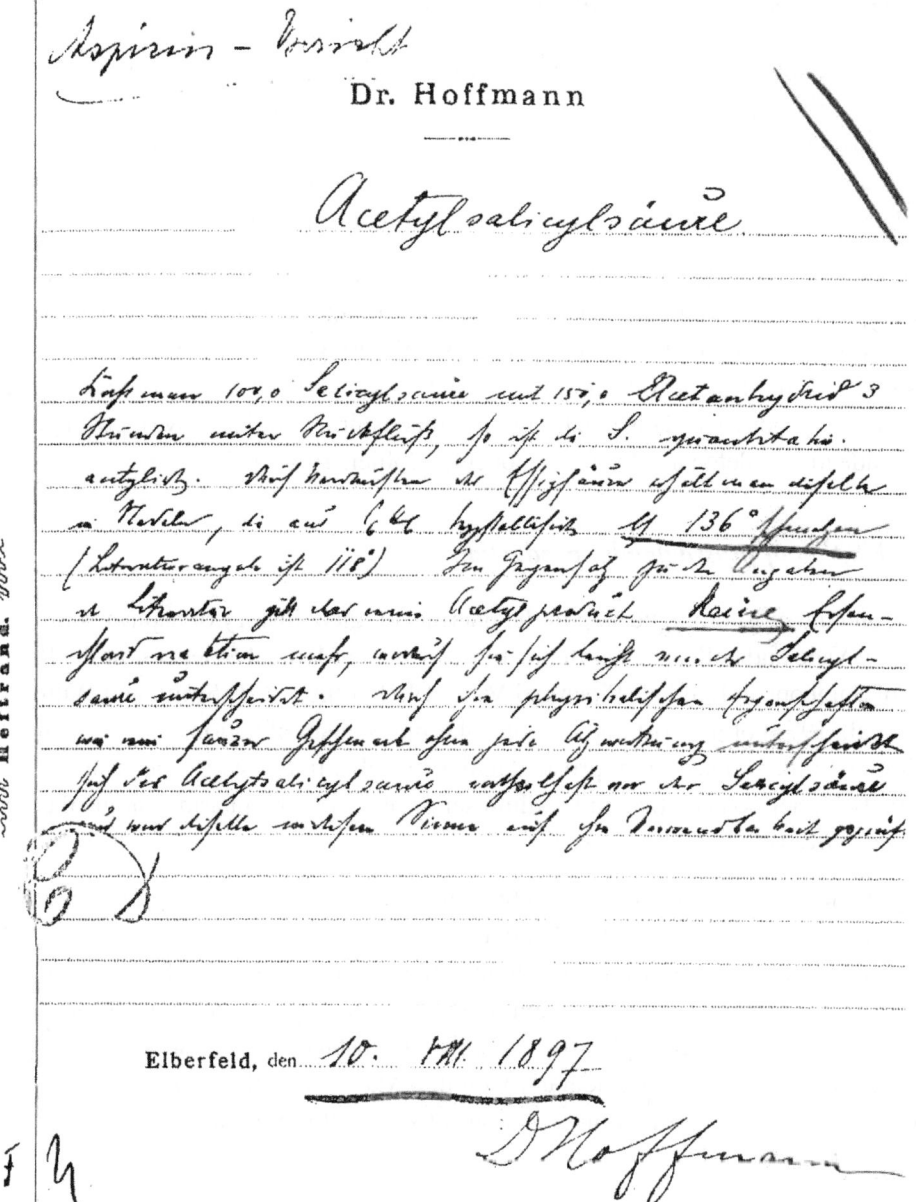

Figure 4.1

Felix Hoffmann's process, which translates as follows: When salicylic acid (100.0 parts) is heated with acetic anhydride (150.0 parts) for 3 hours under reflux, the salicylic acid is quantitatively acetylated. After distilling off the acetic acid one obtains the above in the form of needles, which, when crystallised from benzene, melt at 136° (value in the literature is 118°). In contrast the literature reports my acetyl product no longer gives a reaction with ferric chloride, which readily distinguishes it from salicylic acid. By its physical properties, e.g. its sour taste without being corrosive, the acetylsalicylic acid differs favourably from salicylic acid, and is now being tested in this respect for its usefulness. Elberfeld, 10. VIII 1897.

4.2.4 Aspirin as opponent of local defensive processes

The establishment that aspirin acts in its own right set the stage for investigation of how it acts. Two observations provided the basis of the discovery of its molecular mechanism of action. One of these, was that aspirin was shown, by cross-circulation experiments in dogs, to exert its analgesic action in the periphery, at the site of injection of a noxious substance, rather than in the CNS, as had hitherto been supposed (Lim et al., 1964).

A second basic step was the generalisation that, in all the usual therapeutic uses of aspirin (control of pain, fever and inflammation), it acted as an 'anti-defensive' drug (Collier, 1963). The point was thus made that aspirin could act by inhibiting a single defensive process that manifested itself in different ways in different sites and had become, for some reason, excessive and counterproductive. This meant, in turn, that aspirin could act, by opposing in some way, an unidentified, defensive local hormone(s) (Collier, 1969, 1971b).

4.2.5 Inhibition of prostaglandin production

The next, and the most dramatic step in the pharmacological history of aspirin was the identification by Vane and colleagues at the Institute of Basic Medical Sciences, at the Royal College of Surgeons in London (Piper and Vane, 1969; Vane, 1971; Smith and Willis, 1971; Ferreira et al., 1971) of its most potent molecular mechanism of action. This mechanism was the inhibition of the production of prostaglandins by cells. In this action, aspirin displayed a considerably higher potency than did sodium salicylate, as in the pharmacological comparisons given above (see Section 4.2.3).

Vane argued that this was the mechanism by which aspirin and like-acting drugs exert their main effects, although he was doubtful about including their analgesic action (Vane, 1971). Subsequent work has shown that aspirin inhibits the enzyme prostaglandin synthase (cyclo-oxygenase), which initiates the conversion of arachidonic acid and other twenty-carbon unsaturated fatty acids to prostaglandins and related substances. It has shown, too, that the analgesic action of aspirin fits particularly well into Vane's hypothesis. Difficulties, however, remain in explaining the anti-rheumatic actions of some inhibitors of cyclo-oxygenase in terms of Vane's hypothesis.

A corollary of the discovery at the Royal College of Surgeons was that, if aspirin were truly an anti-defensive drug, then the prostaglandins are very important members of the family of local defensive substances (Collier, 1971a,b, 1974, 1980). This conclusion largely accords both with the pharmacological actions of prostaglandins and with their ease of liberation by any disturbance of the tissues.

A further step within this stage of the aspirin story, yet to be fully evaluated, was the discovery that certain proteins of blood and tissues can also inhibit prostaglandin production from arachidonic acid (Saeed et al., 1977; Hellewell et al., 1980; Collier et al., 1982). Thus, aspirin may be said, in a sense, to mimic natural endogenous inhibitors of prostaglandin production.

4.2.6 Another side of the story

Aspirin has been taken for so many years, by so many different individuals, so often that its low degree of serious toxic risk cannot be gainsaid. Moreover, sufferers from rheumatoid arthritis have lived on high daily doses of aspirin for many years, without having to abandon the drug for reasons of toxicity. Nonetheless, a certain pattern of toxic responses to aspirin has emerged and this has helped to determine the pharmaceutical and medical development of the drug.

Probably the most common toxic effect of aspirin is gastric mucosal irritation or erosion. This is expressed subjectively as indigestion and objectively as faecal blood loss. Pharmaceutically, these effects have led to the development of highly buffered effervescent preparations, in which such effects are minimized. These have taken a large market; but an even more significant commercial consequence has been the rise of paracetamol, which appears to be innocent of gastro-intestinal side-effects.

4.2.7 Rebirth of aspirin

The last stage in the history of aspirin today is the opening up of new uses for this old drug, through understanding its mode of action. For example, the ability of aspirin at low doses to inhibit some forms of platelet aggregation has led to the recognition of its probable value in preventing coronary infarctions or strokes in people liable to these (*Lancet,* editorial, 1980; *Drug and Therapeutics Bulletin,* 1983; Lewis et al., 1983).

4.3 Salicylate in rheumatism

4.3.1 Herbal beginnings

Salicylates probably occur in many genera of plants, and three of these genera (*Salix, Spiraea* (*Filipendula*) and *Gaultheria*) participate in their medicinal history (Fig. 4.2). The scientific record begins with the letter of the Rev. Mr. Edward (or Edmund) Stone to the Earl of Macclesfield, then President of the Royal Society of London, which was published in 1763 in the *Philosophical Transactions of the Royal Society* (Stone, 1763).

This letter, entitled '*An Account of the Success of the Bark of the Willow in the Cure of Agues'* was read to the Society on June 2, 1763. Essentially it reports that, because willow bark, like Cinchona (or Peruvian) bark, tasted bitter and because willows grow in wet land, where agues are also common, and where, therefore, Providence would be expected to have

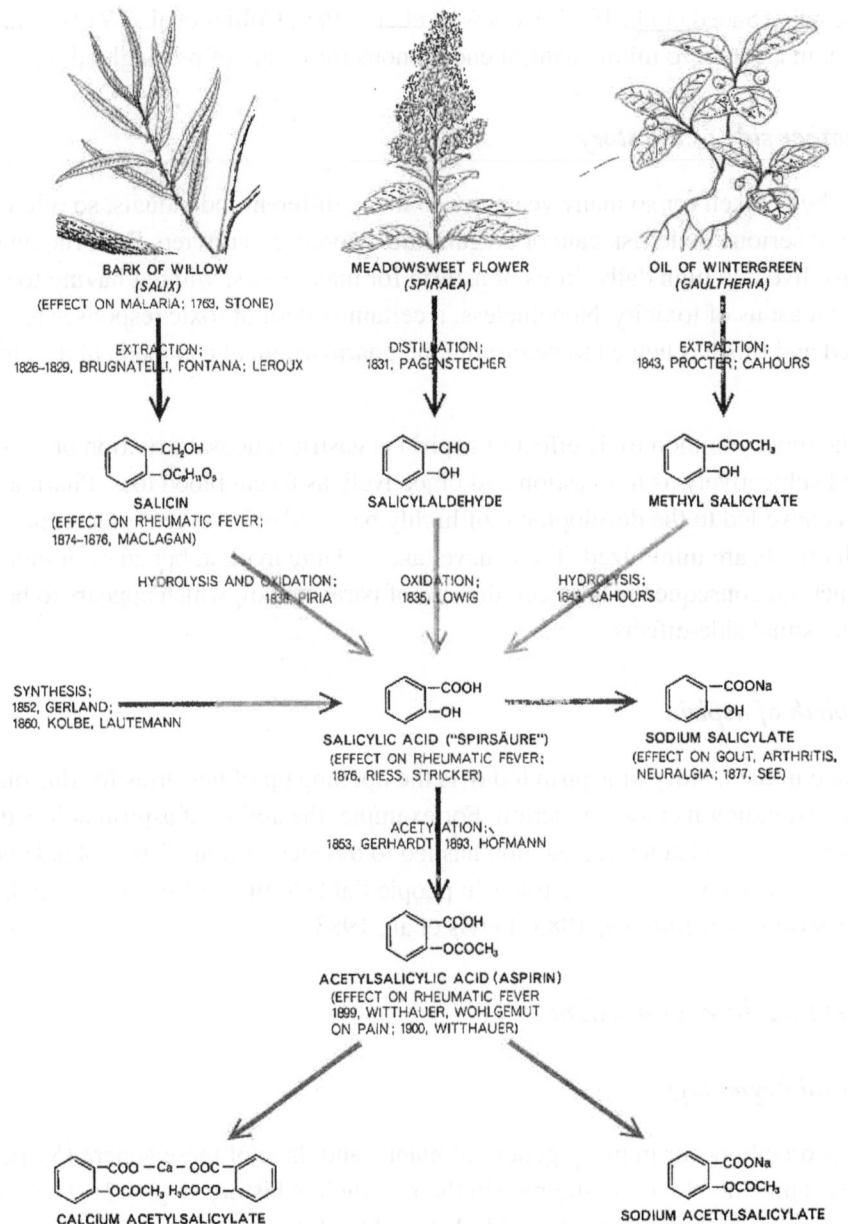

Figure 4.2

Chemical ancestry of acetylsalicylic acid, the chemical now known as aspirin, is traced to plants in which salicylates were found. formulae for the chemical relatives of salicylic acid are given below, with techniques used in isolating it, the chemists who performed the steps and physicians who reported medical uses of the drug. A method of acetylating salicylic acid to weaken its acidity was devised as early as 1853, but only in the last decade of the century was the process refined to make possible large-scale manufacture. The salts of aspirin (bottom) are more soluble, are more quickly absorbed into the bloodstream and are less injurious to the digestive tract. *Reproduced from Collier (1963) with kind permission.*

placed the remedy for the indigenous disease, Stone was led to give the bark to people with fevers.

Stone obtained about a pound of bark from trees of *Salix alba* in summer, hung it in a bag outside a baker's oven to dry, and then pulverised it. He gave the powder, with water, tea or small beer, usually in doses of 2 scruples (2.6 grams) as often as every four hours to persons suffering from 'agues and intermitting disorders'. In all, he studied the bark 'for five years successively and successfully' in about 50 persons. It seldom failed to cure, except in a few obstinate autumnal and quartan agues. For these cases, he 'added one fifth part of the Peruvian bark to it, and with this small auxiliary it totally routed its adversary'. Stone concluded that the willow bark was 'a powerful . . . febrifuge in intermitting cases'.

Stone's description suggests that some at least of the fevers he treated were malarious. Whether he actually treated rheumatic fever is uncertain. At least he demonstrated an antipyretic action in his powdered bark, at the same time providing unscrupulous traders with a cheap diluent for Peruvian bark.

Stone's letter contains an anomaly, which is still unexplained (Collier, 1963). At the beginning of the letter the author is named 'Edmund' and, at the end, 'Edward' (Fig. 4.3). This arose because, in his signature, Stone used the abbreviated form ('Edwd.' or 'Edmd.'), and it was impossible to be sure whether the penultimate letter was 'w' or 'm'. Since, at this time, there was a Fellow of the Society named Edmund Stone, it seems probable that the printer of this letter began by confusing the two Stones.

Edmund Stone was a much more distinguished man than the author of the letter on willow bark. As a young man, he had been a gardener of the Duke of Argyll. The Duke, finding his young gardener reading and understanding Newton's *Principia,* had arranged for him to be trained as a mathematician. In this capacity he was outstanding enough to be elected a Fellow of the Society and to achieve a place in the *Dictionary of National Biography.* The life of the author of the letter on willow bark is more obscure; but pharmaceutical history has allotted him the name Edward, which conveniently distinguishes him from the mathematician, Edmund.

Willow bark contains salicin, which, as Leroux showed in 1829, is a glycoside of salicylic acid. From salicin, as Piria reported nine years later, salicylic acid can be liberated by hydrolysis. It was, however, salicin itself that was used in 1874 in a dramatic therapeutic experiment by the Dundee physician, T.J. MacLagan. MacLagan argued, much as Stone had done more than a century before, that:

> 'Nature seeming to produce the remedy under climatic conditions similar to those which give rise to the disease . . . among the Salicaceae . . . I determined to search for a remedy for acute rheumatism [rheumatic fever]. The bark of many species of willow contains a bitter principle called salicin. This principle was exactly what I wanted.

[195]

XXXII. *An Account of the Succefs of the Bark of the Willow in the Cure of Agues. In a Letter to the Right Honourable* George *Earl of* Macclesfield, *Prefident of R. S. from the Rev. Mr.* Edmund Stone, *of* Chipping-Norton *in* Oxfordfhire.

My Lord,

Read June 2d, 1763. AMong the many ufeful difcoveries, which this age hath made, there are very few which, better deferve the attention of the public than what I am going to lay before your Lordfhip.

There is a bark of an Englifh tree, which I have found by experience to be a powerful aftringent, and very efficacious in curing aguifh and intermitting diforders.

About fix years ago, I accidentally tafted it, and was furprifed at its extraordinary bitternefs; which immediately raifed me a fufpicion of its having the properties of the Peruvian bark. As this tree delights in a moift or wet foil, where agues chiefly abound, the general maxim, that many natural maladies carry their cures along with them, or that their remedies lie not far from their caufes, was fo very appofite to this particular cafe, that I could not help applying it;

[200]

cinnamon or lateritious colour, which I believe is the cafe with the Peruvian bark and powders.

I have no other motives for publifhing this valuable fpecific, than that it may have a fair and full trial in all its variety of circumftances and fituations, and that the world may reap the benefits accruing from it. For thefe purpofes I have given this long and minute account of it, and which I would not have troubled your Lordfhip with, was I not fully perfuaded of the wonderful efficacy of this Cortex Salignus in agues and intermitting cafes, and did I not think, that this perfuafion was fufficiently fupported by the manifold experience, which I have had of it.

I am, my Lord,

with the profoundeft fubmiffion and refpect,

Chipping-Norton, Oxfordfhire, April 25, 1763. your Lordfhip's moft obedient humble Servant

Edward Stone.

Figure 4.3

Uncertain authorship of first paper to describe medicinal effects of willow-bark extract can be traced to a printer's error in the *Philosophical Transactions of the Royal Society,* 1763. At top of paper (left) the author is named Edmund Stone. At bottom (right) the name is Edward. 'Doctriene of signatures' is synopsized in the proposition that 'many natural maladies carry their cures along with them . . .' *Reproduced from Collier (1963) with kind permission.*

I had at that time under my care a well-marked case of the disease which was being treated by alkalies but was not improving. I determined to give him salicin; but, before doing so, took myself first five, then ten and then thirty grains [about 2 grams, H.O.J.C.] without experiencing the least inconvenience or discomfort. I gave the patient referred to twelve grains every three hours. The results exceeded my most sanguine expectations'.

The main results of MacLagan's treatment were a lowering of body temperature and a reduction of pain and swelling; in other words, the antipyretic, analgesic and anti-inflammatory effects for which salicylates were to be used for a century to come.

In the same year (1874) in Germany, Kolbe and Lautemann worked out a practical synthesis for salicylic acid (Friend, 1974). By the time that MacLagan's papers appeared in *The Lancet,* in March 1876, others had entered the field using the synthetic product. In January of that year, S. Stricker (1876) announced in Berlin that salicylic acid was effective in rheumatic fever. Also in Germany, L. Riess reported comparable results. Nonetheless, history has recognised the experimental priority of MacLagan, who recorded the first use of salicin late in 1874.

MacLagan moved from Dundee to London, where he continued to practice medicine. Despite his momentous discovery, his colleagues in London never elected him to Fellowship of the Royal College of Physicians, but allowed him to remain a humbler Member of the College, until his death in 1906 (Sharp, 1915).

Another line in the herbal ancestry of salicylic acid, important to the naming of Aspirin, derives from the meadowsweet flower (Fig. 4.2). As Pagenstecker showed in 1831, meadowsweet contains salicylaldehyde, which Lowig in 1835 oxidised to salicylic acid. At this time, meadowsweet had been placed in the genus *Spiraea* and the acid derived from it thus became 'Spirsäure' in German. Acetylation of spirsaure, gave 'Acetylspirsäure', from which 'aspirin' was a natural shortening. Later, meadowsweet was moved from the genus *Spiraea* to *Filipendula*. Had this occurred before Aspirin was named, we might perhaps now be saying 'Asfilin' instead.

4.3.2 New, synthetic remedy

Soon after the therapeutic effectiveness of salicin and salicylic acid in rheumatic fever had been established, sodium salicylate was recognised as the preparation to be preferred, because of its solubility, low toxicity and relatively easy manufacture. Its therapeutic effectiveness was soon extended to chronic rheumatoid arthritis and gout (Sée, 1877). The success of sodium salicylate required a steady source of supply of a pure compound from the pharmaceutical industry. It seems that this need was fulfilled by the Heyden Chemical Company, using Kolbe's process (Friend, 1974).

To conclude the first stage of the aspirin story, by 1877 one of the earliest effective synthetic drugs, sodium salicylate, had been introduced into medicine and had been provided as a commercial product by the German chemical industry. Although German industry manufactured sodium salicylate, the discovery of the anti-rheumatic action of salicin, its forerunner, was made in Britain. This pattern – of British discovery, followed by foreign exploitation – was to continue for many years. Might it fairly be callen 'la folie anglaise'?

4.4 Aspirin as a pro-drug for salicylate

4.4.1 Manufacturing process for acetylsalicylate

Although, by the end of 1877, the therapeutic efficacy of sodium salicylate had been demonstrated in fever, rheumatism and gout, it was twenty years before a successful improvement was made. The work that led to Aspirin started soon after 1895, when Arthur Eichengrün was appointed Head of the chemical research laboratories of the dyestuff manufacturer, Friederich Bayer, of Elberfeld, Germany (Eichengrün, 1949).

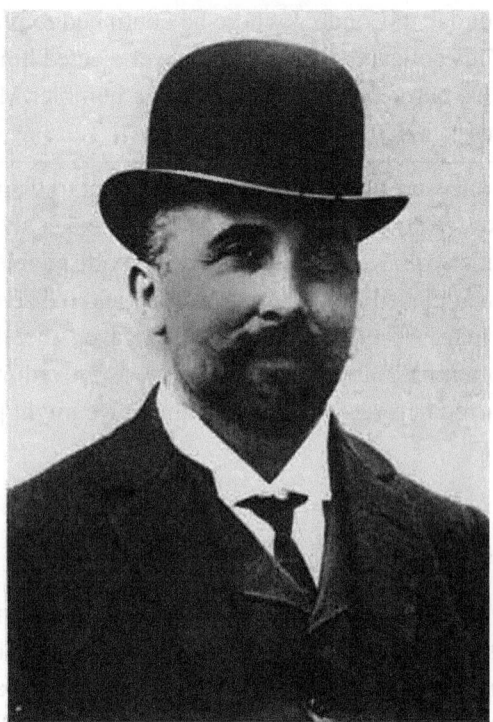

Figure 4.4
Dr. Felix Hoffmann born 21.1.1868 in Ludwigsburg, died 8.2.1946 in Lausanne.

According to Eichengrün's memoirs, written in 1944 in the concentration camp at There-sienstadt, he assigned the synthesis of derivatives of salicylic acid that might be better than sodium salicylate to a young research chemist in his department, Felix Hoffmann (Fig. 4.4). Tradition says that Hoffmann's father was an arthritic, who had come to dislike taking his daily dose of sodium salicylate, which he found, to say the least, nauseating. Be that as it may, Hoffmann, in 1897, found a way to acetylate the hydroxyl group on the benzene ring of salicylic acid (Fig. 4.1) that could be operated on a manufacturing scale.

Acetylsalicylic acid, along with other derivatives of salicylic acid, was passed for biological testing to Hermann Dreser, Head of the first industrial pharmacological laboratory in the world, set up by Bayer in 1890 (Fig. 4.5). Dreser was a pupil of Oswald Schmiedeberg, co-founder of *'Naunyn Schmiedebergs Archivs'* and one of the founding fathers of pharmacology.

Dreser's studies on the pharmacology of acetylsalicylic acid led him to conclude that it was readily reconverted into salicylic acid after absorption into the body. Dreser (1899) added: 'It is self-evident that only a salicylate compound that is split as soon as possible in the blood with liberation of salicylic acid has medicinal value'. Thus, Dreser established a dogma that

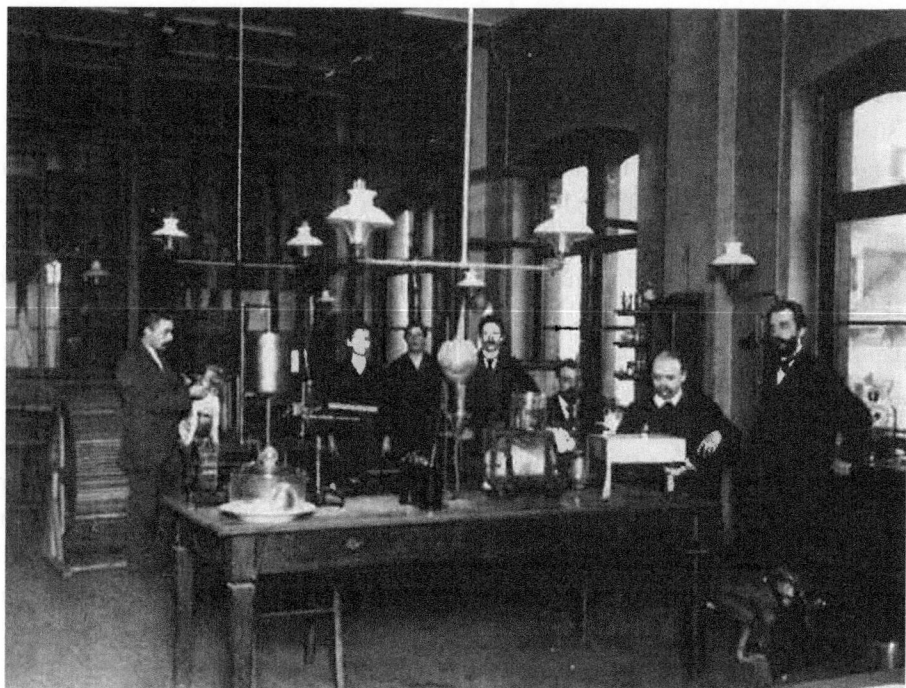

Figure 4.5
Professor Herman Dreser (second from right) in his laboratory. Friederich Bayer & Co., 1897.

had to be overturned before the next step towards understanding the mechanism of action of aspirin could be taken (see Section 4.5 below).

Dreser was responsible, too, for another dogma that was later overturned. He claimed that aspirin was less damaging to the gastric mucosa than was sodium salicylate. It was many years before aspirin-induced loss of blood from the digestive tract with resulting anaemia in heavy and frequent consumers, was identified as quite a common condition.

4.4.2 Launch of Aspirin and after

Simultaneously with Dreser's experimental studies on acetylsalicylic acid, clinical tests were done by Kurt Witthauer, Julius Wohlgemuth and several others. The first reports of these tests appeared early in 1899, the year of Dreser's paper (Witthauer, 1899 and Wohlgemuth, 1899). In these early trials, it was already evident to those taking acetylsalicylic acid that it was a better analgesic than was salicylic acid (Eichengrün, 1949). In fact, aspirin was found to be so good for relieving headache that a writer named a book on the period between the two world wars 'The Aspirin Age', with the explanation that (Leighton, 1950):

'During these throbbing years we searched in vain for a cure-all (for the headaches of the world situation) coming no closer to it than the aspirin bottle'.

We have seen that the German Patent Office refused to grant a patent for the acetylation of salicylic acid. This refusal had unpleasant consequences for the chemists who had invented it, since both Eichengrün and Hoffmann had contracts with Bayer, whereby they would receive a royalty on any patented product that they had invented (Eichengrün, 1949). As there was no patent, neither received any royalty on Aspirin sales in Germany. Patents of Aspirin in foreign countries were, however, allowed; but Eichengrün is silent on how these affected his own or Hoffmann's income. Dreser, on the contrary, had an agreement with Bayer under which he would receive a royalty on any product that he introduced. He therefore received one for Aspirin, which became so large that he was able to retire early.

Friend (1974) has recounted another story of the early days of Aspirin. The son and heir of the last Czar of Russia suffered from haemophilia, with resulting pains from bleeding into the joints, followed by inflammation. For these pains his doctors are thought to have prescribed Aspirin; but, since this drug tends to promote bleeding in haemophilia, the treatment was worse than useless.

Rasputin then came forward to persuade the Czar to abandon modern drugs and allow him to treat the boy by faith healing. Without Aspirin, the boy's bleeding and pain diminished and his health improved, and, with this improvement, Rasputin's power and reputation grew. Thus Aspirin participated in Rasputin's achievement of an ascendancy at the Russian Court, which later affected the fate of the monarchy.

4.5 Distinction between acetylsalicylate and salicylate

4.5.1 Superiority of acetylsalicylate as an analgesic

The superior analgesic action of Aspirin, relative to sodium salicylate, implied that Aspirin acts in its own right as an analgesic. The force of Dreser's dogma, that Aspirin acted by conversion to salicylic acid, was, however, so great that this implication was hardly perceived for nearly fifty years. Probably the first to provide strong evidence for the possibility that aspirin acted differently from sodium salicylate were Lester, Lolli and Greenberg (1946), who investigated the extent to which acetylsalicylate occurred in the blood after a dose of aspirin.

Lester and colleagues found that for a period of up to 1 to 2 hours after absorption of acetylsalicylate, as much as one-quarter of the total salicylate existed in the blood plasma as the acetyl compound. This observation, coupled with their knowledge of the time-course of its analgesic action, led these authors to propose that 'the analgesic action of acetylsalicylate is exercised mainly by the unhydrolyzed acetylate fraction in the plasma' (Lester et al., 1946).

To support this proposition experimentally, it would be necessary to show that aspirin was a more potent analgesic than sodium salicylate and that it could not possibly, therefore, act by being converted to the less potent compound. The difficulties of human experimentation are so great that such tests would have to be done in animals. It was more than ten years later that suitable tests in animals were devised.

A direct test of the proposition of Lester, Lolli and Greenberg (1946) could be based on quantitative comparison of the potencies of aspirin and sodium salicylate in suppressing nociception induced by noxious stimuli in experimental animals. Unfortunately most of the noxious stimuli used in antinociceptive tests at that time failed to show any appreciable activity in aspirin, although they worked well for opioids (Collier, 1964). Even in early tests, where aspirin was effective, it showed very low potency. For example, in one of the first antinociceptive tests consistently to respond to aspirin, in which a radiant heat stimulus was applied to a dark-skinned guinea-pig, the drug gave only a moderate effect at an intraperitoneal dose of 239 mg/kg (Winder, 1947).

In tests in which a noxious chemical was injected into the peritoneal cavity of mice, resulting in nociception expressed by an 'abdominal constriction' or 'writhing' response, aspirin had, however, a higher absolute potency, being effective at about 40–70 mg/kg parenterally. In early comparisons, in tests of this type, aspirin was between 4 and 7 times more potent than was sodium salicylate (Hendershot and Forsaith, 1959; Keith, 1960). The errors were, however, large and the conclusion that aspirin was truly more potent was uncertain. Later, as these tests were refined, the higher potency of aspirin was shown to be statistically significant (Collier et al., 1968a).

4.5.2 Prevention of bronchoconstriction in the guinea-pig

Meanwhile, a higher absolute potency and a larger difference between aspirin and sodium salicylate had come to light. When bradykinin was injected intravenously into an anaesthetized guinea-pig, a powerful and prolonged bronchoconstriction followed. Prior treatment of the animal with a small intravenous dose of aspirin completely prevented this response, although injection of aspirin after bradykinin was ineffective. Much higher doses of aspirin did not prevent the bronchoconstrictor responses to histamine, acetylcholine or 5-hydroxytryptamine (Collier and Shorley, 1960).

The effect of aspirin in preventing bradykinin-induced bronchoconstriction was local, since it occurred after cutting both vagi in the neck (Collier and Shorley, 1960). It was exhibited by all aspirin-like drugs tested, but not by corticosteroids or opiates.

This technique made it possible to place aspirin and like-acting drugs in rank order of potency (Table 4.1). When this was done, aspirin was 32 times more potent than was sodium salicylate. These experiments thus overturned Dreser's dogma, that aspirin must be converted to

Table 4.1: Potencies in suppressing bronchoconstriction due to intravenous bradykinin or srs-a in guinea-pigs.

The minimal effective dose (MED) is the smallest dose of drug to reduce by more than half a standard response to the agonist, without reducing the response to histamine (Collier and Shorley, 1960; Berry and Collier, 1964; Collier et al., 1968b; Saeed et al., 1977).

Drug	MED (mg/kg i.v.)	
	vs. bradykinin	vs. SRS-A
Acetylsalicylate	2	1–2
Salicylate	64–128	64
Indomethacin	0.025	NT
Paracetamol	16	64
Phenylbutazone	4	1
Amidopyrine	8	4
Phenazone	8	16
Mefenamate	1	1
Meclofenamate	0.05	NT
Hydrocortisone	>32	>16
Dexamethasone	>16	>16
Paramethasone	>64	>64
Morphine	>32	>32

NT, not tested: early tests with indomethacin were unreliable owing to its instability.

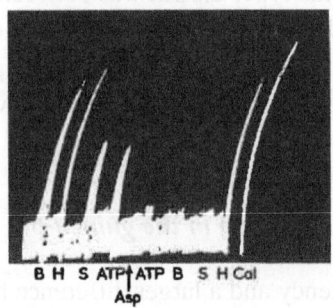

B H   S ATP ATP B   S H Cal
       Asp

Figure 4.6a

Konzett-Rössler preparation of guinea-pig lungs *in vivo*. Antagonism by aspirin of ATP-induced bronchoconstriction. The guinea-pig, 350 g, was pretreated with pronethalol, 10 mg/kg intraperitoneally + 5 mg/kg intravenously; and the brain and spinal cord were destroyed. B, 1 μg of bradykinin; H, 0,25 μg of histamine; S, 0.2 mg of SRS-A; ATP, 0,6 mg; Asp, 4 mg/kg of sodium acetylsalicylate; all given intravenously. Cal, maximum air overflow volume; time, 30 sec. *Reproduced from Collier et al. (1966) with kind permission.*

salicylate in order to act, and showed instead that it is a potent drug in its own right and could not in this situation act by being converted to salicylate.

Continued use of this method revealed that aspirin also potently prevented the bronchoconstriction elicited by slow-reacting substance of anaphylaxis (SRS-A) (Berry and Collier, 1964) and by ATP (Collier et al., 1966), as Fig. 4.6a shows. Moreover, aspirin also lessened

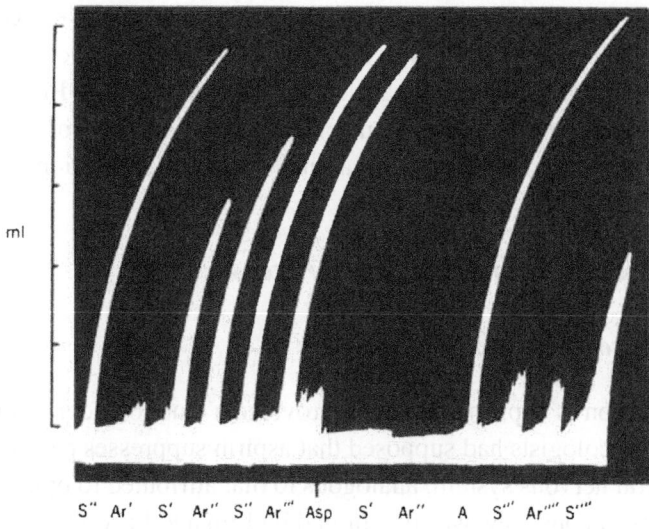

S″ Ar′ S′ Ar″ S″ Ar‴ Asp S′ Ar″   A S‴ Ar⁗ S⁗

Figure 4.6b
Antagonism by acetylsalicylate of responses to arachidonic acid and SRS-A of the Konzett-Rössler preparation of guinea-pig lungs in vivo. Responses are expressed as increase of air overflow volume, calibrated in milliliters; time scale, 10 sec; guinea-pig, 420 g S′, 9 units; S″, 18 units; S‴, 90 units of SRS-A. Ar′, 0.5 mg; Ar″, 1 mg; Ar‴, 5 mg of arachidonic acid. Asp, 2 mg/kg of sodium acetylsalicylate. A, 5 μg of acetylcholine. All doses were given intravenously at 5-minute intervals.
Reproduced from Berry (1966) with kind permission.

anaphylactic bronchoconstriction induced by antigen challenge in sensitized guinea-pigs (Collier et al., 1963). In the course of this work we showed also that aspirin did not suppress the bronchoconstrictor action of prostaglandin $F_{2\alpha}$ (Berry and Collier, 1964), but that aspirin did suppress bronchoconstriction induced by arachidonic acid (Berry, 1966; Fig. 4.6b).

Since bradykinin, SRS-A and ATP acted on different bronchial receptors, we concluded that (Collier et al., 1966):

'Aspirin and like-acting drugs block a route leading to or from the specific receptors for the agonists, rather than the receptors themselves'.

These effects were later attributed to the blockage by aspirin and like-acting drugs of the release of bronchoconstrictor prostaglandins in guinea-pig lungs (Palmer et al., 1973).

4.5.3 Suppression of platelet aggregation

Before the end of the 1960s, it was shown in a third way, also, that aspirin was far more potent than was sodium salicylate. After ingestion of a small dose of aspirin (150 mg) in man, the aggregation of platelets in shed blood in response to certain stimuli, was markedly inhibited; but no such effect was seen after ingestion of the largest dose of sodium salicylate (2 g) tested

(O'Brien, 1968a, b). This effect, which is seen after even smaller doses of aspirin (30 or 40 mg) than O'Brien used, is now attributed to its potent inhibition of the cyclo-oxygenation stage of the synthesis of platelet thromboxane A_2 (Hanley et al., 1982; Remuzzi et al., 1983). Such observations now provide a basis for one of the most important potential new uses of aspirin – the prevention of obstructive cardiovascular disease (see Section 4.9 below).

4.6 Aspirin opposes a local defensive process

4.6.1 Local antinociceptive action

The high analgesic action of aspirin once more provided a clue to understanding its mechanism of action. Pharmacologists had supposed that aspirin suppresses pain sensation through an action in the central nervous system, analogous to that attributed to opiates, but relatively weaker. This erroneous view was overturned by Lim and his colleagues, using cross-circulation experiments in conscious dogs (Lim et al., 1964).

In these experiments, nociception was elicited by injecting noxious substances into the splenic artery. If, in a dog receiving a splenic noxa, the brain were circulated with blood containing an aspirin solution, no lessening of nociception occurred. If, on the contrary, aspirin were administered to the body and not to the head, and thus reached the spleen into which noxious substances were injected, a powerful antinociceptive effect of aspirin could be recorded. With morphine, on the contrary, the suppressive effect was central. With such experiments, Lim's group established that aspirin acts locally to suppress nociception (Fig. 4.7).

4.6.2 Aspirin as opponent of local defensive hormone(s)

Once it had been established that, at least in some actions, aspirin acted in its own right and, that it acted against local stimuli, the way was open for an analysis of its mechanism of action. The questions that needed to be answered were: What local process did aspirin act upon and how did it modify that process? The answers to such questions came in a series of closer and closer approximations.

One step in this approach to understanding the mechanism of aspirin action was the generalization that aspirin is an 'anti-defensive' drug (Collier, 1963, 1969). In other words, all the main bodily conditions for which aspirin is taken – fever, pain and inflammation – constitute parts of the body's system of defensive reactions. The benefits of aspirin could be attributed to the control of such defensive reactions, which had been misdirected or had become excessive (Collier, 1974, 1980). This generalization made it possible to envisage the mode of action of aspirin as the opposition and control of a single defensive process, with various manifestations.

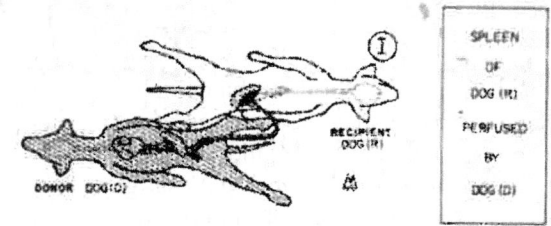

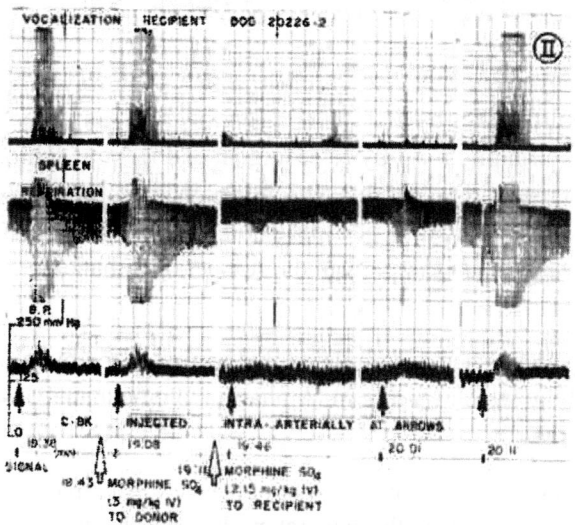

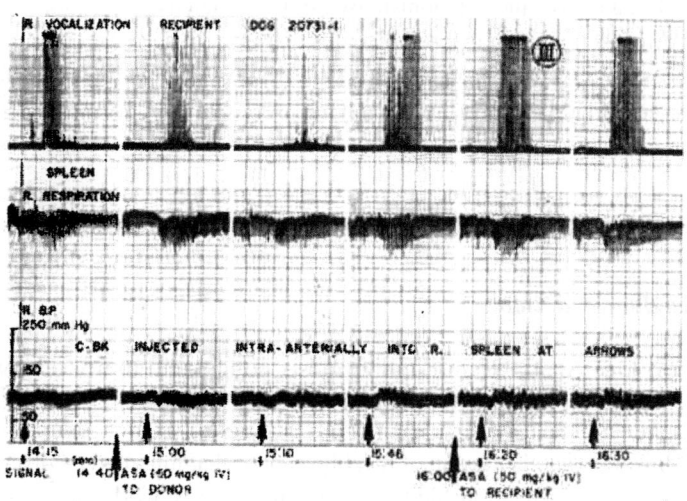

←

Figure 4.7

(i) Diagram showing cross-perfusion of spleen of recipient dog (R), with nerve connections intact, by femoral vessels of donor dog (D). (ii) Morphine sulphate, a central analgesic, failed to block the manifestations of visceral pain (vocalization, respiratory and blood pressure changes) evoked by intra-arterial injection of bradykinin (C-BK) into spleen, when 3 mg/kg IV was given to donor dog (D), but blocked successfully when 2.15 mg/kg IV was given to recipient dog (R). (iii) Aspirin or ASA, a peripheral analgesic, blocked bradykinin-evoked vocalization, etc., when 50 mg/kg IV was given to donor dog (D), but not when the same dose was given to recipient dog (R). *Reproduced from Lim et al. (1964).*

Natural defensive processes can be controlled in two main ways - by direct opposition of some phase of the process or by activating its endogenous inhibitor. Some research workers believed that aspirin might act by releasing an endogenous inhibitor, such as a catecholamine or corticosteroids. That this notion was incorrect was however evident from the divergences between some actions of aspirin and those of catecholamines or corticosteroids. Thus, in 1969, it was evident that aspirin did not act by enhancing a known 'anti-defensive' mechanism.

On the contrary, evidence had accumulated that aspirin acted by opposing some local defensive process, about which I wrote in 'A pharmacological analysis of aspirin' (Collier, 1969):

> 'The balance of evidence now lies in favour of the view that aspirin acts mainly by interfering with one or more of the humoral mechanisms that mediate defensive reactions' [p. 394] - 'In the last analysis, the antagonism by aspirin of defensive reactions may be attributable to a direct action upon macromolecules that operate one or more important biochemical processes. Such a macromolecule could be the receptor site of the carrier for a mediator molecule or it could be some enzyme involved in defensive processes' [p. 395].

4.7 Inhibition of prostaglandin synthase

4.7.1 Anti-prostaglandin action

Among the local hormones that aspirin might oppose, considered in my review were the prostaglandins. As I wrote at the time (Collier, 1969):

> 'The prostaglandins form another group of local hormones that might be involved in some defensive reactions, but their relationship to aspirin remains to be worked out' [p. 385].

At that time, however, a partly misleading clue appeared. In human bronchial muscle in vitro, aspirin and like-acting drugs potently antagonized the bronchoconstrictor action of $PGF_{2\alpha}$ (Collier and Sweatman, 1968). This observation clearly implicated prostaglandins in the mechanism of aspirin action, as we said at the time, but it directed attention away from the inhibition of the enzyme, prostaglandin synthase, which produces prostaglandins.

The misleading part of this finding – a direct antagonism of prostaglandin by aspirin – may perhaps be due to $PGF_{2\alpha}$, liberating in human bronchial muscle a more potent product of cyclo-oxygenase, such as thromboxane A_2. Be that as it may, the upshot of these observations is covered by Tennyson's immortal phrase 'So near and yet so far'.

Such was the scientific background and the position reached in 1968. It explains why, when John Vane, early in 1971, told me privately in advance of publication that aspirin potently inhibits prostaglandin production, I wrote to him:

> 'If you prove to be, as probably you will, the Jesus Christ of aspirin, I think I may claim to be its John the Baptist'.

4.7.2 Aspirin as inhibitor of prostaglandin synthase

In 1971, John Vane (Fig. 4.8) and his colleagues at the Institute of Basic Medical Sciences, Royal College of Surgeons, London, announced that aspirin and like-acting drugs potently inhibit the production of prostaglandins in several biological preparations (Vane, 1971; Smith and Willis, 1971; Ferreira et al., 1971).

To pharmacologists, who had not been thinking about how aspirin acted, and who possibly still accepted Dreser's dogma, this discovery came as a stunning surprise. To those, who were already addressing the problem, it came rather as an elegant answer to the question: what defensive local hormone does aspirin oppose and how does it do it?

To Vane the discovery of the inhibition by aspirin and like-acting drugs of the synthesis of prostaglandins; was in a sense a second step. For two years earlier, Piper and Vane (1969) had shown that aspirin inhibited the release from guinea-pig lungs, during anaphylaxis, of an unidentified substance that powerfully contracted blood-vessels. They named this 'rabbit aorta contracting substance (RCS)'. Some years later, RCS was identified as largely thromboxane A_2 (Hamberg et al., 1976).

Fig. 4.9 gives the essence of the discovery at the Royal College of Surgeons in 1971. In it, indomethacin, aspirin and sodium salicylate, in descending order of potency, and at concentrations attainable in the body during therapy, inhibited the production of prostaglandin by a preparation of prostaglandin synthase (or cyclo-oxygenase as it is now more often called) from guinea-pig lung. The relative potencies of the three non-steroidal anti-inflammatory drugs in this experiment were comparable with those previously obtained in the inhibition of bradykinin-induced bronchoconstriction in the guinea-pig (Table 4.1), in which the same prostaglandin synthase may be supposed to operate.

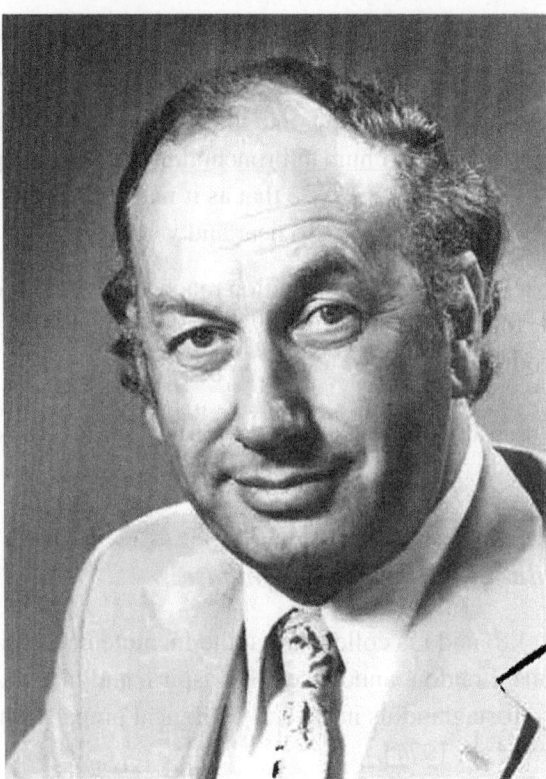

Figure 4.8
Dr. John R. Vane.

The approach of the workers at the Royal College of Surgeons was broad. They not only showed, as in Fig. 4.9, that aspirin and like-acting drugs inhibited prostaglandin synthesis by the cyclo-oxygenase of guinea-pig lung; but also that, in two other situations, these drugs acted in the same way.

Thus, Smith and Willis (1971) in the same issue of *Nature New Biology* in work that was 'initiated independently', showed that platelets from the blood of volunteers who had taken aspirin could no longer produce prostaglandins. Thus, the effect could be seen in man.

Lastly, in another paper in the same issue of *Nature New Biology,* Ferreira et al. (1971) showed that aspirin and indomethacin abolished prostaglandin release from the spleen of dogs. To show this, they used the technique, developed by Vane, of superfusing blood or other fluid from an animal or isolated organ in a cascade over a series of different isolated test tissues, selected to respond only to one of the substances sought (Fig. 4.10). In these particular experiments, the tissues chosen that responded sensitively to prostaglandins were chick rectum and rat stomach. Ferreira et al. showed that these tissues responded to blood from

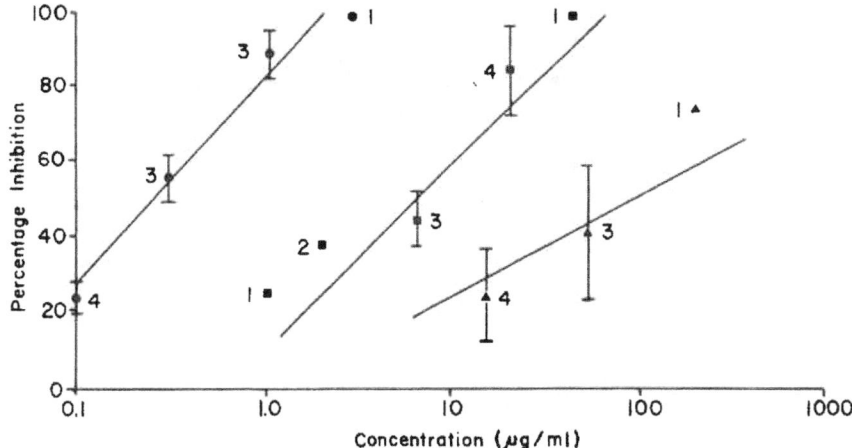

Figure 4.9

Inhibitory effect in vitro of varying concentrations of indomethacin (●), aspirin (■), and sodium salicylate (▲) on prostaglandin synthesis (assayed as $PGF_{2\alpha}$, on rat colon) by guinea-pig lung homogenates. The lines are those calculated for best fit. Numbers by the points indicate number of experiments. *Reproduced from Vane (1971) with kind permission.*

the spleen in dogs untreated with aspirin or indomethacin. After administering either drug, however, the test tissues no longer responded to splenic blood, although they still contracted to addition of preformed prostaglandin.

Since prostaglandins are both readily liberated by any form of stimulation of tissues and readily destroyed after liberation, there is little doubt but that, without Vane's 'blood bathed organ' technique, a convincing demonstration of this potent action of aspirin and like-acting drugs would have rested solely on the work of Smith and Willis (1971) on the platelet production of prostaglandin, which were extracted and measured differently.

These observations were naturally followed up in several directions, both at the Royal College of Surgeons and in other laboratories. Soon after the publications appeared in *Nature New Biology*, J.G. Collier and Flower (1971) showed that aspirin actually inhibited prostaglandin synthesis in man, by measuring the level of prostaglandin in the semen of volunteers, when taking or not taking aspirin.

In another direction it was shown that the particularly potent effect of aspirin on cyclo-oxygenase was due to its ability to acetylate the enzyme both in cells (Roth et al., 1975) and in blood platelets (Burch et al., 1978).

4.7.3 Pain, prostaglandins and aspirin

In his paper in 1971, *Nature New Biology,* Vane (1971) had written: 'Analgesic action is less easily explained . . . by inhibition of prostaglandin synthesis'.

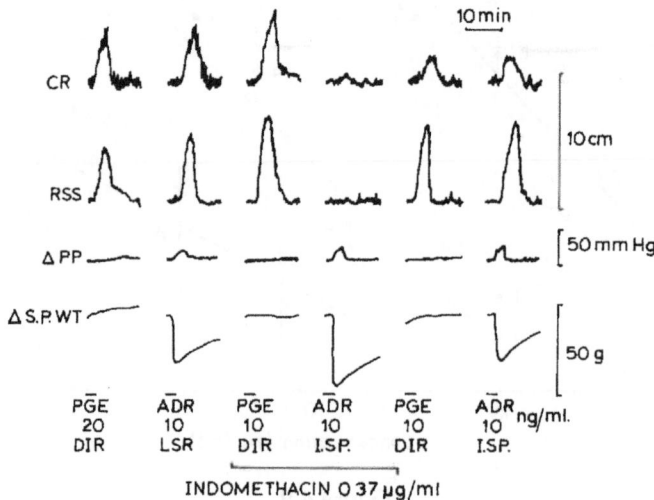

Figure 4.10

A spleen from an 8.5 kg dog was perfused with Krebs-dextran solution at a rate of 20 ml/min. A continuous sample (10 ml/min) of the splenic outflow, with combined antagonists added, was used to superfuse the assay tissues. The figure shows the effects of prostaglandins on a chick rectum (CR; top) and a rat stomach strip (RSS). The next two tracings (bottom) show changes in perfusion pressure (PP) and spleen weight (SP. wt.). Except when infused into the spleen indomethacin was added to the splenic outflow to give a concentration of 0.37 ng/ml. The first panel shows contractions of CR and RSS induced by prostaglandin E_2 (20 ng/ml, DIR). Next an adrenaline infusion into the spleen (ADR 10 ng/ml 1 SP) induced a rise in perfusion pressure, a fall in spleen weight and an output of prostaglandins equivalent to PGE_2 at about 20 ng/ml. Indomethacin (0.37 μg/ml) was then infused into the spleen. During the next 25 min the assay tissues relaxed (not shown) and were then more sensitive to PGE_2 (10 ng/ml, DIR). Adrenaline (40 min after start of indomethacin) now caused a greater increase in perfusion pressure, a greater decrease in spleen weight, but no output of prostaglandin. After stopping the indomethacin infusion into the spleen, the reactivity of the assay tissues gradually decreased and the output of prostaglandin induced by adrenaline infusion into the spleen gradually returned. The adrenaline stimulation shown was made 70 min after stopping the indomethacin. The rise in perfusion pressure was still larger, but the fall in spleen weight had returned to the original size. *Reproduced from Ferreira et al. (1971).*

This anomaly proved a challenge to several groups of workers, including those at the Royal College of Surgeons. Work was set in motion that ultimately showed that, of all the pharmacological actions of aspirin, analgesia was probably one of the most easily explained by the inhibition of prostaglandin synthesis (see Atkinson and Collier, 1980).

In summary, what was shortly to be shown was that prostaglandins infused intravenously or injected intra-muscularly cause pain in man (Karim, 1971; J.G. Collier et al., 1972; Gillespie, 1972). Furthermore, Collier and Schneider (1972) showed that prostaglandins induce abdominal constrictions when injected intraperitoneally in mice and that morphine, but not aspirin, readily blocks this effect. Aspirin, however suppresses similar constrictions elicited by other irritants, including arachidonic acid (Collier et al., 1973).

Such observations demonstrated that prostaglandins in pharmacological experiments, induced nociception. It was necessary, however, to explain why and how small amounts of prostaglandins liberated naturally in tissues during inflammation or injury would also cause nociception. This was achieved by Ferreira (1972), Ferreira et al. (1973), Moncada et al. (1975) and confirmed by Lembeck's group (Juan and Lembeck, 1974, 1977; Lembeck and Juan, 1974; Lembeck et al., 1976). These workers showed that E prostaglandins cause hyperalgesia, which is readily converted to overt nociception by other stimuli, such as pressure or a noxious chemical. If prostaglandin release were blocked by aspirin, other agents, in the absence of hyperalgesia, were much less potent at inducing overt nociception. Among the best candidates as causes of hyperalgesia in pains of short duration was prostacyclin (PGI_2), whereas in long-lasting pain, E prostaglandins might well be involved (Ferreira et al., 1978).

4.7.4 Anti-rheumatic action

Aspirin has therapeutic actions at three different dosage levels, differing by a factor of about ten. Thus, at an oral dose in man of 30–50 mg, aspirin blocks platelet aggregation in response to arachidonic acid in subsequently shed blood (Hanley et al., 1982; Remuzzi et al., 1983). At a dose of 300–600 mg, aspirin controls headache and other pains. Only at a dose of 4–8 g daily, however, is aspirin effective against rheumatoid arthritis or lupus erythematosus. It is difficult to imagine how a single molecular mechanism, the inhibition of cyclooxygenase, could account for all three levels of dosage.

The difficulty that arises from differences in the therapeutic doses of aspirin arises in another way, when we consider the therapeutic activities of various drugs that inhibit cyclo-oxygenase. Why, for example, do drugs such as amidopyrine and paracetamol, which are more potent than sodium salicylate as inhibitors of bradykinin-induced bronchoconstriction in the guinea-pig (Table 4.1), as antinociceptive agents (Collier et al., 1968b) or as inhibitors of prostaglandin biosynthesis (Flower and Vane, 1972; Collier, 1974), fail to show antirheumatic action?

The explanation of such differences, originally proposed by Vane, was that different cyclo-oxygenases display different sensitivities to drugs. Thus, according to Vane's suggestion, the cyclo-oxygenase of platelets is highly sensitive to aspirin, but is sensitive neither to paracetamol nor to sodium salicylate. Cyclo-oxygenases concerned with headache or other pains or with fever are susceptible to inhibition by aspirin or paracetamol but that of dog spleen is not (Flower and Vane, 1972, 1974). Again, the cyclo-oxygenase concerned with rheumatoid processes is not only relatively insensitive to inhibition by aspirin, but is also unresponsive to

Table 4.2: Potencies of anti-rheumatic drugs effective in inhibiting the peroxidation by human blood platelets of 12-HPETE to 12-HETE; and anti-rheumatic doses of drugs in man. Potencies are expressed as concentrations that reduced by half the production of 12-HETE (Siegel et al., 1980). Anti-rheumatic doses are based on Martindale (1982).

Drug	Inhibition of peroxidation	Daily anti-rheumatic dose (mg)
Acetylsalicylate	500	4000–8000
Salicylate	100	4000–8000*
Indomethacin	25	50–200
Paracetamol	Inactive	Ineffective
Phenylbutazone	50	200–600
Ibuprofen	200	600–1200
Naproxen	200	400–1000
Sulindac	1000	400–600

* 600–2000 mg daily in rheumatic fever.

paracetamol. This doctrine, of the capricious responses of various cyclo-oxygenases in different situations, coupled with the differing accessibility to drugs, would probably explain these discrepancies; but it needs several subsidiary hypotheses, each of which requires experimental support.

Although this doctrine may well explain some of these difficulties, an alternative explanation, useful for other difficulties, is that a second process, not the synthesis of prostaglandins, is also involved in producing the symptoms of connective tissue disease (rheumatism and lupus). It is against this process that prostaglandin synthesis inhibitors must also be active if they are to be effective in rheumatism.

What progress has been made in support experimentally of this second hypothesis? The best evidence so far obtained seems to be that of Cuatrecasas' group, who have found that the anti-rheumatic drugs, aspirin, indomethacin, sodium salicylate, phenylbutazone, ibuprofen, naproxen and sulindac, which to varying extents inhibit cyclo-oxygenase, also inhibit the peroxidation of another product of arachidonic acid metabolism (12-HPETE) to a pro-inflammatory substance (12-HETE) (Siegel et al., 1979, 1980).

As Table 4.2 shows, the doses at which these drugs inhibit the peroxidation of 12-HPETE roughly correspond with their anti-rheumatic doses, with the exception of sulindac, with which medical experience is limited. In this table, the high potencies of indomethacin and phenylbutazone and the ineffectiveness of paracetamol, both against peroxidase in vitro and as anti-rheumatic treatments are striking. The dose of sodium salicylate used in acute rheumatism corresponds better with its anti-peroxidase activity than that recommended, but seldom used, in rheumatoid arthritis.

So far, the hypothesis of Siegel et al. appears to offer the best explanation of the therapeutic action of aspirin in rheumatism, apart from its well-known analgesic action, which is also valuable in rheumatoid arthritis. Recent experiments on the effects of aspirin on platelet aggregation in plasma and in a buffer solution support the concept that aspirin has a weak second antiaggregatory action on platelets, not through inhibiting the production of an aggregatory prostaglandin (thromboxane A_2), which it does with high potency, but through inhibiting the peroxidation of 12-HPETE to the pro-aggregatory 12-HETE, which it does at much higher concentrations (W.J. McDonald-Gibson, R. McDonald-Gibson and H.O.J. Collier, unpublished).

4.7.5 Aspirin and the arachidonate defence system

A corollary of the discovery at the Royal College of Surgeons was that, if aspirin were truly an 'anti-defensive' drug, as I had first argued in 1963, then the prostaglandins are important members of the body's local defensive system (Collier, 1971a, 1974, 1980). Although certain prostaglandins have other functions and certain prostaglandins act to restrain rather than promote defensive reactions, as agents they are excellent candidates for the role of defence substances. Both the circumstances of their liberation, in response to any disturbance of tissues, and the catalogue of their effects, such as pain, cough, bronchoconstriction, diarrhoea, vomiting, inflammation, fever, haemostasis and abortion, accord very well with a defensive role.

Continued exploration of the role of aspirin in defensive reactions, coupled with study of corticosteroids, has revealed that arachidonic acid, and probably related long-chain fatty acids, form the backbone of an extraordinarily far-reaching and important defensive system.

Fig. 4.11 summarizes the metabolic transformation of arachidonic acid, leading to the production, by various enzymes, of many substances involved in defensive reactions, including leukotrienes, 12-HETE, prostaglandins, thromboxanes and prostacyclin. Controlling this elaborate system of defence are (i) the corticosteroids, which block the release of arachidonic acid from a state of inactivity in store as phospholipids; (ii) aspirin, which strongly blocks cyclo-oxygenase and weakly also blocks peroxidase and (iii) certain other drugs that have been shown experimentally to inhibit lipoxygenase. It seems probable, although not shown in this diagram, that platelet activating factor (PAF) also belongs to this defensive system (Benveniste et al., 1981).

The arachidonate defensive system is activated in rheumatism, allergy and cardiovascular disease, as well as in frank injury and by bacterial toxins. Thus it is that a study of the mechanism of action of aspirin has led to the discovery of a vast network of defensive mechanisms of the body, which in excess or when misdirected may be responsible for some of our commonest physical afflictions.

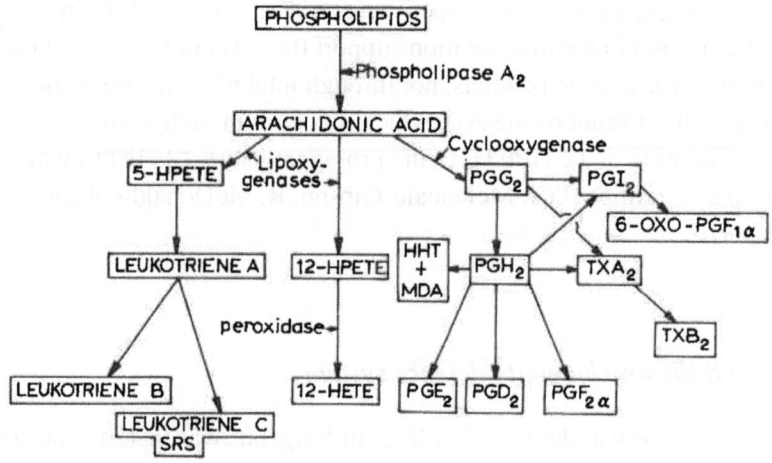

Figure 4.11

A summary of the known metabolic pathways of arachidonic acid.

4.7.6 Aspirin as mimic of endogenous substances

It seemed hardly possible, to some of us, that this vast and potentially dangerous system based on arachidonic acid would exist in the body without several mechanisms of internal control. The rapid catabolism of prostaglandins, when formed, was for long the only mechanism of their control that was recognised. Since, however, 'Nature wears a belt as well as braces' this mechanism would hardly be adequate to ensure that the defensive system did not needlessly get out of hand.

These considerations led us to seek endogenous inhibitors of prostaglandin synthase and of lipoxygenase, and proteins with such activities were demonstrated in plasma, other body fluids and tissue extracts (Saeed et al., 1977, 1980; Collier et al., 1981, 1982; Saeed et al., 1981, 1982). These inhibitors were termed, respectively EIPS (endogenous inhibitors of prostaglandin synthase) and EILOS (endogenous inhibitors of lipoxygenase). As might be expected, tissue extracts can also contain endogenous stimulators of prostaglandin synthase (Saeed et al., 1981).

A single example of the control of prostaglandin synthesis by an endogenous protein must suffice. If human blood platelets are suspended in buffer solution, they aggregate readily in response to addition of arachidonic acid. This aggregation can readily be prevented by addition to the suspension of a low concentration of plasma albumin (Collier and McDonald-Gibson, 1980). Thus plasma albumin may have an important function in controlling unwanted platelet aggregation induced by a rise in blood arachidonic acid. Naturally, an additional effect of albumin is not seen when it is added to platelet-rich plasma, in which a more than maximal inhibitory concentration is already present (Whittle, 1978).

Our concept was confirmed and extended by Robin Hoult's group at King's College, London, who also showed that not only does an endogenous polypeptide inhibit prostaglandin synthetase, but a reciprocal factor also exists, which activates prostaglandin breakdown dehydrogenase (Moore and Hoult, 1980; Hellewell et al., 1980; Hoult and Moore, 1981).

An interesting effect of corticosteroids in our experiments was that they markedly increased the level of EIPS in the blood (Saeed et al., 1977). More recently, other endogenous mechanisms by which corticosteroids control the arachidonate-based defensive system have been discovered.

Two groups of workers have found endogenous polypeptides controlling the release of arachidonic acid from its storage sites in phospholipids (Fig. 4.11) and involved in corticosteroid action. The mechanism appears to be that corticosteroids act by releasing polypeptide inhibitors of phospholipase A_2, whose activity liberates arachidonic acid. Blackwell et al. (1980) have named one of these 'macrocortin' and Hirata et al. (1980, 1981) have named a protein with comparable activity, 'lipomodulin'. Corticosteroids act by inhibiting the induction of these polypeptides, as well as by increasing the levels of plasma EIPS. Thus the mode of action of aspirin, although on the arachidonate defensive system, is at a different level (see also Chapt. 10, Part 2).

These observations emphasize the great importance of the arachidonate system of defence, and point to the probability that the escape of the arachidonate system of defence from its natural controls is a causative factor in diseases such as rheumatism, allergy and arterial occlusion (coronaries and strokes). They also make the point that aspirin is so valuable because it represents a chemically simple and cheap mimic, of relatively low toxicity, of some of these endogenous controlling substances.

4.8 Other sides of the story

4.8.1 Aspirin safety and risk

So far, we have concentrated on how the molecular mechanism of aspirin action has been partly unravelled, and on the consequences of what has so far been discovered. Let us now turn to other aspects of the aspirin story, important in other ways. One side of this story has centred round the safety and toxicity of aspirin.

Although aspirin is clearly regarded by licensing authorities throughout the world as a drug that can safely be sold to the public directly, without medical prescription, and with only minimal warnings against possible side-effects, a pattern of aspirin toxicity has emerged from the vast trials of this drug against cardiovascular disease, which have recently been completed or are now in progress.

Table 4.3: Sales of acetylsalicylate and paracetamol in the united kingdom.
Estimated numbers of tablets (in millions) sold to the public and percentages of total number of both types of tablet are given (Fryers, 1977).

Year	Acetylsalicylate		Paracetamol	
	No. tablets	Percent	No. tablets	Percent
1973	3156	56	2524	44
1974	2983	53	2654	47
1975	3147	52	2868	48
1976	3450	55	2872	45

From such trials, individuals with known hypersensitivity to aspirin were naturally excluded. The many thousands of other subjects, receiving medium to large doses of aspirin daily for several years provide a very exacting chronic toxicity test of aspirin in man. An analysis of the toxicity emerging from these trials was given in a leader in *The Lancet* of 31 May 1980. The writer, himself concerned with the management of such a trial, concluded:

> 'The dose of 1000 mg/day employed in most trials caused dyspepsia, nausea or even vomiting in 10–20% of patients, caused constipation, gout and melaena each in about 1%/year, and caused haematemesis in about 0.1%/year.'

These observations focus the side-effects of aspirin on the alimentary canal, particularly on the stomach. It is to be expected, therefore, that the main pharmaceutical counter-measures have been taken to protect the stomach.

Two such counter-measures are widely used. The older and probably still the best is to give aspirin in highly buffered solution, in which form its toxicity to mucous membranes is minimal. An example of such a preparation is Alka-Seltzer, which commands a wide market.

An alternative manoeuvre has been to develop slow-release preparations of aspirin, which do not supply the drug in the acid conditions of the stomach, but release it lower down in the alkaline part of the intestine. When this is done, the peak of blood aspirin reached is lower, and the absorption is delayed (P.N. Bennett, personal communication); but for some purposes it may be adequate.

4.8.2 Rise of paracetamol

Another possible reaction to aspirin gastric toxicity in a small percentage of people has been the rise of paracetamol. This is equally as good as aspirin in pains, such as headaches, but is not of appreciable use in rheumatic pain. Table 4.3 gives figures for the consumption of aspirin and paracetamol in the United Kingdom in recent years.

Table 4.3 makes two important points. First, it shows the enormous number of mild analgesic tablets taken in the United Kingdom today. Secondly, it shows a gradual growth in the relative number of paracetamol tablets used.

That a drug such as aspirin, more than 80 years after its introduction, is still so widely used says much for its general efficacy and lack of serious toxicity. That it may become even more commonly used, because of its particular ability to inhibit prostaglandin synthase, coupled with its low risk in general use, will be discussed below (see Section 4.9).

4.9 New vistas for the use of aspirin

4.9.1 Future of aspirin

The last stage of the aspirin story concerns its future, rather than its past. Will aspirin continue to be used only for its conventional indications, with its analgesic market eaten away by paracetamol and its anti-rheumatic market by other drugs? Or will new uses for aspirin be developed, in which, perhaps, it becomes even more widely used than before? This section discusses these questions, attempts to read the auguries of current clinical trials, and to project new uses from aspirin's known mechanism of action. Aspirin is particularly suitable for development because it has been taken so widely for so long that its risks are known and manageable.

Since the most potent action of aspirin is to inhibit prostaglandin synthase and since prostaglandins form an important element in the arachidonate defence system, it follows that new uses may exist for aspirin wherever prostaglandin production may be dangerous, as in the arteries, or excessive, as in diarrhoea.

We have seen that in rheumatism and allied diseases, some other factor than aspirin is probably also involved. This second factor is as yet unidentified, but may be 12-HETE, the production of which from 12-HPETE aspirin weakly inhibits (Siegel et al., 1980). Whatever this factor may be, it probably also participates in diseases other than rheumatic disease; and therefore scope exists here, too, for new uses for aspirin. Senile cataract may provide an example of such a potential new use.

4.9.2 Cardiovascular disease

That aspirin may protect against coronary infarction and stroke follows from its ability to prevent the formation by blood platelets of thromboxane A_2 from arachidonic acid. Thromboxane A_2 elicits platelet aggregation, which in turn forms a white thrombus, obstructing coronary or cerebral arteries, and leading to a heart attack or stroke.

At very low doses (30 or 40 mg orally) aspirin prevents platelet aggregation and might thus be effective in preventing these forms of cardiovascular disease (Hanley et al., 1982; Remuzzi et al., 1983). The side-effects of such a low dose are negligible (Patrono et al., 1982).

Unfortunately, we have as yet no appreciable clinical information on the protective value of such a small daily dose of aspirin. Probably the lowest daily dose on which information is at present available is 324 mg aspirin. When this was given in a highly buffered solution, daily to men with unstable angina, a high degree of protection against morbidity and death was obtained (Lewis et al., 1983). At this dose, with these pharmaceutical preparations, no increased gastro-intestinal symptoms were reported.

Many other trials have been carried out, in which considerably higher daily doses of aspirin were given. When these are appropriately analysed, a very highly significant reduction of cardiovascular morbidity is seen (*Lancet*, 1980). Hence it is established that daily aspirin protects men against coronaries and strokes, but we do not know how little needs to be taken to achieve its maximal effect.

4.9.3 Diarrhoea

The clinical trials of aspirin against cardiovascular disease have also shown that constipation is one of the side-effects of taking aspirin. This indicates that bowel movement is mediated at least in part by prostaglandins and opens the way to the use of aspirin in the treatment of diarrhoea, as predicted for cholera by Bennett (1971) for other diarrhoeas by Collier (1971a, 1974). So far, aspirin has been found clinically useful in controlling the diarrhoea of abdominal radiation (Mennie et al., 1975) of infantile gut infections (Burke et al., 1980) and of specific food intolerance (Buisseret et al., 1978).

4.9.4 Senile osteoporosis

A common feature of ageing in men and women is the loss of bone. In women, who have a smaller bone mass than men, this rarefaction soon becomes dangerous, leading to fractures. In men, who start with a larger bone mass, the rarefaction becomes dangerous somewhat later. Since there is much evidence that prostaglandins cause bone resorption, it seems possible that a daily dose of aspirin would protect not only against coronary occlusion and stroke, but also against senile osteoporosis. It is hoped that in some of the trials of aspirin now going on against cardiovascular disease, observations on bone density can also be made.

4.9.5 Senile cataract

The observations of Cotlier and Sharma (1981) have shown that, in patients with rheumatoid arthritis treated with large doses of aspirin, the incidence of senile cataract in the eyes is greatly reduced. It seems possible, therefore, that cataracts may be products of the factor involved in rheumatism, which aspirin controls. This possibility, too, is now being studied.

There are many other possibilities also for the future development of new uses of aspirin, based on our understanding of its mode of action and of the pathological importance of the arachidonate defence system. Space does not allow us to explore more of these possibilities, but this section illustrates the idea that the value of understanding history is to foresee and control the future.

4.10 Summary and conclusions

4.10.1 Aspects of the story studied

The story of aspirin has many sides; for example, its longevity as a drug, its widespread use and its promise for the future; but this chapter has largely been concerned with the discovery of its molecular mechanism(s) of action and the consequences that flow from these. Below, the main conclusions reached and the steps by which this was done are summarized.

4.10.2 Salicylate and acetylsalicylate

One of the earliest synthetic drugs was sodium salicylate, which by 1877 had been established as an effective treatment for rheumatic fever and rheumatoid arthritis. Sodium salicylate for pharmaceutical use was first manufactured by the Germany chemical industry.

Twenty years after the introduction of sodium salicylate, Felix Hoffmann, a research chemist in Bayer at Elberfeld, devised a manufacturing process for acetylsalicylic acid. After pharmacological and clinical studies, Bayer introduced acetylsalicylic acid under the name of 'Aspirin', as an improvement on sodium salicylate (Dreser, 1899).

Dreser presented Aspirin as a derivative of salicylic acid that was pleasanter and less injurious to take than was the parent substance, to which it was converted in the body. Subsequent experience has not endorsed the views that aspirin is less damaging to the gastric mucosa than is sodium salicylate nor that it is solely a pro-drug for sodium salicylate.

It was not until nearly half-a-century after the introduction of Aspirin that the concept was firmly proposed on the basis of experimental evidence that acetylsalicylate acts as an analgesic in its own right and not by being converted to salicylate in the body (Lester et al., 1946). This concept was supported by the new antinociceptive test of abdominal constriction in mice, in which aspirin appeared to be 4 to 7 times more active than sodium salicylate (Hendershot and Forsaith, 1959; Keith, 1960). The concept remained unproven, however until 1960, when aspirin was shown to be 32 times more potent than sodium salicylate in a newly discovered action – the prevention of bronchoconstriction elicited by intravenous bradykinin in the guinea-pig (Collier and Shorley, 1960). Eight years later, the independent activity of aspirin was confirmed, when aspirin was shown at a low oral dose (2 mg/kg) in man to inhibit platelet aggregation in shed blood ex vivo, whereas sodium salicylate, at up to 27 mg/kg by mouth, was inactive (O'Brien, 1968a, b). Despite the higher activity of aspirin in these actions, the doses of aspirin and sodium salicylate required to control joint inflammation in gout or rheumatoid arthritis are equally large.

Two important consequences followed from these observations. First, that aspirin acts in its own right in certain actions, as well as probably being a prodrug for salicylate in others. Second, that, after aspirin has been taken, the measurement of salicylate levels alone in blood or other body fluids is no guide to the potential effectiveness of the treatment.

4.10.3 Molecular mechanisms of action

By 1969, evidence had accumulated that aspirin acts by opposing local hormones mediating pain and other defensive reactions (Collier and Shorley, 1960; Collier 1963, 1969; Lim et al., 1964). In 1971, essentially by use of the 'blood-bathed organ' technique, these hormones were identified as prostaglandins and the mechanism of aspirin action found to be the inhibition of the first stage (cyclo-oxygenation) of prostaglandin synthesis from arachidonic and closely related eicosaenoic acids (Vane, 1971; Smith and Willis, 1971; Ferreira et al., 1971).

The inhibition of cyclo-oxygenase by aspirin provides a convincing explanation of its more potent actions – the inhibition of platelet aggregation induced by arachidonic acid in shed human blood, its analgesic action and the inhibition of bradykinin-induced bronchoconstriction in the guinea-pig. Probably also the antipyretic action of aspirin can be explained in terms of the inhibition of prostaglandin synthase. The anti-rheumatic action of aspirin, however, which requires relatively enormous doses of the drug, does not easily fit into this simple explanation, especially since other drugs, such as paracetamol, which inhibit cyclo-oxygenase, do not have anti-rheumatic action, whereas a weaker inhibitor of this enzyme, such as sodium salicylate, is a good anti-rheumatic.

This difficulty has been met by supposing that a second local hormone is involved in rheumatic inflammation, which also has to be inhibited if an antirheumatic drug is to work. The best candidate for this second local hormone is 12-HETE, as indicated by Siegel et al. (1979, 1980).

4.10.4 Defensive system based on arachidonate

Like prostaglandins, 12-HETE is a product of arachidonic acid, and this exploration of the mechanism of action of aspirin has revealed the enormous importance of the defensive system of local hormones produced by arachidonic acid, which include not only prostaglandins and 12-HETE, but also the leukotrienes and platelet-activating factor. Exploration of the mechanism of action of corticosteroids has recently revealed that these, too, act by controlling arachidonate-based defensive system (Flower and Blackwell, 1979; Blackwell et al., 1980; Hirata et al., 1980, 1981).

4.10.5 Endogenous inhibitors

The existence of such a powerful system of defence based on arachidonic acid constitutes a serious potential threat to the body. Excessive or misdirected activation of this system entails serious risks of arterial obstruction through platelet aggregation, allergy, rheumatism and chronic pain. It is not surprising therefore that a system of endogenous inhibitors of the various enzymes participating in the arachidonate defensive system can be found in body fluids and cells (Saeed et al., 1977, 1980; Collier et al., 1980, 1982; Moore and Hoult, 1980; Hoult and Moore, 1981; Blackwell et al., 1980; Hirata et al., 1980, 1981). These endogenous control mechanisms are still largely unexplored and, indeed, largely neglected or misunderstood by some research workers (Whittle, 1978). They indicate, however, that aspirin can be regarded as a simple mimic of endogenous inhibitors.

4.10.6 Past, present and future

If I were asked to summarize the significance of the history of aspirin in one sentence, I would say: 'Aspirin has helped to reveal the immense medical importance of the arachidonate-based local defence system, which is life-saving when under control, but the cause of disease and death when out of control.' To its inhibitory action on enzymes of this system, aspirin owes its enormous and long-continued use as an analgesic, antipyretic and anti-rheumatic drug. Because some of these enzymes probably play a part in many other conditions, such as coronary infarction, stroke, diarrhoea, osteoporosis and cataract, aspirin promises to have a future even more extensive than its past.

References

Atkinson, D.C., Collier, H.O.J., 1980. Adv. Pharmacol. Chemother. 17, 233–288.

Bennett, A., 1971. Nature 231, 536 only.

Benveniste, J., Jouvin, E., Pirotzky, E., Arnoux, B., Mencia-Huerta, J.M., Roubin, R., Vargaftig, B.B., 1981. Int. Arch. Allergy 66 (Suppl. 1), 121–126.

Berry, P.A., 1966. Ph.D. Thesis. Council for National Academic Awards, London.

Berry, P.A., Collier, H.O.J., 1964. Br. J. Pharmacol. 23, 201–216.

Blackwell, G.J., Carnuccio, R., Di Rosa, M., Flower, R.J., Parente, L., Persico, P., 1980. Nature 287, 147–149.

Buisseret, P.D., Youlten, L.J.F., Heinzelmann, D.I., Lessof, M.H., 1978. Lancet I, 906–908.

Burch, J.W., Stanford, N., Majerus, P.W., 1978. J. Clin. Invest. 61, 314–319.

Burke, V., Gracey, M., Suharyono, Sunoto, 1980. Lancet i, 1329–1330.

Collier, H.O.J., 1963. Aspirin Sci. Am. 209, 97–108.

Collier, H.O.J. 1964. In: Evaluation of Drug Activities: Pharmacometrics, (Laurence, D., Bacharach, A.C., Eds.), Academic Press, London, pp. 183–203.

Collier, H.O.J., 1969. Adv. Pharmacol. Chemother. 7, 333–405.

Collier, H.O.J., 1971a. Nature 232, 17–19.

Collier, H.O.J., 1971b. New Scientist 51, 107.

Collier, H.O.J., 1974. In: Prostaglandin Synthetase Inhibitors, (Robinson, H.J., Vane, J.R., Eds.), Raven Press, New York, NY, pp. 121–133.

Collier, H.O.J., 1980. In: Prostaglandin Synthetase Inhibitors: New Clinical Applications (Ramwell, P.W., (Ed.), Alan R. Liss, Inc., New York, NY, pp. 87–105.

Collier, H.O.J., Denning-Kendall, P.A., McDonald-Gibson, W.J., Saeed, S.A., Brennecke, S.P. and Mitchell, M.D., 1982. In: Role of Chemical Mediators in the Pathophysiology of Acute Illness and Injury (McConn, R., (Ed.), Raven Press, New York, NY, pp. 65–80.

Collier, H.O.J., Dinneen, L.C., Johnson, C.A., Schneider, C., 1968a. Br. J. Pharmacol. 32, 295–310.

Collier, H.O.J., Drew, M., Hammond, M.D. and Saeed, S.A., 1981. In: SRS-A and Leukotrienes (Piper, P.J., Ed.), John Wiley, London, pp. 181–195.

Collier, H.O.J., Hammond, A.R., Whiteley, B., 1963. Nature 200, 176–178.

Collier, H.O.J., James, G.W.L., Piper, P.J., 1968b. Br. J. Pharmacol. 34, 76–87.

Collier, H.O.J., James, G.W.L., Schneider, C., 1966. Nature 212, 411–412.

Collier, H.O.J., McDonald-Gibson, W.J., 1980. J. Physiol. 308, 93–94P.

Collier, H.O.J., Saeed, S.A., Schneider, C., Warren, B.T., 1973. Adv. Biosci. 9, 413–418.

Collier, H.O.J., Schneider, C., 1972. Nature 236, 141–143.

Collier, H.O.J., Shorley, P.G., 1960. Br. J. Pharmacol. 15, 601–610.

Collier, H.O.J., Sweatman, W.J.F., 1968. Nature 219, 864–865.

Collier, J.G., Flower, R.J., 1971. Lancet ii, 852–853.

Collier, J.G., Karim, S.M.M., Robinson, B., Somers, K., 1972. Br. J. Pharmacol. 44, 374–375P.

Cotlier, E., Sharma, Y.R., 1981. Lancet i, 338–339.

Discussion, 1980. Lancet. i, 1172–1173.

Dreser, H., 1899. Pflügers Arch. Ges. Physiol. 76, 306–318.

Drug and Therapeutics Bulletin, 1983. Drug Ther. Bull. 21, 33–35.

Eichengrun, A., 1949. Pharmazie 4, 582–584.

Ferreira, S.H., 1972. Nature 240, 200–203.

Ferreira, S.H., Moncada, S., Vane, J.R., 1971. Nature 231, 237–239.

Ferreira, S.H., Moncada, S., Vane, J.R., 1973. Br. J. Pharmacol. 49, 86–97.

Ferreira, S.H., Nakamura, M., Castro, M.S.A., 1978. Prostaglandins 16, 31–37.

Flower, R.J., Blackwell, G.J., 1979. Nature 278, 456–459.

Flower, R.J., Vane, J.R., 1972. Nature 240, 410–411.

Flower, R.J., Vane, J.R., 1974. Biochem. Pharmacol. 23, 1439–1450.

Friend, D.G., 1974. Arch. Surg. 108, 765–769.

Fryers, G.R., 1977. Proc. R. Soc. Med. 70 (Suppl. 7), 1–3.

Gillespie, A., 1972. Br. Med. J. i, 150–152.

Hamberg, M., Svensson, J. and Samuelsson, B., 1976. In: Advances in Prostaglandin and Thromboxane Research (Samuelsson, B. and Paoletti, R., Eds.), Raven Press, New York, NY, Vol. I, pp. 19–27.

Hanley, S.P., Bevan, J., Cockbill, S.R., Heptinstall, S., 1982. Br. Med. J. 285, 1299–1302.

Hellewell, P.G., Berry, C.N., Moore, P.K., Hoult, J.R.S., 1980. Eur. J. Pharmacol. 68, 509–511.

Hendershot, L.C., Forsaith, J., 1959. J. Pharmacol. Exp. Ther. 125, 237–240.

Hirata, F., Del Carmine, R., Nelson, C.A., Axelrod, J., Schiffmann, E., Warabi, A., De Blas, A.L., Nirenberg, M., Manganiello, V., Vaughan, M., Kumagai, S., Green, I., Decker, J.L., Steinberg, A.D., 1981. Proc. Natl. Acad. Sci. U.S.A. 78, 3190–3194.

Hirata, F., Schiffmann, E., Venkatasubramanian, K., Salomon, D., Axelrod, J., 1980. Proc. Natl. Acad. Sci. U.S.A. 77, 2533–2536.

Hoult, J.R.S., Moore, P.K., 1981. Br. J. Pharmacol. 74, 485–487.

Juan, H., Lembeck, F., 1974. Naunyn-Schmiedeberg's Arch. Pharmacol. 283, 151–164.

Juan, H., Lembeck, F., 1977. Br. J. Pharmacol. 59, 385–391.

Karim, S.M.M., 1971. Ann. N.Y. Acad. Sci. 180, 483–498.

Keith, E.F., 1960. Am. J. Pharmacol. 132, 202–230.

Lancet (Editorial), 1980. Lancet i, 1172–1173.

Leighton, I., 1950. Editor's preface in The Aspirin Age. Bodley Head, London.

Lembeck, F., Juan, H., 1974. Naunyn-Schmiedeberg's Arch. Pharmacol. 285, 301–313.

Lembeck, F., Popper, H., Juan, H., 1976. Naunyn-Schmiedeberg's Arch. Pharmacol. 294, 69–73.

Lester, D., Lolli, G., Greenberg, L.A., 1946. J. Pharmacol. Exp. Ther. 87, 329–342.

Lewis, H.D., Davis, J.W., Archibald, D.G., Steinke, W.E., Smitherman, T.C., Doherty, J.E., Schnaper, H.W., LeWinter, M.M., Linares, E., Pouget, J.M., Sabharwal, S.C., Chesler, E., DeMots, H., 1983. New Engl. J. Med. 309, 396–403.

Lim, R.K.S., Guzman, F., Rodgers, D.W., Goto, K., Braun, C., Dickerson, G.D., Engle, R.J,, 1964. Arch. Int. Pharmacodyn. 152, 25–58.

MacLagan, T.J., 1876. Lancet i (342), 383.

Mennie, A.T., Dalley, V.M., Dinneen, L.C., Collier, H.O.J., 1975. Lancet ii, 942–943.

Moncada, S., Ferreira, S.H., Vane, J.R., 1975. Eur. J. Pharmacol. 31, 250–260.

Moore, P.K., Hoult, J.R.S., 1980. Nature 288, 271–273.

O'Brien, J.R., 1968a. Lancet i, 779–783.

O'Brien, J.R., 1968b. Lancet i, 894–895.

Palmer, M.A., Piper, P.J., Vane, J.R., 1973. Br. J. Pharmacol. 49, 226–242.

Patrono, C., Patrignani, P., Filabozzi, P., Ciabattoni, G., Pugliese, F., 1982. Abstract, Acetylsalicylic Acid Meeting. Rome, p. 18.

Piper, P.J., Vane, J.R., 1969. Nature 223, 29–35.

Remuzzi, G., Benigni, A., Dodesini, P., Schieppati, A., Livio, M., De Gaetano, G., Day, J.S., Smith, W.L., Pinca, E., Patrignani, P., Patrono, C., 1983. J. Clin. Invest. 71, 762–768.

Roth, G.J., Stanford, N., Majcrus, P.W., 1975. Proc. Natl. Acad. Sci. U.S.A. 72, 3073–3076.

Saeed, S.A., Drew, M., Collier, H.O.J., 1980. Eur. J. Pharmacol. 67, 169–170.

Saeed, S.A., Drew, M., Denning-Kendall, P.A., McDonald-Gibson, W.J., Collier, H.O.J., 1981. Biochem. Soc. Trans. 9, 92–93.

Saeed, S.A., McDonald-Gibson, W.J., Cuthbert, J., Copas, J.L., Schneider, C., Gardiner, P.J., Butt, N.M., Collier, H.O.J., 1977. Nature 270, 32–36.

Saeed, S.A., Strickland, D.M., Young, D.C., Dang, A., Mitchell, M.D., 1982. J. Clin. Endocrinol. 55, 801–803.

See, G., 1877. Bull. Acad. Med. (Paris) 6, 926–933.

Sharp, G., 1915. Pharm. J. 94, 857–858.

Siegel, M.I., McConnell, R.T., Cuatrecasas, P., 1979. Proc. Natl. Acad. Sci. U.S.A. 76, 3774–3778.

Siegel, M.I., McConnell, R.T., Porter, N.A., Cuatrecasas, P., 1980. Proc. Natl. Acad. Sci. U.S.A. 77, 308–312.

Smith, J.B., Willis, A.L., 1971. Nature 231, 235–237.

Stone, E., 1763. Phil. Trans. R. Soc. 53, 195–200.

Stricker, 1876. Berl. Klin. Wochenschr. 13, 1–2 15–16, 99–103, Abstract in Dublin J. Med. Sci. *52*, 395–396 (1876).

Vane, J.R., 1971. Nature 231, 232–235.

Whittle, B.J.R., 1978. J. Pharm. Pharmacol. 30, 467–468.

Winder, C.V., 1947. Arch. Int. Pharmacodyn. 74, 219–232.

Witthauer, K., 1899. Ther. Mh. 13, 330.

Wohlgemuth, J., 1899. Ther. Mh. 13, 276–278.

Commentary on Histamine receptor antagonists by Madeleine Ennis and Wilfried Lorenz

Madeleine Ennis[a] and Katerina Tiligada[b]

[a]The Wellcome-Wolfson Institute for Experimental Medicine, School of Medicine, Dentistry and Biomedical Sciences, The Queen's University of Belfast, Belfast, United Kingdom [b]Department of Pharmacology, Medical School, National and Kapodistrian University of Athens, Athens, Greece

In many ways, the field of histamine receptor antagonists has grown dramatically since the publication of our original chapter in 1984. Only two histamine receptors were discussed in the paper and now there are four histamine receptors, all of which belong to the G-protein coupled receptor (GPCR) family. They are named chronologically in the order of their discovery as histamine H_1–H_4 receptors. Interestingly, the H_3 receptor was the last histamine receptor to be identified using classic pharmacological approaches, whereas the H_4 receptor was described through GPCR de-orphanization in the year 2000 (Tiligada and Ennis, 2020). In contrast, the use of a combination of H_1 and H_2 receptor antagonists as a pre-medication to avoid adverse reactions to drugs has hardly progressed.

Scientific and technological progress over the last 4 decades has provided tools such as computational modeling, molecular dynamics, and molecular screening that have advanced our understanding of the genetic/genomic, molecular, structural, and functional characteristics of the histamine receptors, ligand binding at the receptor level and exploitation of histamine receptors as targets for the management of allergies and other pathologies (Tiligada and Ennis, 2020). Notably, all 4 histamine receptors have been cloned; their encoding genes *HRH1*, *HRH2*, *HRH3*, and *HRH4* being located at 3p25.3, 5q35.2, 20q13.33, and 18q11.2, respectively (Chazot et al., 2021). Histamine receptor pharmacological heterogeneity has been attributed, at least in part, to alternative splicing that may generate functional and non-functional splice variants of yet-to-be-established pharmacological and therapeutic relevance (Tiligada and Ennis, 2020).

Discoveries in Pharmacology, Volume 3, Hemodynamics and Immune Defense.
DOI: https://doi.org/10.1016/B978-0-443-18442-0.00007-0

H_1 *receptor antagonists*

Among the histamine receptors, the H_1 has the highest number of associated approved drugs, the majority being used to relieve the symptoms of allergic reactions by antagonizing histamine-mediated smooth muscle contraction and increasing vascular permeability, but also to treat nausea and vomiting (Tiligada and Ennis, 2020).

Several of the originally described "first generation" H_1 receptor antagonists are still on the market including for example mepyramine and dimetindene (for bites and sting relief), promethazine (for allergy, insomnia, and vomiting) (Tiligada and Ennis, 2020). Since the mid-1980s, many "second generation" H_1 receptor antagonists have been developed and entered the market (Tiligada and Ennis, 2020). They only penetrate the blood–brain barrier to a limited degree and lack the additional activities of the first-generation compounds on other receptors (see Table II in the original paper) (Simons and Simons, 2011). They are referred to as non-sedating but a better term would be minimally sedating. Two agents were subsequently withdrawn from the market: terfenadine because of the risk of cardiac arrhythmia caused by QT interval prolongation and astemizole because of cardiac reactions (Tiligada and Ennis, 2020). However, other second-generation H_1 receptor antagonists do not exhibit cardiotoxicity (Church and Church, 2013).

The emergence of the concept of constitutive receptor activity in the 1990s led to the reclassification of GPCR antagonists as inverse agonists that reduce constitutive activity, or neutral antagonists, which interfere with agonist binding without affecting basal receptor activity (Panula et al., 2015). Since compounds that block H_1 receptors may be inverse agonists or neutral antagonists, this therapeutic drug class is commonly referred to as H_1 antihistamines (Church and Church, 2013).

Further advancements that provide additional critical insight into the selectivity and efficacy of H_1 antihistamines and may guide the drug development process include the discovery, in 2011, of the H_1 receptor crystal structure complexed with its inverse agonist doxepin, and the description of missense variants that affect H_1 receptor activity (Ma et al., 2021).

H_2 *receptor antagonists*

Although ranitidine was on the market (United Kingdom 1981), the original article only described the development of H_2 receptor antagonists up to cimetidine. Cimetidine was revolutionary in the treatment of peptic ulcers, which previously had relied on antacids or surgery. It has been described as the first blockbuster drug with sales of 14 billion dollars whilst under patent (Tiligada and Ennis, 2020). Ranitidine had fewer side effects and by 1986 was the best-selling drug in the world. Two further H_2 receptor antagonists (famotidine and nizatidine) were launched in the mid-1980s. Although all are still on the market, other treatments for ulcer disease and gastro-oesophageal reflux now take precedence such as proton pump inhibitors and eradication of *Helicobacter pylori* in those who test positive. H_2 receptor antagonists are currently available as over-the-counter medications in many countries as short-term relief for heartburn, dyspepsia, and hyperacidity especially when the symptoms are associated with eating or drinking. In a recent review, Jafarzadeh and colleagues described the many immunomodulatory properties of cimetidine, which may lead to other indications for this drug (Jafarzadeh et al., 2019), although this is not a new idea (Hast et al., 1989). Interestingly, reports that famotidine could help treat coronavirus disease 2019 (Covid-19) that emerged in April 2020 led to the drug being tested in related clinical trials (Ennis and Tiligada, 2021). The majority of evidence so far points to the putative positive effects of famotidine in reducing the clinical symptoms of Covid-19 being due to H_2 receptor-mediated actions in the host pathophysiology, rather than to a direct action on severe acute respiratory syndrome coronavirus 2 (SARS–CoV–2).

H_3 receptor antagonists

Histamine as a neurotransmitter in the brain was mooted by J.C. Schwartz in 1975 (Schwartz, 1975) and the H_3 receptors were first described in 1983 (Arrang et al., 1983). It is now known that H_3 receptors are present both pre- and post-synaptically, and regulate not only histamine release but also the release of other neurotransmitters (Panula, 2021). Although there are many studies in different disorders, to date only one drug targeting the H_3 receptor has been brought to the market (Schwartz, 2011). Pitolisant (Wakix®) is an antagonist/inverse agonist which can be prescribed for the treatment of narcolepsy with or without cataplexy in adults (Kollb-Sielecka et al., 2017). Currently, there are ongoing trials with H_3 receptor antagonists/inverse agonists in idiopathic hypersomnia, alcohol use disorder, and excessive daytime sleepiness in patients with myotonic dystrophy 1 (ClinicalTrials.gov).

H_4 receptor antagonists

The H_4 receptor was cloned and characterized by a number of independent groups in the year 2000 (Tiligada and Ennis, 2020). In common with the H_3 receptor, the H_4 receptor has a high affinity for histamine. H_4 receptor receptors are found on many immune cells as well as other cells such as epithelial cells (Schirmer and Neumann, 2021), and are involved in chemotaxis, differentiation, and immune crosstalk. This led to research demonstrating the effects of H_4 receptor antagonists in a variety of different animal models of inflammatory diseases such as asthma, dermatitis, pruritus, arthritis, colitis, etc. (Thurmond, 2015). JNJ7777120 was the prototype compound used for the characterization of the physiological role of the H_4 receptor and the first histamine receptor ligand described in 2011 to display ligand-biased signaling, a property that is currently being investigated for other histamine receptor ligands including the standard of care H_1 antihistamines in allergies (Burghi et al., 2021). Although there have been several trials with different H_4 receptor antagonists for conditions such as atopic dermatitis, rheumatoid arthritis, psoriasis, and asthma; none have yet reached the market (Table 5.1).

Table 5.1: Some clinical trials of H_4 receptor antagonists.

Study number	Title	Result
NCT03517566	A study to assess the safety and efficacy of ZPL389 in patients with moderate to severe atopic dermatitis.	Terminated lack of efficacy.
NCT03948334	A study to assess the safety and efficacy of ZPL389 with TCS/TCI in atopic dermatitis patients (ZESTExt).	Terminated (core terminated due to lack of efficacy).
NCT02424253	A study to determine the efficacy of ZPL-3893787 in subjects with atopic dermatitis.	Results posted and published, ZPL-3893787 improved inflammatory skin lesions in patients with AD (Werfel et al., 2019).
NCT01497119	A study of JNJ-39758979 in adult Japanese patients with moderate atopic dermatitis.	Terminated (this study was terminated prematurely due to 2 cases of agranulocytosis) (Murata et al., 2015).
NCT05117060	Efficacy and safety of LEO 152020 tablets for the treatment of adults with moderate to severe atopic dermatitis.	Active, not recruiting.
NCT00946569	A study of the safety and effectiveness of JNJ-39758979 in the treatment of adults with persistent asthma.	Completed. Potential benefit on lung function and asthma control in eosinophilic asthma patients (Kollmeier et al., 2018).
NCT01823016	A study of JNJ-38518168 in symptomatic adult participants with uncontrolled, persistent asthma.	Completed no results posted.
NCT00856687	A study to assess the effect of PF-03893787 on lung function following an allergen challenge in asthmatic subjects.	Completed no results posted.
NCT01493882	Study of JNJ-39758979 in symptomatic adult patients with uncontrolled asthma.	Withdrawn (study was withdrawn due to 2 cases of agranulocytosis in a different clinical trial with this same drug).
NCT01260753	Proof of activity study of UR-63325 in allergic rhinitis induced by nasal challenge.	Completed no results posted.
NCT01679951	A dose range finding study of JNJ-38518168 in patients with active rheumatoid arthritis in spite of treatment with methotrexate.	Terminated (the decision was made to prematurely discontinue this trial due to lack of efficacy).
NCT01862224	A synovial biopsy study of JNJ-38518168 in participants with active rheumatoid arthritis despite methotrexate therapy.	Terminated (the study was stopped due to lack of efficacy in a study conducted in a similar population, 38518168ARA2002-NCT01679951) (Boyle et al., 2019).
NCT00941707	An efficacy and safety study of JNJ-38518168 in adult participants with rheumatoid arthritis.	Terminated (due to a single, unexpected serious event, the trial was stopped).
NCT01679951	A dose range finding study of JNJ-38518168 in patients with active Rheumatoid arthritis in spite of treatment with methotrexate.	Terminated (the decision was made to prematurely discontinue this trial due to lack of efficacy).
NCT04853992	Trial to assess the efficacy and safety of LEO 152020 in adult patients with cholinergic urticaria.	Completed July 11, 2022 (no results posted yet).

(continued on next page)

Table 5.1: Some clinical trials of H$_4$ receptor antagonists—cont'd

Study number	Title	Result
NCT02295865	A study to evaluate safety and efficacy of Toreforant (JNJ-38518168) in participants with moderate to severe plaque-type psoriasis.	Completed did not achieve predefined success criterion (https://clinicaltrials.gov/).
NCT02618616	A study to determine the efficacy of ZPL-3893787 in subjects with plaque psoriasis.	Results posted, no significant difference between groups in primary outcome measure.

From: ClinicalTrials.gov (https://clinicaltrials.gov/) *and literature searches.*

Mast cell heterogeneity and responses to histamine receptor antagonists

There have been major developments in our knowledge about human mast cells; their development, their mediators, their role in non-allergic diseases, etc. We now know that the (micro)environment (e.g. cytokines etc.) can cause mast cells to change their phenotype (for further information about mast cells see the following reviews (Valent et al., 2020; Levi-Schaffer et al., 2022). In a study with human mast cells (HMC-1, LAD-2, and primary cord blood-derived CD34+ human mast cells), Jemima and colleagues demonstrated that both mepyramine and JNJ7777120 were able to inhibit mast cell activation (Jemima et al., 2014). The H$_1$ antihistamines azelastine, desloratadine, and cetirizine, as well as the H$_2$ receptor antagonist ranitidine, can inhibit cytokine release from HMC-1 cells (Lippert et al., 2000). In both studies, the degree of inhibition depended on the cytokines measured. However, there has been debate as to whether these inhibitory effects and those found in other studies are due to binding to the histamine receptors (MacGlashan, 2003). Although there have been many studies on human mast cells, very few have examined the effect of histamine receptor antagonists on mast cell mediator release.

Histamine diseases for histamine receptor antagonists—their place in anesthesia and surgery

Many drugs were shown to cause histamine release in man and the use of a pre-medication of both H$_1$ and H$_2$ receptor antagonists to prevent adverse drug reactions in anesthesia and surgery was proposed. Over 35 papers were led by the late Wilfried Lorenz on this topic, including an elegant study which clearly demonstrated the use of histamine antagonists as prophylaxis for perioperative histamine release (Lorenz et al., 1994). Despite the clear data, few studies seem to have been performed by others. Recently, a small trial found that pre-treatment with desloratadine and ranitidine reduced the number of moderate or severe adverse reactions to peanut oral immunotherapy but was without effect on mild adverse reactions (Chu et al., 2022). Recent reviews of pre-medications to prevent adverse reactions to chemotherapy recommended the use of second-generation H$_1$ receptor antagonists but were not clear on the advantage of also including an H_2 receptor antagonist (Cox et al., 2021; ALMuhizi et al., 2022). An international consensus on drug allergy only mentioned pretreatment with gluco-corticosteroids and H_1 receptor antagonists as useful for non-allergic drug hypersensitivity reactions; with no mention of H_2 receptor antagonists (Demoly et al., 2014).

Conclusion

Histamine research has developed since the original publication with the discovery of two more histamine receptors. It is hoped that discoveries such as the H_1 receptor crystal structure complexed with its inverse agonist doxepin, and the description of missense variants that affect H_1 receptor activity may result in even more effective and selective H_1 antihistamines. Although their use as anti-ulcer medications has declined, several studies indicate that H_2 receptor antagonists may have immunomodulatory properties which should be further investigated (Tiligada and Ennis, 2020). As yet only one drug targeting the H_3 receptor is commercially available, there are ongoing studies investigating other potential indications. The H_4 receptor holds promise as treatment for inflammatory diseases but so far, no agents have reached the market. Knowledge about human mast cell heterogeneity has increased greatly and the (micro)environment can cause mast cells to change their phenotype. In contrast to the developments in the other areas, few studies have looked at the potential benefits of pretreatment with H_1 and H_2 antagonists to prevent adverse drug reactions and the treatment is not recommended in guidelines. It will be interesting to see what happens to the field of histamine research in the next 40 years.

References

ALMuhizi, F., De Las Vecillas Sanchez, L., Gilbert, L., Copaescu, A.M., Isabwe, G.A.C., 2022. Premedication protocols to prevent hypersensitivity reactions to chemotherapy: a literature review. Clin. Rev. Allergy Immunol. 62 (3), 534–547. https://doi.org/10.1007/s12016-022-08932-2.

Arrang, J.M., Garbarg, M., Schwartz, J.C., 1983. Auto-inhibition of brain histamine release mediated by a novel class (H_3) of histamine receptor. Nature 302 (5911), 832–837. https://doi.org/10.1038/302832a0.

Boyle, D.L., DePrimo, S.E., Calderon, C., Chen, D., Dunford, P.J., Barchuk, W., Firestein, G.S., Thurmond, R.L., 2019. Toreforant, an orally active histamine H4-receptor antagonist, in patients with active rheumatoid arthritis despite methotrexate: mechanism of action results from a phase 2, multicenter, randomized, double-blind, placebo-controlled synovial biopsy study. Inflamm. Res. 68 (4), 261–274. https://doi.org/10.1007/s00011-019-01218-y.

Burghi, V., Echeverría, E.B., Zappia, C.D., Díaz Nebreda, A., Ripoll, S., Gómez, N., Shayo, C., Davio, C.A., Monczor, F., Fernández, N.C., 2021. Biased agonism at histamine H_1 receptor: desensitization, internalization and MAPK activation triggered by antihistamines. Eur. J. Pharmacol. 896, 173913. https://doi.org/10.1016/j.ejphar.2021.173913.

Chazot, P., Cowart, M., Fukui, H., Ganellin, C.R., Gutzmer, R., Haas, H.L., Hill, S.J., Hills, R., Leurs, R., Levi, R., Liu, S., Panula, P., Schunack, W., Schwartz, J.C., Seifert, R., Shankley, N.P., Stark, H., Thurmond, R., Timmerman, H., Young, J.M., 2021. Histamine receptors in GtoPdb v.2021.3. IUPHAR BPS Guide Pharm CITE 2021 (3). https://doi.org/10.2218/gtopdb/F33/2021.3.

Chu, D.K., Freitag, T., Marrin, A., Walker, T.D., Avilla, E., Freitag, A., Spill, P., Foster, G.A., Thabane, L., Jordana, M., Waserman, S., 2022. Peanut oral immunotherapy with or without H_1 and H_2 antihistamine premedication for peanut allergy (PISCES): a placebo-controlled randomized clinical trial. J. Allergy Clin. Immunol. Pract. 10 (9), 2386–2394. https://doi.org/10.1016/j.jaip.2022.05.015.

Church, M.K., Church, D.S., 2013. Pharmacology of antihistamines. Indian J. Dermatol. 58 (3), 219–224. https://doi.org/10.4103/0019-5154.110832.

ClinicalTrials.gov (https://clinicaltrials.gov/ct2/results?cond=&term=pitolosant&cntry=&state=&city=&dist=). (Accessed 9 October 2022).

Cox, J.M., van Doorn, L., Malmberg, R., Oomen-de Hoop, E., Bosch, T.M., van den Bemt, P., Boere, I.A., Jager, A., Mathijssen, R.H.J., van Leeuwen, R.W.F., 2021. The added value of H_2 antagonists in premedication regimens during paclitaxel treatment. Br. J. Cancer 124 (10), 1647–1652. https://doi.org/10.1038/s41416-021-01313-0.

Demoly, P., Adkinson, N.F., Brockow, K., Castells, M., Chiriac, A.M., Greenberger, P.A., Khan, D.A., Lang, D.M., Park, H.S., Pichler, W., Sanchez-Borges, M., Shiohara, T., Thong, B.Y., 2014. International consensus on drug allergy. Allergy 69 (4), 420–437. https://doi.org/10.1111/all.12350.

Ennis, M., Tiligada, K., 2021. Histamine receptors and COVID-19. Inflamm. Res. 70 (1), 67–75. https://doi.org/10.1007/s00011-020-01422-1.

Hast, R., Bernell, P., Hansson, M., 1989. Cimetidine as an immune response modifier. Med. Oncol. Tumor Pharmacother. 6 (1), 111–113. https://doi.org/10.1007/BF02985231.

Jafarzadeh, A., Nemati, M., Khorramdelazad, H., Hassan, Z.M., 2019. Immunomodulatory properties of cimetidine: its therapeutic potentials for treatment of immune-related diseases. Int. Immunopharmacol. 70, 156–166. https://doi.org/10.1016/j.intimp.2019.02.026.

Jemima, E.A., Prema, A., Thangam, E.B., 2014. Functional characterization of histamine H4 receptor on human mast cells. Mol. Immunol. 62 (1), 19–28. https://doi.org/10.1016/j.molimm.2014.05.007.

Kollb-Sielecka, M., Demolis, P., Emmerich, J., Markey, G., Salmonson, T., Haas, M., 2017. The European medicines agency review of pitolisant for treatment of narcolepsy: summary of the scientific assessment by the committee for medicinal products for human use. Sleep Med. 33, 125–129. https://doi.org/10.1016/j.sleep.2017.01.002.

Kollmeier, A.P., Greenspan, A., Xu, X.L., Silkoff, P.E., Barnathan, E.S., Loza, M.J., Jiang, J., Zhou, B., Chen, B., Thurmond, R.L., 2018. Phase 2a, randomized, double-blind, placebo-controlled, multicentre, parallel-group study of an H_4 R-antagonist (JNJ-39758979) in adults with uncontrolled asthma. Clin. Exp. Allergy 48 (8), 957–969. https://doi.org/10.1111/cea.13154.

Levi-Schaffer, F., Gibbs, B.F., Hallgren, J., Pucillo, C., Redegeld, F., Siebenhaar, F., Vitte, J., Mezouar, S., Michel, M., Puzzovio, P.G., Maurer, M., 2022. Selected recent advances in understanding the role of human mast cells in health and disease. J. Allergy Clin. Immunol. 149 (6), 1833–1844. https://doi.org/10.1016/j.jaci.2022.01.030.

Lippert, U., Möller, A., Welker, P., Artuc, M., Henz, B.M., 2000. Inhibition of cytokine secretion from human leukemic mast cells and basophils by H_1- and H_2-receptor antagonists. Exp. Dermatol. 9 (2), 118–124. https://doi.org/10.1034/j.1600-0625.2000.009002118.x. Erratum in: Exp Dermatol. 2002 Aug;11(4):386. PMID: 10772385.

Lorenz, W., Duda, D., Dick, W., Sitter, H., Doenicke, A., Black, A., Weber, D., Menke, H., Stinner, B., Junginger, T., et al., 1994. Incidence and clinical importance of perioperative histamine release: randomised study of volume loading and antihistamines after induction of anaesthesia. Lancet. 343 (8903), 933–940. https://doi.org/10.1016/s0140-6736(94)90063-9.

Ma, X., Segura, M.A., Zarzycka, B., Vischer, H.F., Leurs, R., 2021. Analysis of missense variants in the human histamine receptor family reveals increased constitutive activity of $E410^{6.30 \times 30}K$ variant in the histamine H_1 receptor. Int. J. Mol. Sci. 22 (7), 3702. https://doi.org/10.3390/ijms22073702.

MacGlashan Jr., D., 2003. Histamine: a mediator of inflammation. J. Allergy Clin. Immunol. 112 (4 Suppl.), S53–S59. https://doi.org/10.1016/s0091-6749(03)01877-3.

Murata, Y., Song, M., Kikuchi, H., Hisamichi, K., Xu, X.L., Greenspan, A., Kato, M., Chiou, C.F., Kato, T., Guzzo, C., Thurmond, R.L., Ohtsuki, M., Furue, M., 2015. Phase 2a, randomized, double-blind, placebo-controlled, multicenter, parallel-group study of a H_4 R-antagonist (JNJ-39758979) in Japanese adults with moderate atopic dermatitis. J. Dermatol. 42 (2), 129–139. https://doi.org/10.1111/1346-8138.12726.

Panula, P., 2021. Histamine receptors, agonists, and antagonists in health and disease. Handb. Clin. Neurol. 180, 377–387. https://doi.org/10.1016/B978-0-12-820107-7.00023-9.

Panula, P., Chazot, P.L., Cowart, M., Gutzmer, R., Leurs, R., Liu, W.L., Stark, H., Thurmond, R.L., Haas, H.L., 2015. International Union of Basic and Clinical Pharmacology. XCVIII. Histamine receptors. Pharmacol. Rev. 67 (3), 601–655. https://doi.org/10.1124/pr.114.010249.

Schirmer, B., Neumann, D., 2021. The function of the histamine H_4 receptor in inflammatory and inflammation-associated diseases of the gut. Int. J. Mol. Sci. 22 (11), 6116. https://doi.org/10.3390/ijms22116116.

Schwartz, J.C., 1975. Histamine as a transmitter in brain. Life Sci. 17 (4), 503–517. https://doi.org/10.1016/0024-3205(75)90083-1.

Schwartz, J.C., 2011. The histamine H_3 receptor: from discovery to clinical trials with pitolisant. Br. J. Pharmacol. 163 (4), 713–721. https://doi.org/10.1111/j.1476-5381.2011.01286.x.

Simons, F.E., Simons, K.J., 2011. Histamine and H_1-antihistamines: celebrating a century of progress. J. Allergy Clin. Immunol. 128 (6), 1139–1150. https://doi.org/10.1016/j.jaci.2011.09.005.

Thurmond, R.L., 2015. The histamine H_4 receptor: from orphan to the clinic. Front. Pharmacol. 6, 65. https://doi.org/10.3389/fphar.2015.00065.

Tiligada, E., Ennis, M., 2020. Histamine pharmacology: from Sir Henry Dale to the 21st century. Br. J. Pharmacol. 177 (3), 469–489. https://doi.org/10.1111/bph.14524.

Valent, P., Akin, C., Hartmann, K., Nilsson, G., Reiter, A., Hermine, O., Sotlar, K., Sperr, W.R., Escribano, L., George, T.I., Kluin-Nelemans, H.C., Ustun, C., Triggiani, M., Brockow, K., Gotlib, J., Orfao, A., Kovanen, P.T., Hadzijusufovic, E., Sadovnik, I., Horny, H.P., Arock, M., Schwartz, L.B., Austen, K.F., Metcalfe, D.D., Galli, S.J., 2020. Mast cells as a unique hematopoietic lineage and cell system: from Paul Ehrlich's visions to precision medicine concepts. Theranostics 10 (23), 10743–10768. https://doi.org/10.7150/thno.46719.

Werfel, T., Layton, G., Yeadon, M., Whitlock, L., Osterloh, I., Jimenez, P., Liu, W., Lynch, V., Asher, A., Tsianakas, A., Purkins, L., 2019. Efficacy and safety of the histamine H4 receptor antagonist ZPL-3893787 in patients with atopic dermatitis. J. Allergy Clin. Immunol. 143 (5), 1830–1837. https://doi.org/10.1016/j.jaci.2018.07.047.

Histamine receptor antagonists by Madeleine Ennis and Wilfried Lorenz

Madeleine Ennis and Wilfried Lorenz

Contents

5.1 Discovery of H_1-receptor antagonists

The pharmacological effects of histamine were first described by Barger and Dale, 1910; Dale and Laidlow, 1910 and Dale and Laidlow, 1918–1919, and Popielski (1920). Against these effects functional and specific antagonists were discovered, a distinction summarized

Disclaimer: The original text that follows is reproduced from the first edition and carries errors and omissions from it. The editors and publisher agreed to retain them and honor the original authors and challenges they had to deal with in publishing back in those times.

Discoveries in Pharmacology, Volume 3, Hemodynamics and Immune Defense.
DOI: https://doi.org/10.1016/B978-0-443-18442-0.00065-3
© 1984, Elsevier Science Publishers B.V.

by Rocha e Silva (1955). Functional antagonists of histamine where the drug and the antagonist have opposing effects, were known for many years. For example some of the effects caused by histamine, e.g. stimulation of the smooth muscle in the alimentary tract and the bronchioli or blood pressure lowering, can be antagonized by adrenaline which relaxes these muscles and elevates blood pressure. In this type of antagonism the drug and antagonist act on different receptors. Specific antagonists, however, block the drug receptors before the drug can act pharmacologically. Specific antagonists for histamine (later defined as H_1-receptor antagonists) were first described in the late 30s and even they were not able to block all actions of histamine. Only in the 70s were a second type of antihistamines described which were able to antagonize the other actions of histamine. In this section an outline of the discovery of the H_1-receptor antagonists will be described.

The first specific antihistamine was described by Ungar, Parrot and Bovet (1937). For many years Ungar and Parrot had been studying anaphylaxis in isolated organs (Parrot, personal communication). They had extended the 'Schultz-Dale' test to enable them to study anaphylaxis in non-contractile tissues. An organ from a sensitized animal was suspended in a physiological solution and challenged with antigen, some of this solution was then added to an organ bath containing guinea-pig ileum (Ungar and Parrot, 1936). They investigated the mediators released and concluded that at least one of them was histamine. However, at that time no specific antagonists for histamine were known but they believed that such compounds should exist. Then, collaborating with Bovet who had this idea, they studied many compounds that had been synthesized in the laboratories of Prof. Fourneau from the Pasteur Institute Paris. These compounds had originally been synthesized as possible antagonists of adrenaline. Only by a systematic search was the first synthetic antihistamine discovered (Parrot, personal communication; Ungar et al. 1937). This compound was 2(1-piperidinomethyl)-1,4-benzodioxane, Fourneau compound F933.

In 1939 Staub (Staub, 1939a, b) published two comprehensive articles on her researches with synthetic antagonists of histamine. The benzodioxane (F933) had only feeble antihistamine activity, therefore Staub studied related open-chain ethers prepared by Lestrange and Fourneau. The two most successful compounds were the thymol ether (F929) and the diamine (F1571). These compounds were the prototypes for the diphenhydramine and phenbenzamine classes of antihistamines. Staub compared the toxicology and the 'indice antihistaminique' (a measure of the protection afforded by the compound to in vivo histamine administration) for 19 different compounds from the Fourneau series. Many of these compounds were able to protect the guinea-pig against 2–3 times the lethal dose of histamine. The strength of this early work was based on the many compounds available to the pharmacologists. Huttrer (1948) in his review listed 36 Fourneau compounds of which 20 were active as antihistamines and 16 were either inactive or almost inactive. Several classes of H_1-receptor antagonists can be distinguished:

5.1.1 Ethylene diamines

The first clinically useful antihistaminic drug phenbenzamine was discovered by Halpern, while studying a series of derivatives of N'-dialkylamino-N-phenylethylene diamines. These were able not only to protect animals against histamine shock but also against anaphylaxis. In clinical studies phenbenzamine was found to help patients with urticaria, oedema, hay fever and certain types of asthma (Halpern, 1942, 1952). Heterocyclic compounds began to be examined in France in 1942 and in America in 1943 (Huttrer, 1948). This led to the independent development of mepyramine and pyribenzamine (Bovet et al., 1944; Huttrer et al., 1946). In the late 40s various changes in structure were made producing methapyrilene, chlorpyriline etc. Table 5.1 illustrates some commonly prescribed antihistamines.

5.1.2 Tertiary aminoalkyl ethers

Loew (1947) states that the availability of benzhydryl derivatives synthesized by Rieveschl and Huber (1946) which were structurally similar to F929, prompted him to test these compounds for antihistaminic actions. Diphenhydramine and related compounds exerted both an antihistamine and an anticholinergic activity. Dimethhydrinate, the salt with 8-chlorotheophylline, in addition to its antihistamine activity gave good protection against travel sickness (Casy, 1978). The replacement of a phenyl group with a 2-pyridyl group elevated the potency of the drug (Sperber et al., 1949).

Cyclizine and its analogues can also be considered in this section. They possess benzhydryl or substituted benzhydryl groups (Ehrlich and Kaplan, 1950; P' An et al., 1954). Cyclizine is less potent and chlorcyclizine more potent than diphenhydramine on the guinea-pig ileum.

5.1.3 Phenothiazine derivatives

The phenothiazine derivatives were discovered as a result of bridging the terminal diaryl units of compounds such as phenbenzamine and diphenhydramine (Halpern, 1947; Halpern and Ducrot, 1946). Promethazine is probably the best known member of the group.

5.1.4 Pheniramines

Between the years 1945 – 1949 the alkyl amines were investigated by the Schering group and the pharmacological activities of 70 compounds carefully described by Labelle and Tislow (1955). The activity of the prototype compound pheniramine could be significantly increased by halogenation.

Table 5.1: Names, chemical structures and formulae of some commonly prescribed antihistamines (H$_1$ type).

Name	Chemical structure	Chemical formulae
Antazoline		2-(N-benzylanilinomethyl)-2-imidazoline
Chlorpheniramine		3-(p-chlorophenyl)-N,N-dimethyl-3-pyrid-2-ylpropyl-amine
Clemastine		2-[2-(p-chloro-α-methyl-α-phenyl benzyloxy)ethyl]-1-methylpyrolidine
Cyproheptadine		4-(5-dibenzo[a,d]cyclohepten-5-ylidene-1-methyl piperidine
Dimetindene		[(dimethylamino ethyl)inden-3-ylethyl]-pyridine
Ketotifen		4,9-dihydro-4-(1-methyl-piperid-4-ylidene)-10H-benzo-[4,5]cyclohepta[l,2-b]-thiopen-10-one
Mepyramine		(2-[[2-(dimethylamino)ethyl]-(p-methoxybenzyl)amino]-pyridine

(*continued on next page*)

Table 5.1: Names, chemical structures and formulae of some commonly prescribed antihistamines (H$_1$ type)—cont'd

Name	Chemical structure	Chemical formulae
Phenbenzamine		*N*-benzyl-*N'*,*N'*-dimethyl-*N*-phenylethylene diamine
Pheniramine		2-[α-[2-(dimethylamino)-ethyl] benzyl] pyridine
Promethazine		10-[2-(dimethylamino)-propyl]phenothiazine
Tripelennamine		*N*-benzyl-*N'*,*N'* -dimethyl-*N*-pyrid-2-ylethylienediamine

Haas (1952) in his book listed 95 antihistamine preparations available. The number has certainly grown since that time, Douglas (1971) refers to a needlessly large number of antihistamines. However, they do vary considerably with respect to potency, dosage, type of preparation available and side effects. All of the H$_1$ antihistamines produce side effects in some patients. These will be described in the next section.

5.2 Detection of pharmacological effects of antihistamines other than those at H$_1$-receptors

The first synthetic antihistamines were discovered during a systematic search for antiadrenergic compounds (Ungar et al., 1937), and did indeed possess both activities. Many of the later developed compounds were also relatively non-specific. The most common additional properties are anticholinergic, antiserotonin and antikinin activities (Table 5.2). In addition, Haas (1952) and others have described the influence of a number of antihistamines on the actions of nicotine and on vagal stimulation. The influence differs from antihistamine to antihistamine and both the tissue and species involved are important. A number of the central actions of antihistamines are discussed by Douglas (1971). These include both stimulant and depressive actions on the central nervous system; some compounds are effective against

Table 5.2: Further properties of some commonly used antihistamines (H₁ type).

Drug	Additional activities Anticholinergic	Antiserotonin	Antibradykinin	Antikallidin
Antazoline	+ [b,e] – [j]	n.t.	+ [j]	+ [j]
Chlorpheniramine	+ [d] – [i]	– [i]	n.t.	n.t.
Cyproheptadine	+ [i]	+ [h,i]	+ [g]	n.t.
Dimetindene	+ [j]	+ [j]	+ [j]	+ [j]
Mepyramine	+ [b]	n.t.	+ [a]	n.t.
Phenbenzamine	+ [b,e]	n.t.	n.t.	n.t.
Pheniramine	+ [d,j]	+ [i,j]	+ [j]	+ [j]
Promethazine	+ [b,f,i,j]	+ [c,h,i,j]	+ [g,j]	n.t.
Tripelennamine	– [i]	– [i]	n.t.	n.t.

+ / – indicates the drug has/has not the additional activity described, n.t. that it was not tested in these studies.
[a] Becker et al., 1968.
[b] Haas, 1952.
[c] Hahn, 1978.
[d] Labelle and Tislow, 1955.
[e] Loew, 1947.
[f] Rocha e Silva, 1955.
[g] Rocha e Silva and Lerne, 1963.
[h] Stone et al., 1961.
[i] Tozzi et al., 1974.
[j] Werle and Lorenz, 1970.

travel sickness, others lessen the rigidity and improve spontaneous movement and speech in Parkinson's disease, a few have a clinical role in the control of petit mal etc. Finally H₁-receptor antagonists possess a marked local anaesthetic action which was first detected by Rosenthal and Minard (see Rocha e Silva and Antonio, 1978). Since the nonspecific actions of H₁-receptor antagonists contribute considerably to their effects in vivo they will briefly be described.

5.2.1 Anticholinergic activity (Table 5.2)

Loew (1947) reported that sufficient doses of some of the original Fourneau compounds (F929, F1571) prevented the spasmogenic action of acetylcholine on guinea-pig ileum. Haas (1952) described the anticholinergic effects of a number of antihistamines and found there was a great variation e.g. diphenhydramine and promethazine were potent whereas mepyramine was relatively ineffective. Tozzi and coworkers (1974) compared the anticholinergic activities of the antiallergic drug azatadine with other compounds. Two test systems were employed (i) inhibition of the effect of acetylcholine on the guinea-pig ileum and (ii) the ability of the drug to delay the onset of dyspnoea produced by an aerosol of acetylcholine in the conscious guinea-pig. In the first system azatadine had approximately one third of the activity of atropine and was equipotent with the anticholinergic activities of promethazine and cyproheptadine. In the in vivo system azatadine was equipotent with atropine and significantly more potent than 8 other antihistamines tested. Labelle and Tislow (1955) found that a number of antihistamines including prophenpyridamine and chlorprophenpyridamine were able to relax spasm in rabbit ileum preparations induced by carbamylcholine chloride. Werle and Lorenz (1970) found a significant correlation between the antihistamine and anticholinergic activities of 14 antihistamines tested. The data of several studies were compiled by Rocha e Silva and Antonio (1978) who included 34 drugs for the calculation of the regression lines between the two pharmacological activities ($r = 0.48$, $p < 0.01$).

5.2.2 Antiserotonin activity (Table 5.2)

In 1961 Stone et al. (1961) demonstrated that cyproheptadine not only acted as a potent antihistamine in a variety of test systems but also was a potent antiserotonin agent and blocked the spasmogenic effect of serotonin in the rat uterus or the vasopressor action of serotonin in the anaesthetized ganglionic blocking agent treated dog. Werle and Lorenz (1970) tested 14 antihistamines and observed antiserotonin activity in many of them. However, this activity was not correlated with the antihistamine activity. Mepyramine was a relatively strong antiserotonin agent (Lorenz et al., 1973). The study of Tozzi and coworkers (1974) examined the action of azatadine and 8 other antihistamines on serotonin-induced contractions of rat uterus and their ability to delay the onset of dyspnoea induced by serotonin in the conscious guinea-pig. In the in vitro model azatadine was equipotent with promethazine and only chlorpyrrilene (another antihistamine) and methysergide (a standard antiserotonin drug) were more potent. In the in vivo model only cyproheptadine and methysergide were more effective.

5.2.3 Antikinin activities (Table 5.2)

Werle and Lorenz (1970) tested 14 antihistamines for antibradykinin activity; this was indeed present in all cases but not correlated to the antihistamine activity. Using the guinea-pig ileum assay the antikallidin activity of the 5 antihistamines tested was equal to the antibradykinin activity, however, in the rat uterus model the antikallidin activity was much greater. No correlation was found between the antibradykinin activity on the guinea-pig ileum and the rat uterus. Rocha e Silva and Leme (1963) extending the work of Mariani (1961), who had indicated that promethazine and chlorpromazine had an inhibitory effect against bradykinin on guinea-pig ileum, demonstrated that promethazine and chlorpromazine had a possible potentiating effect at low concentrations but reversibly inhibited the action of bradykinin at higher concentrations but that diphenhydramine was without inhibitory action at concentrations up to 10^{-3} M. Becker et al. (1968) examining the action of antihistamines on the local increase of vascular permeability induced by intradermal application of bradykinin, found that both mepyramine and triprolidine had a marked inhibitory effect. This effect was, however, species dependent being observed in rabbits, rats and mice but not in guinea-pigs.

5.3 Discovery of histamine H_2-receptors and their antagonists

In the sixties it became more and more recognised that histamine exerted its effect through more than one set of receptors. The basis for this idea, was however proposed very early on in the study of H_1-receptor antagonists. In 1948, Folkow et al. (1948) examining the action of histamine on blood pressure found that the sharp decrease in blood pressure caused by histamine could only partially be blocked by the antihistamines they were studying. They suggested that there were two types of receptors sensitive to histamine only one of which could be blocked by diphenhydramine and related drugs.

H_1-receptor antagonists were found not to inhibit the action of histamine in a number of different preparations such as gastric acid secretion, relaxation of uterus and the positive chronotropic effect on the isolated heart. The lack of inhibition caused by these compounds on either basal gastric secretion or the gastric secretory response to histamine, gastrin and the vagus has been demonstrated in a large variety of species including man, dog, cat, mouse and guinea-pig (Loew, 1947; Huttrer, 1948; Grossman et al., 1952; Lin et al., 1962; Tozzi et al., 1974) (for a comprehensive survey see Ivy and Bachrach (1966). Also the action of histamine on the rat uterus was neither inhibited by phenbenzamine nor by mepyramine. Using the isolated guinea-pig uterus a number of antihistamines including phenbenzamine, antazoline, tripelennamine were excitory stimuli whereas promethazine and mepyramine were not (Haas, 1952). Finally, although antihistamines had been reported to block the positive chronotropic action of histamine on the isolated atrium (Greef and Bokelmann, 1959; Mannaioni, 1960), this was later proved to be a nonspecific effect (Bartlet, 1963; Mannaioni, 1972; Brimblecombe et al., 1975).

The key study which quantitatively described histamine receptor heterogeneity was published in the mid-sixties by Ash and Schild (1966), who examined the histamine receptors in three test systems, the guinea-pig ileum, rat uterus and rat stomach. They concluded that there were at least two types of histamine receptors one set of which were denoted as H_1-receptors but that further classification of the other histamine receptors required the discovery of specific antagonists.

In 1964 work began at Smith Kline and French to try to design antagonists of histamine-stimulated acid secretion. The basic plan was to start with histamine and then modify the structure in order to obtain a suitable antagonist. The first assay system used was a modification of the Ghosh and Schild (1958) technique, where gastric acid secretion was measured in the anaesthetised rat stomach stimulated by histamine infusion. To make the system more

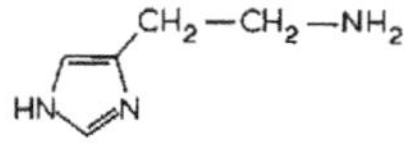

(a) Histamine

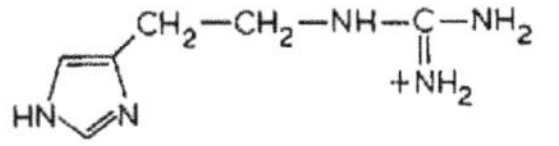

(b) *N*-α-guanylhistamine

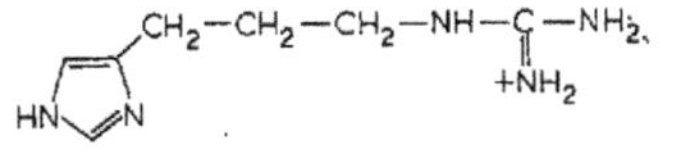

(c) SK&F 91486

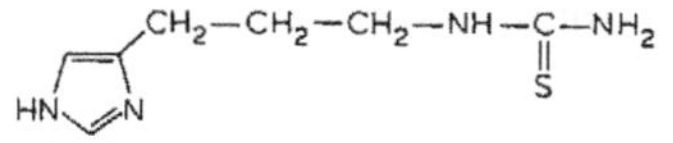

(d) Thiourea analogue

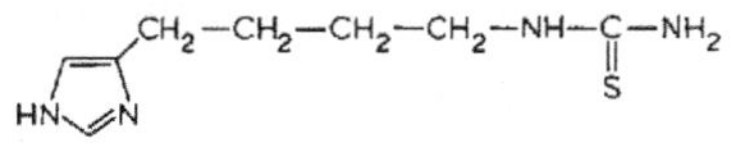

(e) SK&F 91863

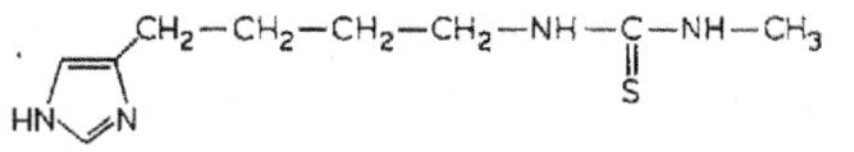

(f) Burimamide

Figure 5.1
Development of the H_2 receptor antagonist Burimamide.

insensitive, and hence avoid detecting non-specific antisecretory compounds, approximately 30 – 40% of the maximum secretion was selected. For the next couple of years many compounds were produced but none had the required activity.

However, on increasing the dose of infused histamine an inhibition was observed with some of the test substances, as one of the members of the SKF team has described in his thesis (Parsons, 1969, 1982). Some of the compounds, especially side-chain modified histamine derivatives, were then re-evaluated using the more sensitive assay. Thus, a compound which acted as a partial agonist and a weak antagonist, was uncovered when injected during a histamine plateau: *N-α-guanylhistamine* (Fig. 5.1b). The molecule was then modified to increase its antagonistic activity. First by a simple extension of the side chain (Fig. 5.1c) the antagonistic activity was increased by 6–8 fold (Ganellin, 1978). Then making the thiourea derivative (Fig. 5.1d) removed the partial agonist activity but still left the compound a weak antagonist. A further extension of the side chain (Fig. 5.1e) increased the antagonist activity and led finally to burimamide (Fig. 5.1f). The pharmacology of burimamide was described by Black et al. (1972) and it was shown to be a competitive antagonist of histamine at the histamine H_2-receptors which were defined in this extraordinary article both by the antagonist and by a set of methylated histamines as H_1 and H_2-agonists. Using similar concentrations of

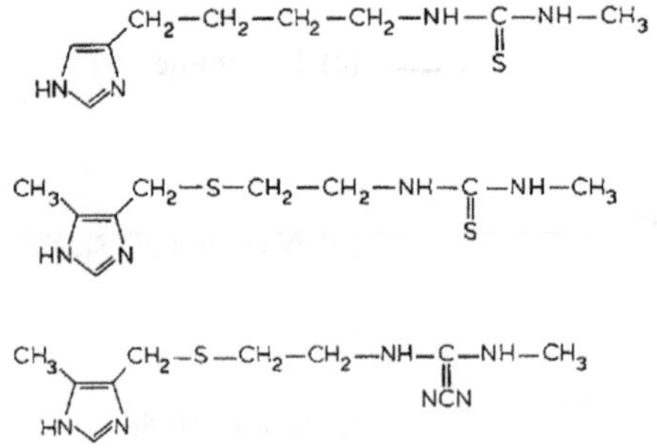

$$CH_2-CH_2-CH_2-CH_2-NH-\underset{\underset{S}{\|}}{C}-NH-CH_3$$

(a) Burimamide

$$CH_3 \quad CH_2-S-CH_2-CH_2-NH-\underset{\underset{S}{\|}}{C}-NH-CH_3$$

(b) Metiamide

$$CH_3 \quad CH_2-S-CH_2-CH_2-NH-\underset{\underset{NCN}{\|}}{C}-NH-CH_3$$

(c) Cimetidine

Figure 5.2

Development of the H_2 receptor antagonist Cimetidine.

burimamide with other autocoids no significant interactions were observed with β-adrenergic receptors, histamine H_1-receptors or muscarinic receptors. In human volunteers burimamide decreased not only the histamine stimulated but also the pentagastrin stimulated gastric acid secretion.

Although burimamide (Fig. 5.2a) was a specific histamine H_2-receptor antagonist, it did not have sufficient oral activity and so a more potent compound was required. In 1973 metiamide (Fig. 5.2b) was offered to the public by Black et al. (1973). It was shown to be 5–10 times more active than burimamide in a number of different test systems. However in chronic toxicity tests some animals developed kidney damage and agranulocytosis (Black et al., 1973). Then during the clinical testing of metiamide two cases of agranulocytosis were reported (Forrest et al., 1975). Fortunately, the continuing search for antagonists which did not have the thiourea group in the molecule considered responsible for the toxicity, turned up a thione with a cyanoguanidine group, later known as *cimetidine* (Fig. 5.2c), was shown to be a specific histamine H_2-receptor antagonist. It was a highly effective inhibitor of gastric acid secretion in animals and in man similar to metiamide and in toxicity studies behaved differently to metiamide, demonstrating that the development of agranulocytosis was not due to an inherent property of H_2-receptor antagonists (Brimblecombe et al., 1975).

In the search for an effective H_2-receptor antagonist some 700 compounds were synthesized leading to the discovery of metiamide (Durant et al., 1973). A large team of chemists and pharmacologists were dependent on each other for information. The development of new drugs using structure-activity relationships required people of different disciplines who could interact and communicate. Sir James Black (1982) in the postscript of the book describing the discovery of histamine H_2-receptors and their antagonists says:

'Even a lifetime in research generates such a tiny base of direct experience that we need to find ways to enlarge our knowledge, however vicariously, of the pitfalls as well as the triumphs of effective drug research'. [In a personal comment (Black, personal communication, 1983) he summarized the story of the discovery of the H_2-antihistamines which should not be made into something mysterious:] 'Two things about which I am completely certain are that I was there and that I could not have done it on my own.'

5.4 Histamine receptor antagonists and histaminocytes – the mast cell heterogeneity

Histamine receptor antagonists do not only compete with histamine at the target cells of histamine action, but interfere with histamine storage and release and with histamine catabolism (for a survey see Lorenz et al., 1983). These effects were observed with varying doses and concentrations in vitro and in vivo in human subjects, animals, isolated tissues and cells. Thus it is mandatory to be critical of any interpretations of clinical relevance if the effects have been observed in conditions which largely differ from those in physiological or pathophysiological situations in man.

One of the main reasons for the difficulty in extrapolating the data from one system to another is the heterogeneity of the histaminocytes in species and tissues, especially that of mast cells. These cells were defined for the first time by Paul Ehrlich in 1879, and as Selye (1965) has pointed out, it seems reasonable to follow Ehrlich's description since already 25 definitions were collected for these cells in Selye's fundamental book *'The Mast Cells'*. Thus a mast cell is a connective-tissue element which possesses cytoplasmatic granules that stain metachromatically under *ordinary conditions* (Lorenz et al., 1981b). Riley and West (1966) demonstrated the occurrence of histamine in mast cells.

Most in vitro studies on histamine release since that time have employed rat peritoneal mast cells as the model system, since these cells are readily available and easily purified to near homogeneity (Kazimierczak and Diamant, 1978). However it has been known for some time (Giertz and Hahn, 1966; Mota, 1966; Rothschild, 1966) that both species and organ variability are factors which can influence the functional properties of mast cells. More recent studies employing mast cells isolated from different tissues have further emphasized this point (Schmutzler et al., 1977; Pearce and Ennis, 1980; Ennis and Pearce, 1980; Barrett et al., 1983; Church et al., 1982; Ennis, 1982; Heymanns et al., 1982; Pearce, 1982; Pearce et al., 1982). Immunological mechanisms including reaginic antibodies and antigen and many hundreds of compounds are able to release histamine from mast cells but only two will be discussed to illustrate the species and tissue variability.

First, compound 48/80 which is a synthetic polyamine and the condensation product of *p*-methoxy-phenethylmethylamine with formaldehyde (Kazimierczak and Diamant, 1978). More than 30 years ago Paton (Paton, 1951) described its ability to elevate plasma histamine levels in the cat and to cause a marked hypotensive response. He concluded that the compound was a strong histamine releaser and since that time it has been widely studied. There is however a marked species and tissue specificity. It is a potent secretagogue in the rat, cat and

Table 5.3: Histamine release from isolated mast cells treated with compound 48/80 (10 μg/ml).

Source of mast cells	Corrected histamine release (% total)	
Rat peritoneal cavity	85.1 + 2.0	($n = 5$)
Rat mesentery	34.5 ± 2.7	($n = 4$)
Rat intestine	0.9 ± 1.0	($n = 5$)
Guinea-pig mesentery	9.5 ± 1.8	($n = 6$)
Guinea-pig lung	0.0 ± 0.0	($n = 4$)
Human lung	2.2 ± 1.1	($n = 5$)

Values are means ± S.E.M. for the number (n) of experiments noted. Data taken from: Ennis and Pearce, 1980; Barrett et al., 1983; Ennis, 1982; Pearce, 1982.

dog (Dews et al., 1953, Feldberg and Talesnik, 1953; Smith, 1953) but only weakly or inactive in the rabbit, mouse and guinea-pig (Enerbäck, 1966; Rothschild, 1966). The variation in organ specificity is well illustrated with the rat. When 48/80 is administered systemically, there is a marked degranulation of mast cells and a depletion of mast cells in the skin, mesentery, omentum, skeletal muscle, heart, lung, diaphragm and tongue (Feldberg and Talesnik, 1953; Smith, 1953; Lorenz et al., 1969) but the mast cells in the mucosa of the gastrointestinal tract are unresponsive (Enerbäck, 1966). Using in vitro models (isolated cells) similar results are obtained (Table 5.3).

Second, cremophor El is a non-ionic detergent used clinically as a solvent for a number of drugs including anaesthetics, steroids and vitamins (Lorenz et al., 1977b). It is a liberator of histamine in the dog and the cat but ineffective in the pig (on first exposure), the rabbit, and man (Lorenz et al., 1971). In combination with other drugs, however, it is highly effective in human subjects (Lorenz et al., 1982b). In the dog significant histamine release is seen in the submandibular and parotid glands, the gastric mucosa in the corpus and fundic regions, the gastric musculature of the antrum, the jejunum, the ileum, the colon, the pancreas and the skin but not from the lung, liver, spleen or diaphragm (Lorenz et al., 1981a).

From the data of these prototypes of histamine releasers it is not surprising that histamine receptor antagonists also show a marked species and tissue variability concerning histamine release by these drugs or inhibition of histamine release. In isolated tissues of human subjects and animals and in isolated cells a fairly multifaceted picture of observations was obtained. Diphenhydramine and antazoline liberated histamine from human and guinea-pig lung (Arunlakshana, 1953), diphenhydramine and mepyramine from chopped dog skin (Tasaka, 1957), 11 histamine H_1-receptor antagonists from a variety of rat and guinea-pig tissues including skin, diaphragm, mesentery and lung (Mota and Dias de Silva, 1960) and 5 classical antihistamines of the H_1-type from guinea-pig and rat mesenteric mast cells (Vugman, 1969). Histamine release by H_1-receptor antagonists was cytologically accompanied by damage of mast cells similar to that produced by the surfactant octylamine. In low concentrations H_1-receptor antagonists inhibited antigen-induced histamine release (Mota and Dias de Silva, 1960; Lichtenstein et al., 1973; Church and Gradidge, 1980). Histamine H_2-receptors at the surface of basophils and tissue mast cells were postulated to be involved in the autoregulation of histamine release (Lichtenstein and Gillespie, 1973; Chakrin et al., 1974;

Dulabh and Vickers, 1978; Kazimierczak et al., 1981), but it should be emphasized that the concentrations of the histamine H_2-receptor antagonists used in these experiments were very high and far beyond those realized in clinical practice.

However, histamine H_1- and H_2-receptor antagonists were shown to release histamine in human subjects and dogs in vivo by a mechanism which has not been fully elucidated (Lorenz et al., 1973, 1980). Inhibition of histamine release by clinical doses of H_1- + H_2-receptor antagonists was also demonstrated in dogs (Lorenz and Doenicke, 1985a,b). Thus species and tissue variability of histamine release or inhibition of histamine release by H_1- and H_2-receptor antagonists have to be taken into account if the effects and side-effects of these drugs are analysed in clinical conditions.

5.5 Histamine diseases for histamine receptor antagonists – their place in anaesthesia and surgery

In the field of histamine we suffer from the curious situation that powerful histamine antagonists are available to prevent or treat human diseases, but that histamine-induced human diseases have not yet been identified unequivocably. Mastocytosis is a rare disease and antihistamines have not been shown to prevent more than some of the minor symptoms of this disorder. Some of the immunological processes, especially type I immediate hypersensitivity reactions, are associated with more or less histamine release. But many paradigms in this research area do not hold true when analysed in clinical conditions (Lorenz, 1983). Especially in anaphylaxis research trends and fashions have swung over to 'serotonin, kinins, prostaglandins and to the leukotrienes, and so on' (Lorenz, 1981) leaving undefined the quantitative role of histamine in this important human state of disease.

In the last 10–15 years this frustrating situation has been changed by the development of highly sensitive and reliable histamine assays (Lorenz et al., 1970; Beaven et al., 1972) and by the discovery of the H_2-receptor antagonists. Only in this way could the classical demands for defining a causal relation in disease be fulfilled: (1) presence in disease in sufficient amounts to induce the disease, (2) absence in large amounts in good health, (3) ability to elicit the disease when administered exogenously, (4) ability to block its effect by specific antagonists *and* preventing or healing the disease. The first cases where these demands could be fulfilled occurred in anaesthesia and surgery.

A large variety of drugs nowadays in common use during anaesthesia and surgery are able to elicit histamine release in man, when given in *clinical doses* and using the *clinical route* of application (Table 5.4) (Neugebauer and Lorenz, 1981; Lorenz et al., 1982a). All drugs which have a '+' in the 'Result of testing' column fulfilled the criteria for histamine release in man (Lorenz et al., 1981a), when tested in controlled clinical trials in human volunteers and patients or in a few of the examples in single patients (Lorenz, 1975;

Table 5.4: Drugs used in anaesthesia and surgery, which have been demonstrated to release histamine in man or to elevate plasma histamine levels to pathological values (> 1 ng ml^{-1}).

Substance	Number of subjects	Dose (mg/kg i.v.)	Result of testing
(1) *Anaesthetics and hypnotics*			
Propanidid, volunteers	56	5–7	+
patients	2	7	+
Althesin, volunteers	8	0.075	+
patients	18[a]	0.07	+
Etomidate	43	0.3	–
Thiopentone	15	5	+
Methohexitone	10	1.5	+
Diazepam	10	0.15	–
Flunitrazepam	10	0.02	+
Lormetazepam	10	0.015	+
(2) *Muscle relaxants*			
Succinylcholine, volunteers	8	1.0	+
patient	1[b]	1.0	+
Alloferin	8	0.1	+
Pancuronium	8	0.06	+
(3) *Analgesics*			
Morphine, patients	15[c]	1.0	+
patients	10[d]	0.05 i.th.	+
Fentanyl, patients	15[c]	0.05	–
patients	10[e]	0.002	+
volunteers	22	0.02	+
Alfentanil	22	0.016	–
(4) *Local anaesthetics*			
Mepivacain (0.5%), patient	1[f]	1 wheal s.c.	+
Impletol® (Procaine, caffeine)	1[f]	1	+
(5) *Drug combinations*			
Etomidate-pancuronium	8	0.2, 0.1	+
Etomidate-lormetazepam	10	0.2, 0.015	(+)***
(6) *Premedication*			
Saline	48	0.2 ml/kg	+
Atropine	36	0.01	+
Methylprednisolone	7	15	+
(7) *Antihistamines*			
Pimethpyrindene (H$_1$)	7	0.1	–
Promethazine (H$_1$)	10	0.4	–
Chlorpheniramine (H$_1$)	7	0.3	+
Cimetidine (H$_2$)	12[g]	5, 10	+
Ranitidine (H$_2$)	5[g]	1.0	+
(8) *Plasma substitutes*			
Haemacel® *, volunteers	80	6 ml/kg	+
patients	600[h]	6 ml/kg	+
Haemacel-35**, patients	150[i]	6 ml/kg	–
Oxypolygelatin, volunteers	10	6 ml/kg	+

(continued on next page)

Table 5.4: Drugs used in anaesthesia and surgery, which have been demonstrated to release histamine in man or to elevate plasma histamine levels to pathological values (> 1 ng ml^{-1})—cont'd

Substance	Number of subjects	Dose (mg/kg i.v.)	Result of testing
patients	1[f]	ca. 20 ml	+
Modified fluid gelatin	25	6 ml/kg	+
Dextran-60 (Macrodex), volunteers	35	6 ml/kg	+
patients	2	ca. 20 ml	–
Dextran-70 (Fisons)	10	6 ml/kg	+
Dextran-75 (Salvia)	5	6 ml/kg	+
Dextran-40 (Salvia)	5	6 ml/kg	+
Hydroxyethyl starch (400/0.7)	20	6 ml/kg	+
(250/0.5)	25[f]	6 ml/kg	–
Human albumin, patient	1	3 ml/kg	+
(9) *Blood transfusion*			
Erythrocyte concentrates, patients	14[j]	6 ml/kg	+

Unless otherwise stated, all studies used human volunteers. Controlled trials with volunteers and patients were conducted by A. Doenicke and W. Lorenz (1968–1983) with the following exceptions:

[a] Johnson, J., Thornton, J.A., Watkins, J. and Lorenz, W. in Watkins and Thornton, 1982.

[b] Scöning, B. and Lorenz, W. (unpublished).

[c] Philbin et al., 1982.

[d] Berg-Seiter et al., 1985.

[e] Asbury, J., Watkins, J. and Lorenz, W. in Watkins and Thornton, 1982.

[f] Lennartz, H., Lorenz, W., Röher. H.D. and Dudziak, D. (unpublished).

[g] Parkin et al., 1982.

[h] Schöning, B. and Lorenz, W. In Lorenz et al., 1981c; Lorenz et al., 1982c.

[i] Schöning and Lorenz, 1980.

[j] Röher et al., 1982.

* Haemacel® = 'classical' now outdated polygeline.

** Haemacel-35 = 'purified' Haemacel.

*** Only symptoms of a cutaneous anaphylactoid reaction, no increase in plasma histamine levels greater than 1 ng/ml.

Lorenz and Doenicke, 1978a, b). Those indicated as a '(+)' only exhibited symptoms but had no significant (> 1.0 ng/ml) elevation of plasma histamine levels (Lorenz et al., 1981a).

Although histamine release is caused by a variety of drugs, an important question is how high is the incidence of histamine release in patients during anaesthesia and surgery. In a controlled clinical trial on 600 orthopaedic patients it was tested whether anaphylactoid reactions and histamine release were associated with the routine i.v. infusion of different batches of the plasma substitute polygeline in its now outdated formulation (Lorenz et al., 1980). Thirty of the patients (5%) exhibited systemic anaphylactoid reactions following infusion and of these 26 had more than 1 ng histamine per ml of plasma. Similar incidences of histamine-release response in man were obtained with other drugs (Basta et al., 1981; Philbin et al., 1981; *Klin. Wochenschr.,* 1982; Moss et al., 1982).

In view of the above information it is interesting to consider the effect of a combined premedication using H_1- and H_2-receptor antagonists since both types of receptors are found in the cardiovascular and respiratory system.

During the first International Symposium on histamine H_2-receptor antagonists in London 1973, Lorenz et al. (1973) presented data that the pretreatment of dogs with both H_1- and H_2-receptor antagonists (dimetindene and metiamide) prevented the histamine-induced severe hypotension in this species and put forward the idea, in the general discussion (Lorenz, 1973), that a combination of H_1- and H_2-receptor antagonists should be given when plasma substitutes were infused in clinical situations. In reply, Lichtenstein (1973) mentioned that as H_1-antagonists were no good in anaphylaxis it would not be a winning suggestion.

However, in 1977 Lorenz et al. (1977a) posed the question 'does a combination of dimetindene and cimetidine inhibit either partially or completely the anaphylactoid side effects of polygeline in man?' Following infusion with polygeline six systemic anaphylactoid and nine cutaneous anaphylactoid reactions were observed in the control group but none in the group receiving the combined antihistamine pretreatment thus further supporting the idea that premedication with H_1- and H_2-receptor antagonists before anaesthesia or surgery would be appropriate at least in high risk patients (e.g. those with carcinoma, allergic diathesis or a history of anaphylactoid reactions (Doenicke and Lorenz, 1982). Since 1979, an improved form of polygeline (Haemacel-35) has been available. In studies involving dogs, volunteers and patients the new purified version demonstrated a dramatic reduction in the anaphylactoid reactions and histamine release (Lorenz et al., 1982a). Philbin et al. (1981) examined the effect of pretreatment with an H_1-(diphenhydramine), and H_2-(cimetidine) receptor antagonist alone or in combination, on changes in plasma histamine and blood pressure caused by the administration of morphine. Morphine alone produced increases in plasma histamine and decreases in systemic vascular resistance and diastolic blood pressure. In the presence of both the H_1- and H_2-receptor antagonists the haemodynamic alterations were significantly attenuated although the plasma histamine levels remained elevated. The authors showed that prior administration of both types of antihistamines provided greater protection from the response to morphine than either drug given alone.

In June 1981 a symposium entitled 'Histamine and Antihistamines in Anaesthesia and Surgery' was held in Munich. Specialists from throughout the world came and reported on the mechanism, incidence, significance and treatment of adverse reactions in the two medical disciplines (Klin. Wochenschr., 1982). For the first time histamine release by surgical manoeuvres and administration of exogenous histamine in blood transfusion was shown in the course of standard operations (Röher et al., 1982). Using tissue models, Levi et al. (1982) examined dysrhythmias caused by histamine release and demonstrated that a combination of H_1- and H_2-antagonists was required to block the effects. Owen et al. (1982) found that although the immediate response to histamine in the circulatory systems of the cat, the dog and man were due to H_1-receptors, the sustained response involved H_2-receptors and abolition of the response to histamine throughout the infusion period required the administration of both H_1- and H_2-receptor antagonists. Finally Doenicke and Lorenz (1982) discussed premedication with H_1- and H_2-receptor antagonists: (i) the alternatives, (ii) the problems to be clarified and (iii) the indications. (i) Obviously the best alternative is for the pharmaceutical companies to design drugs that do not release histamine. Thus etomidate (a barbiturate-free hypnotic) is used in preference to propanidid because although causing myoclonia and vein pain, it does not release histamine (Doenicke et al., 1973). If the drugs do release histamine then the manufacturers should try to modify the compound so that it is no longer active as discussed above with polygeline (Doenicke et al., 1973). Drugs which do release histamine should be administered slowly to minimize the effects (Lorenz et al., 1972; Moss et al., 1982). The application of glucocorticoids in combination with an H_1-receptor antagonist ten minutes before the start of anaesthesia completely inhibits the effects of histamine release and is considered as a possible premedication in allergic patients, bearing in mind the well known side effects of these drugs. (ii) There is still a need for a prospective controlled clinical trial involving 5–10 departments of anaesthesiology to determine whether premedication with H_1- and H_2-receptor antagonists is the ideal pretreatment in a variety of operative situations. The incidence of anaphylactoid reactions in anxious and poor risk patients should also be further investigated. (iii) At present the indications for the use of H_1- and H_2-receptor antagonists as premedications include: hypersensitivity reactions during previous anaesthesia or after the administration of contrast media or plasma substitutes, second exposure to the drug within a few days (Watkins and Thornton, 1982), a previous history of allergy and the expectation of heavy blood loss during the operative procedure.

Nine years after the London meeting, Ahnefeld (1982) summed up the Munich symposium as follows:

'In this symposium we could not find answers for all questions. On one hand there are already ways of preventing side-effects of anaesthesia and surgery with a combination of H_1- and H_2-receptor antagonists, on the other hand, the incidence of adverse reactions and histamine release in anaesthesia and surgery is not high enough to justify a premedication in all patients. We should look also for other ways which have been successfully pursued in the past decade – the discarding of some histamine-releasing drugs, development of better drugs and solvents, limitation of prescribing indications and avoidance of unduly rapid administration'.

So the idea of H_1- and H_2-receptor antagonists as premedication is no longer 'not a winning suggestion' but a useful tool when drug companies are unable to modify their drugs or the 'poor risk' patient is on the operating table.

Acknowledgement

This work was supported by a grant from the Deutsche Forschungsgemeinschaft (Lo 199/14-1). One of us (M.E.) wishes to thank the Alexander von Humboldt-Stiftung for support.

References

Ahnefeld, F.W., 1982. Histamine and antihistamines in anaesthesia and surgery. Klin. Wochenschr. 60, 871.

Arunlakshana, O., 1953. Histamine release by antihistamines. J. Physiol. (London) 119, 47P–48P.

Ash, A.S.F., Schild, H.O., 1966. Receptors mediating some actions of histamine. Br. J. Pharmacol. 27, 427–439.

Barger, G., Dale, H.H., 1910 Oct. 11. Chemical structure and sympathomimetic action of amines. J. Physiol. 41 (1–2), 19–59.

Barrett, K.E., Ennis, M., Pearce, F.L., 1983. Mast cells from guinea-pig lung: isolation and properties. Br. J. Pharmacol. 75 (S1), 1.

Bartlet, A.L., 1963. The action of histamine on the isolated heart. Br. J. Pharmacol. 21, 450–461.

Basta, S.J., Moss, J., Savarese, J.J., Ali, H.H., Sunder, N., Gionfriddo, B.A., Lineberry, C.G., 1981. Cardiovascular effects of BWA444U: Correlation with plasma histamine levels. Anesthesiology 50, A198.

Beaven, M.A., Jacobsen, S., Horáková, Z., 1972. Modification of the enzymatic isotopic assay of histamine and its application to measurement of histamine in tissues, serum and urine. Clin. Chim. Acta 37, 91–103.

Becker, E.L., Mota, I., Wong, D., 1968. Inhibition by antihistamines of the vascular permeability increase induced by bradykinin. Br. J. Pharmacol. 34, 330–336.

Berg-Seiter, S., Kossmann, B., Dick, W., Lorenz, W., 1985 Aug. The behavior of plasma histamine levels following peridural morphine administration. Anaesthesist. 34 (8):388–391.

Black, J.W., 1982. The Discovery of Histamine H$_2$-Receptors and their Antagonists. Smith Kline & French, Welwyn Garden City, p. 81.

Black, J.W., Duncan, W.A.M., Durant, D.J., Ganellin, C.R., Parsons, M.E., 1972. Definition and Antagonism of Histamine H$_2$-receptors. Nature 236, 385–390.

Black, J.W., Duncan, W.A.M., Emmett, J.C., Ganellin, C.R., Hesselbo, T., Parsons, M.E., Wyllie, J.H., 1973. Metiamide–an orally active histamine H$_2$-receptor antagonist. Agents Actions 3, 133–137.

Bovet, D., Horclois, R., Walthert, F., 1944. Antihistaminic properties of N-p-methoxybenzyl-N-dimethylaminoethyl α-aminopyridine. C. R. Soc. Biol. 138, 99–100.

Brimblecombe, R.W., Duncan, W.A.M., Durant, G.J., Emmett, J.C., Ganellin, C.R., Parsons, M.E., 1975. Cimetidine–A Non-Thiourea H$_2$-Receptor Antagonist. J. Int. Med. Res. 3, 86–92.

Casy, A.F., 1978. Chemistry of Anti-H$_1$ Histamine Antagonist. In: Rocha e Silva, M. (Ed.), Histamine and Antihistamines, XVIII/2. Springer, Berlin, pp. 175–214.

Chakrin, L.W., Krell, L.D., Mengel, J., Young, D., Zaher, C., Wardell, J.R., 1974. Effect of a histamine H$_2$-receptor antagonist on immunologically induced mediator release in vitro. Agents Actions 4, 297–303.

Church, M.K., Gradidge, C.F., 1980. Inhibition of histamine release from human lung in vitro by antihistamines and related drugs. Br. J. Pharmacol. 69, 663–667.

Church, M.K., Pao, G.J., Holgate, S.T., 1982. Characterization of histamine secretion from mechanically dispersed human lung mast cells: effects of anti-IgE, calcium ionophore A23187, compound 48/80, and basic polypeptides. J. Immunol. 129, 2116–2121.

Dale, H.H., Laidlow, P.P., 1910 Dec 31. The physiological action of beta-iminazolylethylamine. J. Physiol. 41 (5), 318–344.

Dale, H.H., Laidlow, P.P., 1919. Histamine shock. J. Physiol. 52, 355–390.

Dews, P.B., Wunck, A.L., Fanelli, R.V., Light, A.E., Tornaben, J.A., Norton, S., Ellis, C.H., De Beer, E.J., 1953 Jan. The pharmacology of No. 48-80, a long-acting vasodepressor drug. J. Pharmacol. Exp. Ther. 107 (1), 1–11.

Doenicke, A., Lorenz, W., 1982. Histamine release in anaesthesia and surgery. premedication with H_1- and H_2-receptor antagonists: indications, benefits and possible problems. Klin. Wochenschrift 60, 1039–1045.

Doenicke, A., Lorenz, W., Beigl, R., Bezecny, H., Uhlig, G., Praetorius, B., Mann, G., 1973. Histamine release after intravenous application of short-acting hypnotics. A comparison of etomidate, Althesin (CT1341) and propanidid. Br. J. Anaesth. 45, 1097–1104.

Douglas, W.W. (1971) In: The Pharmacological Basis of Therapeutics (Goodman, L.S., Gilman, A., Eds.), pp. 621–662, Macmillan, London.

Dulabh, R., Vickers, M.R., 1978. The effects of H_2-receptor antagonists on anaphylaxis in the guinea-pig. Agents Actions 8, 559–565.

Durant, G.J., Emmett, J.C., Ganellin, C.R., 1973 In: International Symposium on Histamine H_2-Receptor Antagonists (Wood, C.J., Simkins, M.A., Eds.), Smith Kline & French, Welwyn Garden City, pp. 13–21.

Ehrlich, N.J., Kaplan, M.A., 1950. An evaluation of perazil in allergic rhinitis. Ann. Allergy 8, 682–683.

Enerbäck, L., 1966. Mast cells in rat gastrointestinal mucosa. 3. Reactivity towards compound 48/80. Acta Physiol. Microbiol. Scand. 66, 313–322.

Ennis, M., 1982. Histamine release from human pulmonary mast cells. Agents Actions 12, 60–63.

Ennis, M., Pearce, F.L., 1980. Differential reactivity of isolated mast cells from the rat and guinea pig. Eur. J. Pharmacol. 66, 339–345.

Feldberg, W., Talesnik, J., 1953. Reduction of tissue histamine by compound 48/80. J. Physiol. 120, 550–568.

Folkow, B., Hjeger, K., Kahlson, G., 1948. Observations on Reactive Hyperaemia as Related to Histamine, on Drugs Antagonizing Vasodilatation Induced by Histamine and on Vasodilator Properties of Adenosinetri phosphate. Acta Physiol. Scand. 15, 264–278.

Forrest, J.A.H., Shearman, D.J.C., Spence, R., Celestin, L.R., 1975. Neutropenia associated with metiamide. Lancet i 392–393.

Ganellin, C.R., 1978. Chemistry and Structure-Activity Relationships of H_2-Receptor Antagonists. In: Rocha e Silva, M. (Ed.), Handbook of Experimental Pharmacology. Histamine and Antihistamines, XVIII. Springer, Berlin, pp. 251–294.

Ghosh, M.N., Schild, H.O., 1958. Continuous recording of acid gastric secretion in the rat. Br. J. Pharmacol. 13, 54–61.

Giertz, H., Hahn, F., 1966. Makromolekulare Histaminliberatoren. Handbook of Experimental Pharmacology. In: Rocha e Silva, M. (Ed.), Histamine and Antihistamines, XVIII. Springer, Berlin, pp. 481–568.

Greeff, K., Bokelmann, A., 1959. [Anaphylactic reactions in the isolated guinea pig heart]. Verh Dtsch Ges Kreislaufforsch 25, 298–302 German. PMID: 13829191.

Grossman, M.I., Robertson, C., Rosiere, C.E., 1952. The effect of some compounds related to histamine on gastric acid secretion. J. Pharm. Exp. Ther. 104, 277–283.

Haas, H., 1952. Histamine and Antihistamine, II. Sandmaier and Sohn, Buchau a.F.

Hahn, F. (1978) Antianaphylactic and Antiallergic Effects. In: Handbook of Experimental Pharmacology, Vol. XVIII,2: Histamine and Antihistamines (Rocha e Silva, M., Ed.), pp. 439–504, Springer, Berlin.

Halpern, B.N., 1942. Synthetic antihistamine substances. Arch. Int. Pharmacodyn. 68, 339–408.

Halpern, B.N., 1947. Research on a new chemical series of bodies endowed with antihistamine and anti-anaphylactic properties; thiodiphenylamine derivatives. Bull. Soc. Chem. Biol. 29 (1–3), 309–318.

Halpern, B.N., 1952 Dec. Histamine and synthetic antihistaminics. C.R. Soc. Biol. 146 (23–24) 1996–2002.

Halpern, B.N., Ducrot, R., 1946. Recherches expérimentales sur une série chimique de corps doués de propriétés antihistaminiques puissantes: Les derivés de la thiodiphénylamine (T.D.A.). C.R. Soc. Biol. 140, 361–363.

Heymanns, J., Behrendt, H., Schmutzler, W., 1982. Comparative studies of mast cells from normal (non-immunized) and actively sensitized dogs. Agents Actions 12, 192–198.

Huttrer, C.P., 1948. Chemistry of antihistaminic substances. Enzymologia 12, 277–332.

Huttrer, C.P., Djerass, C., Beears, W.L., Mayer, R.L., Scholz, C.R., 1946. Heterocyclic amines with antithistaminic activity. J. Am. Chem. Soc. 68 1999–2002.

Ivy, A.C., Bachrach, W.H., 1966. Physiological Significance of the Effect of Histamine on Gastric Secretion. Handbook of Experimental Pharmacology. In: Rocha e Silva, M. (Ed.), Histamine and Antihistamines, XVIII. Springer, Berlin, pp. 810–891.

Kazimierczak, W., Diamant, B., 1978. Mechanisms of histamine release in anaphylactic and anaphylactoid reactions. Prog. Allergy 24, 295–365.

Kazimierczak, W., Szczepaniak, K., Bankowska, K., 1981. A modulation of the anaphylactic basophil histamine release by selective H_2 histamine agonists. Agents Actions 11, 96–98.

Klin. Wochenschr. (1982) 60,871–1062.

Labelle, A., Tislow, R., 1955 Jan. Studies on prophenpyridamine (trimeton) and chlorprophenpyridamine (chlortrimeton). J. Pharmacol. Exp. Ther. 113 (1), 72–88.

Levi, R., Chenouda, A.A., Trzeciakowski, J.P., Guo, Z., Aaronson, L.M., Luskind, R.D., Leo, C., 1982. Dysrhythmias caused by histamine release in guinea pig and human hearts. Klin. Wochenschr. 60, 965–971.

Lichtenstein, L.M., 1973. In: Int. Symp. on Histamine H_2-Receptor Antagonists (Wood, C.J., Simkins, M.A., Eds.), Smith Kline & French, Welwyn Garden City, p. 203.

Lichtenstein, L.M., Gillespie, E., 1973. Inhibition of histamine release by histamine controlled by H_2 receptor. Nature 244, 287–288.

Lichtenstein, L.M., Plant, M., Henney, C., Gillespie, E. 1973 In: Int. Symp. on Histamine H_2-Receptor Antagonists (Wood, C.J., Simkins, M.A., Eds.), pp. 187–198, Smith Kline & French, Welwyn Garden City.

Lin, T.M., Alphin, R.S., Henderson, F.G., Bensley, D.N., Chen, K.K., 1962. The role of histamine in gastric hydrochloric acid secretion. Ann. N.Y. Acad. Sci. 99, 30–44.

Loew, E.R., 1947. Pharmacology of antihistamine compounds. Physiol. Rev. 27, 542–573.

Lorenz, W. (1973) In: Int. Symp. on Histamine H_2-Receptor Antagonists (Wood, C.J. and Simkins, M.A., Eds.), p. 203, Smith Kline & French, Welwyn Garden City.

Lorenz, W., 1975 Dec. Histamine release in man. Agents Actions 5 (5), 402–416.

Lorenz, W., 1981. Histamine and Antihistamines in Anaesthesia and Surgery. Lancet 74–75.

Lorenz, W. (1983) In: Immunotoxicology (Gibson, G.G., Hubbard, R. and Parke, D.V., Eds.), pp. 283–305, Academic Press London, New York.

Lorenz, W., Schauer, A., Heitland, S., Calvoer, R., Werle, E., 1969. Biochemical and histochemical studies on the distribution of histamine in the digestive tract of man, dog and other mammals. Naunyn-Schmiedeberg's Arch. Pharmakol. 265, 81–100.

Lorenz, W., Benesch, L., Barth, H., Matejka, E., Meyer, R., Kusche, J., Hutzel, M., Werle, E., 1970. Fluorometric assay of histamine in tissues and body fluids: Choice of the purification procedure and identification in the nanogram range. Z. Analyt. Chem. 252, 94–98.

Lorenz, W., Meyer, R., Doenicke, A., Schmal, A., Reimann, H.-J., Hutzel, M., Werle, E., 1971. Naunyn-Schmiedebergs Arch. Pharmakol. 269, 417.

Lorenz, W., Doenicke, A., Meyer, R., Reimann, H.-J., Kusche, J., Barth, H., Gesing, H., Hutzel, M., Weissenbacher, B., 1972. An improved method for the determination of histamine release in man: its application in studies with propanidid and thiopentone. Eur. J. Pharmacol. 19, 180–190.

Lorenz, W., Thermann, M., Hamelmann, H., Schmal, A., Maroske, D., Reimann, H.-J., Kusche, J., Schingale, F., Dormann, P. and Keck, P. (1973) In: Int. Symp. on Histamine H_2-Receptor Antagonists (Wood, C.J. and Simkins, M.A., Eds.), pp. 151–165, Smith Kline & French, Welwyn Garden City.

Lorenz, W., Doenicke, A., Dittmann, I., Hug, P., Schwarz, B., 1977a Dec. Anaphylactoid reactions following administration of plasma substitutes in man. Prevention of this side-effect of haemaccel by premedication with H_1- and H_2-receptor antagonists. Anaesthesist 26 (12), 644–648.

Lorenz, W., Reimann, H.-J., Schmal, A., Dormann, P., Schwarz, B., Neugebauer, E., 1977b. Histamine release in dogs by Cremophor E1 and its derivatives: oxethylated oleic acid is the most effective constituent. Agents Actions 7, 63–67.

Lorenz, W. and Doenicke, A. (1978a) Anaphylactoid reactions and histamine release by intravenous drugs used in surgery and anaesthesia. In: Adverse Response to Intravenous Drugs (Watkins, J. and Ward, A.M., Eds.), pp. 83–112, Academic Press, London.

Lorenz, W., Doenicke, A., 1978b. Histamine release in clinical conditions. Mount Sinai J. Med. 45, 357–386.

Lorenz, W., Doenicke, A., Schöning, B., Mamorski, J., Weber, D., Hinterlang, E., Schwartz, B., Neugebauer, E., 1980. H_1 + H_2-receptor antagonists for premedication in anaesthesia and surgery: a critical view based on randomized clinical trials with Haemaccel and various antiallergic drugs. Agents Actions 10, 114–124.

Lorenz, W., Doenicke, A., Schöning, B. and Neugebauer, E., 1981a. The role of histamine in adverse reactions to intravenous agents. In: Adverse Reactions of Anaesthetic Drugs (Thornton, J.A., Ed.), Elsevier/North-Holland, Amsterdam, pp. 169–238.

Lorenz, W., Mohri, K., Reimann, H.-J., Troidl, H., Rohde, H., Barth, H., 1981b. Intramucosal mechanisms: relevance of the mast cell concept. Advances in Ulcer Disease, International Congress Series No. 537, Amsterdam. Excerpta Medica, pp. 176–194.

Lorenz, W., Doenicke, A., Schöning, B., Karges, H., Schmal, A., 1981c. Incidence and mechanisms of adverse reactions to polypeptides in man and dog. Developments in Biological Standardization. In: Hennessen, W. (Ed.), Symposium on Standardization of Albumin, Plasma Substitutes and Plasmapheresis, 48. Karger, Basel, pp. 207–234.

Lorenz, W., Doenicke, A. and Schöning, B., 1982a. In: Complications of Anaesthesia. Operative Risk (Conseiller, C., Ed.), Libraire Arnette, Paris, Excerpta Medica, Amsterdam, pp. 173–190.

Lorenz, W., Schmal, A., Schult, H., Lang, S., Ohmann, Ch., Weber, D., Kapp, B., Lüben, L., Doenicke, A., 1982b. Histamine release and hypotensive reactions in dogs by solubilizing agents and fatty acids: analysis of various components in cremophor El and development of a compound with reduced toxicity. Agents Actions 12, 64–80.

Lorenz, W., Doenicke, A., Schöning, B., Ohmann, Ch., Grote, B., Neugebauer, E., 1982c. Definition and classification of the histamine-release response to drugs in anaesthesia and surgery: studies in the conscious human subject. Klin. Wochenschr. 60, 896–913.

Lorenz, W., Thon, K., Barth, H., Neugebauer, E., Reimann, H.J., Kusche, J., 1983. Metabolism and function of gastric histamine in health and disease. J. Clin. Gastroenterol. 5 (Suppl. 1), 37–56.

Lorenz, W., Doenicke, A., 1985a. H_1 and H_2 blockade: a prophylactic principle in anesthesia and surgery against histamine-release responses of any degree of severity: Part I. N. Engl. Reg. Allergy. Proc. 1, 37–57.

Lorenz, W., Doenicke, A., 1985b. H_1 and H_2 blockade: a prophylactic principle in anesthesia and surgery against histamine-release responses of any degree of severity: Part II. N. Engl. Reg. Allergy. Proc. 2, 174–194.

Mannaioni, P.F., 1960 Dec. Interaction between histamine and dichloroisoproterenol, hexamethonium, pempidine, and diphenhydramine, in normal and reserpine-treated heart preparations. Br. J. Pharmacol. Chemother. 4, 500–505.

Mannaioni, P.F., 1972 Apr. Physiology and pharmacology of cardiac histamine. Arch. Int. Pharmacodyn. Ther. 196 (196 Suppl.), 64–67.

Mariani, L., 1961 Dec. Decrease in tissue and blood histamine by the action of reserpine. Boll. Soc. Ital. Biol. Sper. 37 (24), 1478–1481.

Moss, J., Philbin, D.M., Rosow, C.E., Basta, S.J., Gelb, C., Savarese, J.J., 1982. Histamine release by neuromuscular blocking agents in man. Klin. Wochenschr. 60, 891–895.

Mota, I., 1966. Release of Histamine from Mast Cells. Handbook of Experimental Pharmacology. In: Rocha e Silva, M. (Ed.), Histamine and Antihistamines, XVIII. Springer, Berlin, pp. 569–636.

Mota, I., da Silva, W., 1960 Sep. The anti-anaphylactic and histamine-releasing properties of the antihistamines. Their effect on the mast cells. Br. J. Pharmacol. Chemother. 15 (3), 396–404.

Neugebauer, E., Lorenz, W., 1981. Behring Inst. Mitt. 68, 102–133.

Owen, D.A., Harvey, C.A., Boyce, M.J., 1982 Sep 1. Effects of histamine on the circulatory system. Klin. Wochenschr. 60 (17), 972–977.

P'An, S.Y., Gardocki, J.F., Reilly, J.C., 1954. Pharmacological properties of two new antihistaminics of prolonged action. J. Am. Pharm. Assoc. 43, 653–656.

Parkin, J.V., Ackroyd, E.B., Glickman, S., Hobsley, M. and Lorenz, W. (1982) Release of histamine by H_2-receptor antagonists. Lancet ii, 938–939.

Parsons, M.E. 1969, Quantitative Studies of Drug Induced Gastric Secretion. Ph. D. Thesis, University of London.

Parsons, M.E., 1982. The Discovery of Histamine H_2-Receptors and their Antagonists. Smith Kline and French, Welwyn Garden City, pp. 41–42.

Paton, W.D.M., 1951 Sep. Compound 48/80: a potent histamine liberator. Br. J. Pharmacol. Chemother. 6 (3), 499–508.

Pearce, F.L., 1982. Functional heterogeneity of mast cells from different species and tissues. Klin. Wochenschr. 20, 954–957.

Pearce, F.L., Ennis, M., 1980. Isolation and some properties of mast cells from the mesentery of the rat and guinea pig. Agents Actions 10, 124–131.

Pearce, F.L., Befus, A.D., Bienenstock, J., 1982. Isolation and properties of mast cells from the small bowel lamina propria of the rat. Agents Actions 12, 183–185.

Philbin, D.M., Moss, J., Akins, C.W., Rosow, C.E., Kono, K., Schneider, R.C., VerLee, T.R., Savarese, J.J., 1981. The use of H_1 and H_2 histamine antagonists with morphine anesthesia: a double-blind study. Anesthesiology 55, 292–296.

Philbin, D.M., Moss, J.-., Roscow, C.E., Akins, C.W., Rosenberger, J.L., 1982. Histamine release with intravenous narcotics: protective effects of H_1 and H_2-receptor antagonists. Klin. Wochenschr. 60, 1056–1059.

Popielski, L., 1920. Beta-imidazolyläthylamin und die Organextrakte. I. Beta-imidazolylathylamin als mächtiger Erreger der Magendrüsen. Pflügers Arch. Ges. Physiol. 178, 214–236.

Rieveschl, G.R. and Huber, W.F. (1946) Abstracts, 109th Meeting American Chemical Society, 50 K.

Riley, J.F., West, G.B., 1966. The Occurrence of Histamine in Mast Cells. Handbook of Experimental Pharmacology. In: Rocha e Silva, M. (Ed.), Histamine and Antihistamines, XVIII/1. Springer, Berlin, pp. 116–135.

Rocha e Silva, M., 1955. Histamine its Role in Anaphylaxis and Allergy. C.C. Thomas, Springfield, IL.

Rocha e Silva, M., Leme, J.G., 1963. Antagonistis of bradykinin. Med. Exp. Int. J. Exp. Med. 8, 287–295.

Rocha e Silva, M., Antonio, A., 1978. Bioassay of Antihistaminic Action. Handbook of Experimental Pharmacology. In: Rocha e Silva, M. (Ed.), Histamine and Antihistamines, XVIII/2. Springer, Berlin, pp. 381–438.

Röher, H.D., Lorenz, W., Lennartz, H., Kusche, J., Dietz, W., Gerdes, G., Parkin, J.V., 1982. Plasma histamine levels in patients in the course of several standard operations: influence of anaesthesia, surgical trauma and blood transfusion. Klin. Wochenschr. 60, 926–934.

Rothschild, A.M., 1966. Histamine Release by Basic Compounds. Handbook of Experimental Pharmacology. In: Rocha e Silva, M. (Ed.), Histamine and Antihistamines, XVIII/1. Springer, Berlin, pp. 386–430.

Schmutzler, W., Behrendt, H., Blum, U., Pearce, F.L., Poblete-Freundt, G., Stang-Voss, C., 1977. Histamine release from isolated guinea pig mast cells by anaphylatoxin. Monogr. Allergy 12, 143–144.

Schöning B, Lorenz W. 1980. Prevention of allergoid (cutaneous anaphylactoid) reactions to polygeline (Haemaccel) in orthopaedic patients by premedication with H_1- and H_2-receptor antagonists. Dev. Biol. Stand. 48, 241–249.

Seyle, H., 1965. The Mast Cells. Butterworth, London.

Smith, A.N., 1953. Release of histamine by the histamine liberator compound 48/80 in cats. J. Physiol. 121, 517–538.

Sperber, N., Papa, D., Schwenk, E., Sherlock, M., 1949. Pyridyl-substituted alkamine ethers as antihistaminic agents. J. Am. Chem. Soc. 71, 887–890.

Staub, A.M., 1939a. Recherches sur quelques bases synthetiques antagonistes de l'histamine. Ann. Inst. Pasteur Paris 63, 400–436.

Staub, A.M., 1939b. Recherches sur quelques bases synthetiques antagonistes de l'histamine. Ann. Inst. Pasteur Paris 63, 485–529.

Stone, C.A., Wenger, H.C., Ludden, C.T., Stavorski, J.M., Ross, C.A., 1961. Antiserotonin-antihistaminic properties of cyproheptadine. J. Pharmacol. Exp. Ther. 131, 73–84.

Tasaka, K., 1957. Histamine release and its inhibition by antihistamines. Folia Pharmacol. Jap. 53, 1029–1035.

Tozzi, S., Roth, F.E., Tabachnick, I.I.A., 1974. The pharmacology of azatadine, a potential antiallergy drug. Agents Actions 4, 264–270.

Ungar, G., Parrot, J.L., 1936. Recherches sur le choc anaphylactique in vitro. Mise en liberté d'une substance active par le poumon isolé du cobaye sensibilisé. C.R. Soc. Biol. (Paris). 123, 676–678.

Ungar, G., Parrot, J.L., Bovet, D., 1937. Inhibition des effets de l'histamine sur l'intestineisole du cobaye par quelques substances sympathomime tiques et sympathicolytiques. C.R. Soc. Biol. 124, 445–446.

Vugman, I., 1969. The effect of pH on mast cell damage by antihistamines. Experientia 25, 55–56.

Watkins, J., Thornton, J.A., 1982. Immunological and non-immunological mechanisms involved in adverse reactions to drugs. Klin. Wochenschr. 60, 958–964.

Werle, E., Lorenz, W., 1970. The Antikinin Action of Some Antihistaminic Drugs on the Isolated Guinea-Pig Ileum, Rat Uterus and Blood Pressure of the Anesthetized Dog. In: Sicuteri, F., e Silva, M.R., Back, N. (eds.) Bradykinin and Related Kinins. Advances in Experimental Medicine and Biology, vol. 8. Springer, Boston, MA.

Commentary on Asthma: A long and continuing story by Walter E. Brocklehurst

Peter J. Barnes

National Heart & Lung Institute, Imperial College London, London, United Kingdom

Introduction

W.E. (Bill) Brocklehurst, a pharmacologist working in London, expertly described the understanding of asthma in his 1983 chapter which follows. He had described a mediator that was released in anaphylactic reactions and caused slow and sustained smooth muscle contraction, in contrast to the rapid onset and short duration of histamine, which he termed a slow-reacting substance of anaphylaxis (SRS-A) (Brocklehurst, 1960). SRS-A was subsequently identified as the potent cysteinyl-leukotrienes (LT), LTC_4, LTD_4, and LTE_4, which contribute to bronchoconstriction in asthma. This led to the development of specific leukotriene receptor ($CysLT_1$) antagonists, which were widely used in the management of asthma. However, much has changed in our understanding of asthma pathogenesis and there have been major advances in the management of asthma over the last 40 years.

Mediators of asthma

Anaphylactic shock in guinea pigs was widely used as a model of asthma since it produced bronchoconstriction via the activation of lung mast cells. Histamine is a prominent bronchoconstrictor mediator released from mast cells, yet even potent antihistamines (H_1-receptor antagonists) are ineffective as a treatment for asthma, and Brocklehurst recognized that histamine is not an important bronchoconstrictor in this disease. An experimental SRS-A inhibitor, FPL55712, was mentioned by Brocklehurst, but this drug did not reach clinical trials. More potent and orally active anti-leukotrienes, such as montelukast and zafirlukast, were introduced in the 1990s and proved to be popular asthma therapies (especially for children) as they reduced bronchoconstriction in response to allergen and other triggers of asthma and were well tolerated (Peters-Golden and Henderson, 2007). However, these treatments proved to be somewhat disappointing in improving asthma control compared with other controller therapies, and the recognition that there were neuropsychiatric side effects led to a reduction in their use (Yokomizo et al., 2018). Brocklehurst recognized that other bronchoconstrictor mediators could also be released from mast cells, including kinins, prostaglandins, and platelet-activating factors, suggesting that blocking a single bronchoconstrictor mediator may not be the most effective strategy, particularly as β_2-agonist bronchodilators counteract all bronchoconstrictors. More recently, prostaglandin D_2 from mast cells was shown to be an important bronchoconstrictor and cause inflammation via DP_2-receptors. Potent DP_2-receptor antagonists, while promising in early clinical studies, also proved to be ineffective (Powell, 2021).

Mast cells in asthma

Brocklehurst recognized that mast cells play a central role in allergic asthma as well as in anaphylaxis. It was known that mast cells could be activated to release preformed mediators such as histamine and synthesize new mediators, such as cys-LTs and PGD_2 in response to allergens via IgE bound to their surface. Mast cells are still believed to play a key role in the release of bronchoconstrictors, leading to the symptoms of asthma and contributing to plasma exudation and mucosal oedema, which together contribute to the airway narrowing in asthma. Mast cells induce bronchoconstriction in response to indirect triggers of asthma, including allergens, exercise, and cold air and are activated during acute exacerbations. Since blocking individual mast cell mediators proved to be disappointing as treatments, a more promising approach is to inhibit mast cells with drugs known as mast cell stabilizers. Sodium cromoglycate, derived from the herbal agent khellin, was shown by Altounyan to be very effective in inhibiting induced asthma symptoms and acted through the stabilization of mast cells (Altounyan, 1980). Cromoglycate was given by dry powder inhaler and was widely used in the treatment of allergic asthma, particularly in children, due to its safety but its value as a long-term preventive treatment for asthma is limited by its short duration of action. Even now its molecular mechanism of action is poorly understood and although another inhaled cromone, nedocromil, was introduced, it had no advantage over cromoglycate. Other mast cell stabilizers that were designed for oral administration failed in clinical studies and cromoglycate is no longer recommended for asthma, as it is poorly effective in asthma control compared to more recently developed controllers (Tasche et al., 2000).

Other inflammatory cells

It is now recognized that asthma involves acute and chronic inflammation of the airway mucosa, with the involvement of many inflammatory cells in addition to mast cells, as well as the release of inflammatory mediators from structural cells, such as airway epithelial and smooth muscle cells (Papi et al., 2018). Brocklehurst's chapter says little about eosinophils, which are now recognized to play a key role in airway hyperresponsiveness, symptoms, and exacerbations of asthma and are a major target in therapy. Eosinophilic inflammation is regulated by type 2 (T2) immunity via CD4$^+$ type 2 helper T lymphocytes (Th2) and type 2 innate lymphoid cells (ILC2). Neutrophils may also play a role, particularly in severe asthma and in asthmatic patients who smoke, although their role in symptoms remains uncertain as anti-neutrophilic therapies have so far proved to be disappointing.

Cytokines as key mediators of asthma

Since the publication of Brocklehurst's chapter, it has been recognized that cytokines and chemokines play a critical role in the pathogenesis of asthma and result in the orchestration of chronic mucosal inflammation in the airways. Of particular importance are the cytokines that regulate T2 immunity, including interleukin (IL)-4, IL-5, and IL-13 (Barnes, 2018). T2 cytokines from lymphocytes are regulated by upstream cytokines (alarmins) secreted by airway epithelial cells in asthma, including IL-25, IL-33, and thymic stromal lymphopoietin (TSLP).

The discovery that airway inflammation in asthma is regulated by T2 cytokines has led to the development of anti-cytokine antibodies (biologics), which are now used in the treatment of severe eosinophilic (T2) asthma (Brusselle and Koppelman, 2022). The first T2 cytokine to be targeted in asthma was IL-5 and the antibody mepolizumab was found to markedly reduce eosinophils in the blood and airways of asthmatic patients (Leckie et al., 2000). Anti-IL-5 antibodies include mepolizumab and benralizumab, which reduce exacerbations by ~50% in patients with severe T2 asthma. More recently an antibody dupilumab, which targets the common receptor (IL-4Rα) for IL-4 and IL-13, is even more effective. Antibodies that target TSLP and IL-33 are also in development and are promising, with beneficial effects in non-T2 severe asthma.

Bronchodilators

Inhaled β_2-agonists remain the major bronchodilator therapy for asthma, with short-acting β_2-agonists still used as the most common reliever therapy. The inhaled long-acting β_2-agonists (LABA) salmeterol and formoterol were introduced in the 1990s and have proved to be a very useful add-on therapy to inhaled corticosteroids (ICS); they are given as fixed combination inhalers and are now the most commonly used controller medication (Barnes, 2002). ICS-formoterol combinations are more effective as reliever medication in all patients with asthma, including those with mild asthma (O'Byrne et al., 2018). The rapid relief of symptoms by the bronchodilator is combined with the anti-inflammatory effect of the corticosteroid to prevent the development of exacerbations and provide more effective control of asthma (Reddel et al., 2022).

Anticholinergics have a long history as bronchodilators in asthma but are less effective than β_2-agonists as they counteract increased cholinergic tone and reflex bronchoconstriction, whereas β_2-agonists act as functional antagonists counteracting all bronchoconstrictor mediators. Long-acting muscarinic antagonists, such as tiotropium bromide, are now used as an add-on bronchodilator therapy in poorly controlled severe asthma, although there is relatively little benefit in reducing symptoms and exacerbations (Kerstjens et al., 2012). Theophylline also has a long history as a bronchodilator in asthma therapy and is still widely used as an oral therapy globally as it is inexpensive. It was subsequently found to have anti-inflammatory effects at lower doses than those required for bronchodilatation but is now used much less because of side effects that are due to phosphodiesterase inhibition and adenosine receptor antagonism (Barnes, 2013).

The pivotal role of inhaled corticosteroids

Systemic glucocorticoids have been recognized as effective treatments for severe asthma since their discovery in the 1950s and are still used to treat acute exacerbations and in lower doses as maintenance therapy in the very small number ($\sim$1%) of asthma patients with very severe asthma when no other treatment is sufficient to control the disease. Early on in their use, the endocrine and metabolic side effects of systemic steroids were recognized, so it was clear that this therapy had a limited role in long-term management. ICS, which delivers a topically acting anti-inflammatory to the airways are not mentioned by Brocklehurst, although they have revolutionized asthma management and are now the mainstay of asthma therapy in almost all patients. ICS, such as beclomethasone dipropionate, budesonide, and fluticasone propionate is effective when given twice daily, and more recently once daily ICS, including fluticasone furoate, mometasone, and ciclesonide has been introduced. These ICS are now usually given in a combination inhaler with a LABA and are effective in reducing exacerbations, controlling asthma, and may reduce loss of lung function over time (Barnes, 2017). They are largely free of systemic side effects. Their molecular mechanism of action in asthma is now well understood and their major effect is in switching off activated inflammatory genes, particularly cytokine genes, and suppressing T2 inflammation.

Conclusions

There have been major changes in our understanding of asthma since Brocklehurst wrote his chapter in 1983. Mast cells are still considered important effector cells in causing the bronchoconstriction and symptoms of asthma, but the importance of T2 immunity leading to chronic eosinophilic inflammation of the airways and airway hyperresponsiveness is now recognized to be important in understanding the clinical features of asthma. This has led to a shift from bronchodilator therapies to ICS to suppress the chronic inflammation of the airways, resulting in control of asthma and prevention of exacerbations. More recently biologic therapies to inhibit eosinophilic inflammation in patients with poorly controlled severe asthma have been introduced and several new types of therapy are now in development for the less common non-T2 severe asthma.

References

Altounyan, R.E.C., 1980. Review of clinical activity and mode of action of sodium cromoglycate. Clin. Allergy 10, 481–489.

Barnes, P.J., 2002. Scientific rationale for combination inhalers with a long-acting β2-agonists and corticosteroids. Eur. Respir. J. 19, 182–191.

Barnes, P.J., 2013. Theophylline. Am. J. Respir. Crit. Care Med. 188, 901–906.

Barnes, P.J., 2017. Glucocorticosteroids. Handb. Exp. Pharmacol. 237, 93–115.

Barnes, P.J., 2018. Targeting cytokines to treat asthma and chronic obstructive pulmonary disease. Nat. Rev. Immunol. 18, 454–466.

Brocklehurst, W.E., 1960. The release of histamine and formation of a slow-reacting substance (SRS-A) during anaphylactic shock. J. Physiol. 151, 416–435.

Brusselle, G.G., Koppelman, G.H., 2022. Biologic therapies for severe asthma. N. Engl. J. Med. 386, 157–171.

Kerstjens, H.A., et al., 2012. Tiotropium in asthma poorly controlled with standard combination therapy. N. Engl. J. Med. 367, 1198–1207.

Leckie, M.J., et al., 2000. Effects of an interleukin-5 blocking monoclonal antibody on eosinophils, airway hyper-responsiveness and the late asthmatic response. Lancet 356, 2144–2148.

O'Byrne, P.M., et al., 2018. Inhaled combined budesonide-formoterol as needed in mild asthma. N. Engl. J. Med. 378, 1865–1876.

Papi, A., et al., 2018. Asthma. Lancet 391, 783–800.

Peters-Golden, M., Henderson Jr., W.R., 2007. Leukotrienes. N. Engl. J. Med. 357, 1841–1854.

Powell, W.S., 2021. Eicosanoid receptors as therapeutic targets for asthma. Clin. Sci. 135, 1945–1980.

Reddel, H.K., et al., 2022. Global initiative for asthma strategy 2021: executive summary and rationale for key changes. Am. J. Respir. Crit. Care Med. 205, 17–35.

Tasche, M.J., Uijen, J.H., Bernsen, R.M., de Jongste, J.C., van Der, W., 2000. Inhaled disodium cromoglycate (DSCG) as maintenance therapy in children with asthma: a systematic review. Thorax 55, 913–920.

Yokomizo, T., Nakamura, M., Shimizu, T., 2018. Leukotriene receptors as potential therapeutic targets. J. Clin. Invest. 128, 2691–2701.

Asthma: a long and continuing story

Walter E. Brocklehurst

Contents

6.1 Introduction

The objective study of asthma spans the present century and has been under the continuous influence of the 'scientific method'. Thus, the laboratory data have been interpreted in accordance with Occam's Razor i.e. that any hypothesis should be the simplest that is compatible with established facts: in retrospect this is seen to have been too restrictive. By contrast the clinician has been unhampered in interpreting subjective observations and has often been unduly influenced by enthusiasm. We now know that the asthma attack involves many factors and some substances of quite amazing potency. The previous laudable attempts to keep the story simple were therefore doomed to mislead. Furthermore the lack of methods sufficiently sensitive and specific to detect and separate some of the important pharmacologically active autacoids involved, resulted in long delays and much frustration and confusion.

In hindsight we can eliminate the minor and irrelevant discoveries and arrive at the following list of major advances:

Disclaimer: The original text that follows is reproduced from the first edition and carries errors and omissions from it. The editors and publisher agreed to retain them and honor the original authors and challenges they had to deal with in publishing back in those times.

Discoveries in Pharmacology, Volume 3, Hemodynamics and Immune Defense.
DOI: https://doi.org/10.1016/B978-0-443-18442-0.00066-5
© 1984, Elsevier Science Publishers B.V.

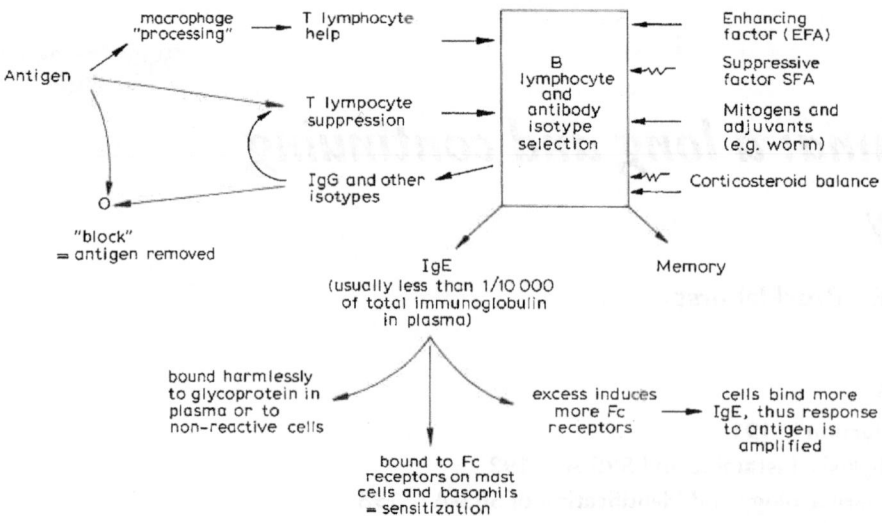

Figure 6.1

IgE production and sensitization of tissue.

Anaphylactic shock in the guinea-pig as a model of asthma involving sensitization by antibody (see Fig. 6.1).

Resemblance between histamine intoxication and anaphylactic shock.

Extraction of histamine from mammalian tissue and from blood during anaphylactic shock.

Synthesis of anti-histamine compounds leading to study of other substances involved in asthma.

Passive long-lasting sensitization and the recognition of IgE.

The mast cell as the source of histamine and the site of the antigen-antibody trigger.

The biochemistry of the trigger process and the complexity of subsequent events.

The factors influencing the production of IgE and its ability to sensitize mast cells and basophils.

Chemical analysis and pharmacology of SRS-A and other substances contributing to the syndrome of asthma.

It has only quite recently become possible to make rational assessments of therapeutic measures in terms of pharmacology and cell biology. Many logical approaches to treatment remain unexplored for lack of suitable drugs.

6.2 Anaphylaxis, histamine and SRS-A

The recognition of an animal 'model' of a human ailment always leads to enthusiasm and speculation, and evidence for the validity of the model is therefore of the utmost importance.

The phenomenon discovered in 1902 by Richet and Portier and christened 'anaphylaxis' was a totally unexpected spin-off from a study intended to illustrate that immunity could be generated to harmful chemical toxins and was not confined to disease-producing microorganisms. Richet firmly believed that a healthy animal reacted quickly in its own defence, so that the blood carried protective substances which were amplified to meet any repetition of the threat to health. He had shown that the blood of animals resistant to certain infections could protect recipient animals from those organisms responsible for the infection, and believed that the protective factors acted by neutralizing the toxic products of the microorganism.

The phenomenon of 'anaphylactic shock' was seen following a non-lethal dose of the toxin collected from the nematocysts of the 'Portuguese Man of War' jellyfish. Some practical outcome of the experiment was envisaged, since these jellyfish are a hazard to bathers on the Cote d'Azure. A range of doses was injected into dogs to assess overt toxic manifestations, and the animals were then rested several days to recover fully before the injection of a narrower range of doses of the same toxin, which Richet expected to be fully neutralized by the animal's protective responses to the earlier injection. To Richet's horror, all the animals died with bizarre symptoms totally unrelated to the previously observed effect of the toxin, and to his further consternation he discovered that even very small second doses could be fatal. Fortunately, Richet was a mature physiologist who not only fully confirmed his discovery of 'anaphylaxis', but also went on to show that it was not a simple consequence of heightened response to the toxin itself, since non-toxic material (e.g. serum) could also generate the anaphylactic state (i.e. the inverse of protection). Understandably, he remained convinced that it was an anomaly to the general rule. He continued to teach the teleological theme that the body reacts in ways affording better future protection, and that this is essential to survival of the species.

The symptoms of anaphylactic shock in the dog did not suggest any causative similarity with asthma; this had to await the phenomenon in the guinea-pig. Anaphylactic shock was so intriguing, and so easy to produce in some species (but not all), that within a few years the overt symptoms and the gross pathology had been described in the rabbit and guinea-pig. The concept of the 'shock organ' quickly emerged, since the symptoms were associated with hepatic and portal system vascular engorgement in the dog, right heart failure in the rabbit, and bronchospasm in the guinea-pig, irrespective of the nature of the antigens used. The syndrome in the guinea-pig was strongly reminiscent of human asthma, and this similarity was reinforced by the specificity of the sensitizing antigen and the need for an existing sensitized state to initiate any response at all to the antigen.

From 1900 onwards the subject of pharmacology was taking shape as a branch of applied physiology, and it was possible to measure and make simple comparisons of the effects of crude drug extracts tested alongside crystalline products or those made artificially, since synthetic chemistry was rapidly advancing at this time. Dale (see *Discoveries in Pharmacology,* Vol. 1, Chapt. 2) was attracted to this field after his clinical training, and became interested in histamine after identifying it as an extraordinarily potent uterine contractant and vaso-depressor factor in ergot. At this time, histamine was known only in plants and as a product of tissue putrefaction, along with several other amines produced by decarboxylation of amino acids: it had not been found in any fresh animal tissue. A data base of pharmacology was almost non-existent prior to 1910, and Dale used a range of species and isolated smooth muscle tissues (in the Magnus bath) to establish a 'pharmacological profile' for histamine. He was sufficiently impressed by the similarity between this and the pattern of anaphylactic shock symptoms in known susceptible species (notably the guinea-pig), that he tentatively drew attention to the similarity 'as a matter of interest and possible significance'. His work with isolated tissues, now immortalized as 'Schultz-Dale' reactions in which sensitized smooth muscle contracts once to antigen, and is thereafter unresponsive, soon provided further support for the 'histamine theory', (see Dale, 1920), and incidentally served to develop ideas concerning the immunology of the anaphylactic state; but it was not until 1927 that Dragstedt demonstrated the presence of histamine in the blood of a dog at the height of anaphylactic shock, and so completed the picture of the involvement of histamine. Up to this time Lewis was obliged to refer to 'H-substance' in pathophysiological reactions in which he believed that histamine was the active agent, because they so strikingly paralleled the pharmacology of synthetic histamine, (see Feldberg, 1941, 1954).

The 'humoral theory' of anaphylaxis ran more or less neck and neck with the 'histamine theory' during the early years up to 1925. This had been built on the fact that 'protein split products' were present in the circulation during serum sickness and anaphylactic shock and that 'anaphylatoxin' could be generated by simple exposure of serum to a charged surface (e.g. kaolin or agar) and produce anaphylactoid (i.e. resembling anaphylactic) shock when given intravenously. After 1930, the 'histamine theory' received more and more support, thanks to improved methods of analysis and many detailed studies, whereas the 'humoral theory' lacked any identifiable causative agents, and seemed to afford no opportunities for therapeutic intervention. Interest was thus lost until quite recently, when the availability of sophisticated methods for separating and identifying proteins has permitted academic studies which link anaphylatoxins with the complement system (see later section).

In the mid 1930s it was confidently expected that drugs able to inhibit the effects of histamine would effectively control asthma. No physiological role other than the triple response in skin, had been ascribed to histamine, and it was regarded as the product of a redundant or quasi-pathological tissue reaction. When Landsteiner and Chase showed that antibodies could be raised to small (hapten) molecules conjugated to carrier proteins, the possibility of raising antibodies able to protect against histamine was quickly recognized. Unfortunately the frequent therapeutic use of antibodies produced in another species carries the double hazard of quickly losing effectiveness, and of generating hypersensitivity, since these antibodies are themselves antigenic. Fortunately this approach was superseded by the discovery of the first antihistamine drugs. These had been synthesized as antagonists of adrenaline (epinephrine), but an astute pharmacologist (D. Bovet) demonstrated that they could inhibit the vasodepressor activity of histamine in the cat (cf. p. 624). The structures of the active substances were simple and bore some similarity to that of histamine; other structurally comparable compounds were quickly synthesized and tested. Recognition of the relationship between the structures of antagonists and agonists (mimetics) of adrenaline and histamine opened the eyes of chemists to the possibility that this might afford a general approach to situations in which active molecules must fit a 'receptor' molecule and could thus stimulate or block. The existence of receptors for acetylcholine had been recognised and studied for many years, but the natural antagonists, atropine and curare had afforded no clues to the manner in which they acted. The existence of a range of substances related to each other and able to exert various degrees of stimulation, or prevention of stimulation, permitted the pharmacologist to separate receptors into different classes (see Ahlquist, 1948). Conceptually similar studies in enzymology have led to major advances in cell biology and biochemistry, even though the actual receptor structure has remained obscure in most instances.

When antihistamine drugs showing good activity in the laboratory were used in man, they were effective against most types of response produced by histamine administered by injection, inhalation, or by iontophoresis into the skin but were generally disappointing in allergies. At first this was ascribed to insufficient potency of the antagonist substance in the face of a flood of histamine acting at short range in 'target' tissues. When more potent drugs proved to be little better, Dale (1950) introduced the term 'intrinsic histamine', which envisaged ultra-short distances between the site of histamine production and action, 'even within a single cell'. Dale also drew attention to histamine-produced phenomena which were resistant to antihistamine drugs, (e.g. gastric secretion of HCl) thus seeming to take place in a site sequestered from the drug. Atropine-resistant cholinergic phenomena were also cited as analogous. Many clinical allergists were more willing to accept a similar 'intrinsic' role for acetylcholine, arguing that an asthma-like syndrome of dyspnoea, increased viscid secretions, and airway irritation was produced by acetylcholine, and that atropine was of definite, though limited virtue in clinical asthma – the dosage being restricted by side effects produced by atropine.

By 1950 clinical experience had convinced most allergists that histamine played an insignificant role in allergy, except in skin reactions of urticarial type, in hay fever, and in the milder forms of childhood asthma, but this downgrading of histamine merely produced a void in the approaches to therapy of asthma. There was no shortage of suggestions for alternative theories or explanations but all of these lacked good data and some were not testable. They included:-

1. The presence of other mediators, such as bradykinin or factors present in inflammation.
2. Direct action of antigen upon antibody fixed to responding cells, with no mediator involved.

3. A fundamental difference between the human ('reaginic') reaction and the antibody-dependent reaction in animal models,
4. A genetic difference in the autonomic physiology of the lung or the reactivity of the smooth muscle in asthmatic subjects,
5. An intrinsic psychological trigger event.

Fortunately the antihistamines could be used as tools to remove the effects of histamine in experimental situations and so to unmask the presence of other substances having less spectacular pharmacological properties. Studies of this nature using the vascular perfusion fluid from organs or the bathing fluid from fragments of sensitised tissue taken before or after challenge with antigen, showed the presence of 'SRS', which had been discovered but not studied ten years earlier, and of tissue kallikrein, suggesting that bradykinin could be produced in vivo. These studies also excluded (in man and guinea-pig) acetylcholine and 5-hydroxytryptamine in the in vitro reaction, although in vivo both might well be acting, acetylcholine as a result of vagal innervation and 5-HT from platelets (Kellaway and Trethewie, 1940; Brocklehurst, 1956; Jonasson and Becker, 1966).

A small number of studies was possible, using surgically removed lung from well-documented human asthmatics, to exclude major differences in the active agents found after antigen challenge compared with those found when guinea-pig lung was used. The similarity was striking, and served to counter the argument that the animal model did not reflect the human reaginic reaction. The asthmatic tissue was also used to shown that the Schultz-Dale reaction was only partly inhibited by massive concentrations of anti-histamine, thus unmasking a non-histamine bronchoconstrictor agent active after challenge (Schild et al., 1951) – or alternatively suggesting totally 'intrinsic' histamine! A Schultz-Dale reaction is the contractile response of a sensitized smooth muscle preparation in vitro, when challenged with antigen: the tissue may be gut, uterus or rings from the larger or small airways etc. Isolated human airway smooth muscle was also used to construct a table of pharmacological reactivity, which could be compared with a similar table for the various laboratory species and so permit a reasonable extrapolation of laboratory studies to the clinical situation and vice versa. Human small bronchioles were shown to be moderately responsive to histamine and acetylcholine, but very responsive to SRS (either from human or guinea-pig lung) (Brocklehurst, 1962). They were poorly responsive to bradykinin and 5-HT. The airways of all other species tested then or since, failed to match the remarkable responsiveness to SRS-A which human tissue exhibits. The nearest laboratory animal was the guinea-pig, which had comparable responsiveness to histamine, rather less to SRS-A, notably more to 5-HT: no other animal studied was at all comparable except the rhesus monkey, which was no better than the guinea-pig and was less reliable.

The chemical identification of SRS-A ('A' for anaphylactic reactions) was not achieved for another thirty years. We now know that SRS-A is produced by 5-oxygenation of arachidonic acid leading to rearrangement, and a 6-thio-ether linkage with cysteine or a cysteine-containing short peptide, usually glutathione, and we now can study its effects directly since all the component products and related structures have been synthesized. Its full potency and importance have been directly shown, and it is evident that the interpretations of the early studies were close to the truth, including the observation that SRS-A enhances the response of smooth muscle to other agonist substances, such as histamine (see Hammarström, 1983; Griffin et al., 1983).

The discovery of 'SRS' during an anaphylactic reaction in lung is attributed to Kellaway and Trethewie (1940), but their experiment was the logical consequence of several previous discoveries. In 1936, Feldberg had shown that when the lung of a sensitised guinea-pig was isolated and perfused through the vascular system with physiological saline alone, the effluent perfusion fluid contained no substance able to contract the smooth muscle of the guinea-pig ileum or cause depression of the cat's blood pressure. However, within one or two minutes of adding antigen to the perfusing fluid, substantial amounts of histamine were present in the effluent. In 1938 Feldberg and Kellaway had done a technically similar experiment, showing that lung damage caused by the venom of the Australian Black Snake produced histamine, phospholipid, and an agent producing a slow but sustained contraction of guinea-pig ileum. The venom also produced a 'slow reacting substance' (SRS) when incubated with yolk of egg. World War II disrupted the partnership between Feldberg and Kellaway, so the study to see if 'SRS' was also produced by an antigen-antibody reaction in lung was done by Kellaway and Trethewie. Although they found that there was undoubtedly some difference between the time-course of the contraction produced by authentic histamine and that produced by lung perfusate, the histamine component was so strong that it masked any contribution that a second substance might have made to the early part of the contraction and prevented any detailed pharmacological study of the non-histamine component. In spite of determined attempts by Kellaway and Trethewie to separate the histamine and non-histamine responses by altering the pH of the bath (pCO_2) and by using tissues other than guinea-pig ileum, they were not successful. The study of SRS was resumed when potent and selective anti-histamine drugs were available, thus permitting a pharmacological profile to be established for SRS and some simple chemical studies to be done (Brocklehurst, 1960). It then became evident that SRS was indeed a substance different from any other so far described, and different from the active substance produced by egg yolk incubated with phospholipase from venom. Since many unidentified substances had been given the 'generic' title of 'SRS' it seemed desirable to distinguish the products of the anaphylactic reaction from these other unrelated materials and the suffix 'A' was proposed. It was quickly shown that SRS-A was produced by human asthmatic lung, and was very active in contracting the isolated muscle of small human bronchioles. Its role in human asthmatic attacks was now apparent and this was seen as the reason for the poor performance of antihistamine drugs. The surprising species-related differences in the airway response to SRS-A, with man the most susceptible, guinea-pig next and all others either weakly or very weakly responsive, was coupled with poor or negligible pharmacological responses to SRS-A from nearly all the usual smooth muscle and cardio-vascular preparations in common use. Indeed, assays of the low-potency, semi-purified SRS-A available were limited to the guinea-pig ileum and human bronchiole chain, thus making comparative pharmacology difficult and depriving the experimentalist of the ability to validate purification procedures by parallel quantitative assay.

6.3 The pharmacology and identification of SRS-A

The big advances in chemical separation and identification of biological materials in the period 1950–1970 were mainly in the field of proteins and were not relevant to SRS-A. It was known by 1960 that SRS-A was an atypical lipid, showing great affinity for charged surfaces and denatured protein, stable in both moderately acid and alkaline pH (Brocklehurst, 1962). However the purity was not adequate to justify analysis, and in any case the quantities available were too small even for the most sensitive analytical methods in use, although these amounted to many thousands of effective 'doses' in the in vitro assay using the guinea-pig ileum. During this period studies on SRS-A moved to the clinical and biological aspects such as the tissue source, the cell biology involved, and lessons for therapeutics. Austen and Orange and their group provided findings showing that the ratio of cyclic AMP to cyclic GMP in the mast cell modulated the release of histamine and the synthesis and release of SRS-A, (Austen, 1973 – review). Thus exposure of the sensitized lung tissue or mast cells to adrenaline or other β adrenergic agonists, caused a rise in cAMP, and a reduction in the yield of mediators when the tissue was challenged with antigen. Pretreatment with a phosphodi-esterase inhibitor served to sustain the rise of cAMP and further reduce the release process. By contrast, treatment with cholinergic agents raised the cGMP, and the amounts of mediator released were increased. The effects on SRS-A were more striking than those on histamine (Kaliner et al., 1972). Recent studies (Holgate et al., 1980; Krilis et al., 1983) have shown that the reduced response of the mast cell when cAMP is raised, is due to reduction in available protein kinase, which it normally activates. The sequence of intracellular effects set off by the membrane trigger includes an increase in cAMP which activates the protein kinase con-trolling the biochemical energy required for the events shown in Fig. 6.2. The whole process is attenuated if any link in the chain of events is already depleted by prolonged low-level activity.

Lichtenstein (1975) working mainly with blood basophils, (which are not entirely comparable to mast cells) extended the studies of Mongar and Schild (1953) to show that calcium acts at a second step in the release process, and that in the absence of calcium the first stage set off by IgE-antigen bridging will decay within a very few minutes and no further changes in the mast cell membrane will occur. The effect of reduced levels of extracellular calcium on this reaction is not seen until the levels are reduced well below those which would be physiologically acceptable. A role for intracellular protease/esterase activity was also established. Austen and Brocklehurst (1961) had shown by the use of inhibitors and alternative ester substrates, that a chymotrypsin-like enzyme was involved in histamine release, and in 1965 Becker had used DFP and related serine-phosphorylating agents to show that somewhat different serine-proteases were essential for the formation of histamine and SRS-A. Austen's group have studied isolated granules from rat mast cells and found a remarkable crystalline structure and a very high internal concentration of esterase pro-enzyme in the granule (Austen (review), 1980; Becker and Henson (review), 1973). The need for energy to drive the biochemical synthesis had been recognized for many years. The systematic studies of Mongar and Schild in the 1950s (see review, 1962) had shown that anaphylactic histamine release was much reduced by modest reductions in temperature, by lack of glucose, or treatment with inhibitors of oxidative metabolism. The use of the metabolic blocking agent deoxyglucose more recently, has provided direct proof that glucose is the source of the energy.

The studies on the essential role of calcium took on new interest when a substance was found in the supernatant from a mould culture which selectively enhanced the passage of ionic calcium across cell membranes. This ionophore substance, Lilly A23187, was used by Mongar's group (Foreman et al., 1973) to cause histamine release from mast cells and tissues, and by Bach and Brashler, (1974, 1978) to show that guinea-pig lung both from normal and sensitized animals would produce SRS-A when calcium ions from the bathing fluid entered

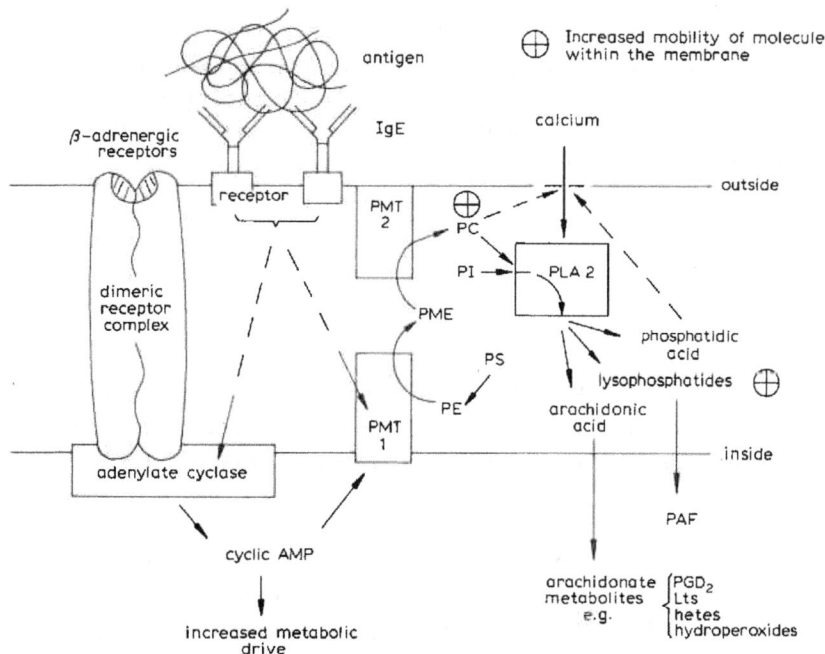

Figure 6.2: All the arrows in Fig. 6.2 indicate forward reactions, i.e. they initiate or promote the changes shown. The sequence of events is as follows:

1. IgE previously attached by the Fc region to specific receptors on the outer surface of the cell initiates membrane activity when two or more receptor sites are linked by antigen-bridging of the Fab regions of IgE molecules.

Phosphomethyl transferase I (PMT1) located at the inner surface of the membrane is activated and adds –CH_3 to phosphatidyl ethanolamine (PE), which is then fully methylated by phosphomethyl transferase 2 (PMT2) to give phosphatidyl choline (PC): fresh substrate is provided by phosphatidyl serine (PS).

2. Phosphatidyl choline increases fluidity of the membrane thus facilitating interaction between enzymes and substrates. It also permits entry of calcium, which activates phospholipase A_2 (PLA2).

3. Phospholipase A_2 splits phosphatidyl choline and phosphatidyl inositol (PI) to give arachidonic acid, lysophosphatides and phosphatidic acid. The lysophosphatides have 'detergent' characteristics and will further increase fluidity of the membrane. They also include the precursor of 'platelet activating factor' (PAF). Phosphatidic acid is a calcium ionophore.

4. Arachidonic acid is metabolized in the endoplasmic reticulum to give: prostaglandin D_2 (notably in human cells) and small amounts of other cyclo-oxygenase products: leukotrienes (LT) C_4, D_4 and E_4: LTB_4 and other HETEs (hydroxy aliphatic metabolites): hydroperoxides.

5. Concurrently with the initial methylation processes there is stimulation of the membrane-associated adenylate cyclase to give a brief burst of cyclic AMP, which activates PMT1 further, and generates protein kinase which enhances cell activity, but it also inhibits entry of calcium. Protein kinase is essential for the phosphorylation processes which constitute the energy sources for movement of granules prior to fusion and then for secretion of their contents: it is also necessary for the biosynthetic production of PGs, LTs. HETEs, PAF, eosinophil chemotactic factor (ECF-A) etc.

6. Prolonged increase of cyclic AMP, as caused by hormonal (catecholamine) stimulation of beta adrenergic receptors, or the use of drugs to inhibit the phosphodiesterase which normally destroys cyclic AMP, shuts down the whole reaction by inhibiting PMT1, by depleting protein kinase in the cell, and by shutting the 'calcium gates' in the membrane. Thus treatment with a beta adrenergic agonist and a phosphodiesterase antagonist will be synergistic and can severely attenuate all the events leading to mediator release.

the tissue. This new reagent permitted the experimenter to avoid the inevitable scatter in levels of sensitization, and start his reactions at a point near the end of the chain of membrane events worked out subsequently by Ishizaka and Axelrod (see Fig. 6.2) (see also Fewtrell and Metzger, 1981).

Parker saw the feasibility, at long last, of using cultured cells in large numbers and the calcium ionophore to produce SRS-A in quantities sufficient for analysis. He was fortunate in that the cell line he chose (the RBL1 rat-adapted mouse mastocyte tumour) produces much more SRS-A than the rat basophil that it is supposed to represent, and that in hindsight we know that an unusually large yield of relatively pure and authentic SRS-A was obtained from the particular sub-line which Parker had to hand. He was thus able to bring to bear his extensive knowledge of purification and analytical procedures to show that SRS-A was derived from arachidonate, and that it contained sulphur as Orange et al., had postulated in 1973, but additionally, he identified nitrogen, which had never been adequately shown, (Parker et al., 1979). The clear finding that arachidonate was the source of SRS-A, was of the utmost importance for future studies. Walker (1973) had observed that blockade of the cyclooxygenase pathway of arachidonate metabolism with indomethacin caused an increase in the yield of SRS-A from guinea-pig lung and had interpreted this as indicating a switch of arachidonate metabolism from the prostaglandins to SRS-A. However, direct studies using ^{14}C-labelled arachidonate and an anaphylactic reaction in guinea-pig lung had produced equivocal results because the amount of label incorporated in the tissue was very small, and any ^{14}C in the perfusate or supernatant fluid did not clearly parallel the biological activity of SRS-A after TLC or other methods of separation from unchanged arachidonic acid (Bach et al., 1978). The RBL1 cell not only gave large yields of SRS-A but it incorporated much more [^{14}C]arachidonate during preincubation, and so gave amounts of SRS-A which after rigorous purification showed radioactivity and biological activity in parallel.

This major break in the mystery surrounding the chemistry of SRS-A was speedily opened wide by others already extensively engaged in prostaglandin research, and thus familiar with sophisticated methods for the study of arachidonate products. Foremost among these was Samuelsson, who in 1979 reported preliminary findings that SRS-A was a 6-thio ether of 5-hydroxy eicosatrienoic acid with cysteine, and coined the name 'leukotriene' (Samuelsson et al., 1980). At practically the same time several other groups reported essentially similar findings by the use of somewhat different methods, and the novel nature of the structure of SRS-A was firmly established. It soon became clear that the thio-ether link formed in vivo was with the cysteine of glutathione which was plentiful in all tissues, although ultimately this tripeptide would lose both glutamic acid and glycine, to give the cysteinyl ether found by Samuelsson. We now know that SRS-A is composed principally of the 20C leukotrienes C_4 (glutathione), D_4 (cysteine-glycine), and E_4 (cysteine) (Bach et al., 1978; Morris et al., 1978, 1979; Murphy et al., 1979; Samuelsson et al., 1979). The structures and biological scheme have now appeared many times (e.g. reviewed by Hammarström, 1983). All these, and many related products of phospholipase action on membrane lipids, have been prepared synthetically and immuno-assays now exist, so an extensive data bank is being accumulated for their pharmacology, their role in normal and pathophysiology, and the dynamics of bio-chemical synthesis and metabolism. The view that SRS-A is responsible for much of the asthmatic bronchospasm has been validated by much more direct studies including human pharmacology (e.g. Griffin et al., 1983) and now awaits final confirmation by the clinical use of a drug able to prevent its formation or its actions. The use of pure material has permitted extensive quantitative studies on the pharmacology of SRS-A components, and has provided

Table 6.1: Pharmacological activity of the leukotrienes (SRS-A) relevant to the asthma syndrome.

	LTC$_4$	LTD$_4$	LTE$_4$
Contraction of large airways	+	+	±
small airways	+ +	+ +	+
Increased pulmonary vascular resistance	+ +	+ +	+
Increased mucus production	+	+	+
Reduced mucus clearance	+	+	+
Increased pulmonary vascular permeability	+	+ +	+
Reduced coronary blood flow	+	+	+
Cardiac function: decreased rate	+	+	+
decreased force	±	±	
Aggregation and margination of neutrophils	+	+	+
Release of secondary mediators e.g. thromboxane, histamine and 5-ht	+	+	+

Note: LTE is the end-product in the above series, and although it is of lower potency than LTC and LTD it is likely to be present in higher concentration and for a longer time. It is therefore believed to contribute at least as much activity in vivo as the other leukotrienes.

some surprises, such as the increase in mucus production in the airways, which was formerly attributed mainly to histamine and vagal activity, and the reduction of ciliary activity resulting in slower and incomplete clearance of mucus from the airways. Details of SRS-A pharmacology relevant to asthma are listed in Table 6.1. Many of these may well be secondary events due to the involvement of different types of cell and local release of other mediators.

The biosynthesis of leukotrienes requires the action of 5-lipoxygenase on arachidonic acid, in contrast to the family of prostaglandins and thromboxane which require cyclooxygenase activity. The lipoxygenase enzymes were recognized rather superficially before the leukotrienes were known, and 5-HETE (via 5-lipoxygenase) and 12-HETE (via 12-lipoxygenase) were known as chemotaxic agents. These enzymes are now under very active study, since effective blockers might be useful therapeutically, both for asthma and chronic inflammation, and at the very least would be tools permitting critical study of the role of their products in both normal and pathophysiology.

6.4 The central role of the mast cell

Mast cells were so called by Ehrlich who believed them to be 'well-fed' because they were packed with granules having strong affinity for basic histological stains. Their function remained a matter for conjecture for many years until it was recognized that they were especially plentiful in tissues rich in heparin, and their strategic location, notably around the points of bifurcation of small arterioles, would suggest a role in preventing coagulation of blood and deposition of leukocytes and platelets at these sites of potential damage.

The discovery that the mast cell granules contained histamine was reported by Riley and West in 1954, and Riley's review (1959) makes fascinating reading. At last the major source of tissue histamine was apparent, and the effects caused when it was released by non-immune means could be considered in a physiological context. Feldberg and Miles (1953) showed the distribution of cutaneous extravasation of plasma which occurred when the poly-cationic histamine-releaser 'substance 48/80' was given intravenously to an animal whose blood proteins had been dyed blue. Blue areas resulting from release of tissue histamine were most marked in sites subject to natural trauma, e.g. ears, snout, paws, nipples and in mucous membranes, and corresponded to the distribution of mast cells. Others showed that both anaphylactic and non-anaphylactic reactions resulted in loss of ability of the mast cell granules to take up stain, and in severe damage the granules were spilled from the cell and became unstainable. The appearance of histamine in the blood, or set free in vitro was correlated with the reduction of numbers of stainable mast cells in tissue (Mota and Humphrey, 1959). The biochemical dynamics of histamine sequestration in the mast cell granules and subsequent release, showed this to be a secretory process rather like that seen in exocrine glands and different from that of mediators at neuronal synapses. The existence of efficient means to inactivate any histamine which had reached the circulation and could thus cause unwanted systemic effects, was shown by Schayer (1959, 1963) and confirmed the view that histamine had a physiological local mediator function other than in gastric secretion. The inactivation was by conjugation or by oxidative deamination. Histamine is synthesized by mast cells from the amino acid histidine, and is immediately bound to the highly acidic polysaccharides of the granule. The enzyme responsible for the synthesis (histidine decarboxylase) shows remarkable adaptation, quickly expanding its activity to restore histamine which has been lost from the cell. Studies with labelled histidine have shown that virtually all the histamine in the granules has been synthesized de novo and no significant amount is acquired by reuptake. This is in sharp contrast to the platelet, which binds rather than synthesizes 5-HT, and the amines of the CNS where active presynaptic reuptake of transmitter is an essential aspect of sustained synaptic transmission. Thus, there is a large store of readily renewed histamine in normal tissue mast cells. The total amount is greatly increased in skin conditions where mast cells are abnormally abundant (e.g. urticaria pigmentosa), and mast cell tumours contain very large quantities (see reviews by Kahlson and Rosengren, 1972; Uvnäs, 1974).

The mast cell was obviously the source of the histamine released in allergic reactions, but what was the nature of the immunological stimulus for release? The Prausnitz-Kustner reaction and passive sensitization in vitro provided strong clues. There was evidently a special type of antibody which would attach very firmly to cells, rendering the tissue sensitive; when this tissue made contact with the specific antigen, an explosive release of histamine occurred in a few seconds, even after the tissue had been thoroughly washed. It was later shown that mast cells obtained by lavage of the peritoneal cavity of the rat and well washed would also release histamine (Keller, 1965) provided that the animal had previously been induced to produce a cell-fixing (homocytotropic) antibody to a given antigen.

The biochemical changes occurring during the release process in the mast cell will be discussed later (see Fig. 6.2).

6.5 IgE – the underlying cause of asthma

The first clear evidence that severely asthmatic subjects possessed circulating antibody of a type not found in non-asthmatics was reported by Prausnitz and Küstner in 1921, and the 'P-K test' came into wide clinical use to confirm the nature of the sensitizing allergen(s). If the serum of an asthmatic is injected intradermally into a non-asthmatic, and after 24 or 48 hours the appropriate antigen is injected at the same site, a local wheal and flare reaction occurs at the site, just as would have been seen if a small amount of antigen had been injected into the skin of the asthmatic donor of the serum. The response in the recipient is specific for whatever antigens the donor was sensitive to, and no response is ever found with the serum of non-asthmatic persons. It was many years before any comparable reaction was produced in animals or by laboratory procedures (see review by Ovary, 1958). It was evident that an unusual type of antibody was present, which could attach itself to the tissue at the injection site for several days, and produce a histamine-like reaction when challenged with a matching antigen. It was christened 'reagin' or 'reaginic antibody', and its existence cast doubt on the clinical relevance of all the studies in animals, in spite of the fact that normal guinea-pigs could be passively sensitized by the i.v. administration of serum from a sensitized animal, and undergo anaphylactic shock when subsequently challenged with antigen and that isolated tissues could be passively sensitized by soaking in antibody-containing serum at room temperature.

It was not until 1960 that methods of separating proteins and identifying them by their physical characteristics had been developed sufficiently to enable the homocytotropic antibody responsible for asthma to be purified and studied. It was called IgE (immunoglobulin type E) and was found to have a different buoyant density from the other Igs, and to have a high anionic charge due to greater carbohydrate content. The reason for so much difficulty in identifying IgE also became clear: it was present in minute amounts in serum, and was remarkably potent in rendering tissue sensitive. Because such small amounts were available, there was yet more delay in studies on its structure and composition, and of course on the mode and dynamics of attachment to mast cells. When highly sensitive assays became available (radioimmunoassay and later the enzyme-linked immunoassay), it was found that IgE was present in the blood of all birds and higher animals, in remarkably similar concentration, except in allergic individuals where the level was sharply raised, sometimes to as much as 100-fold that in normal subjects. In all species studied there was an abnormally high level of IgE in those animals which were chronically infested with intestinal parasites. The tissues of these individuals reacted to worm antigens, and often to unrelated antigens also. High IgE levels and resulting hypersensitivity could be induced by artificial infection with worms, but it could also be induced by sensitization procedures in which the antigen was presented in an unusual physical state (e.g. adsorbed on aluminium hydroxide gel) or in conjunction with certain adjuvant toxins (e.g. *B. pertussis),* or when the body was subjected to particular stresses so that the corticosteroid levels were temporarily deranged (Selye, 1950). Much of the mystery surrounding the peculiar immunological reactivity of the asthmatic subject was thus swept away, and the following picture emerged. A prerequisite for the allergy able to cause asthma was an abnormal level of circulating IgE. Worm infestations could cause this, so genetic factors were not of dominant importance. Incidentally, the IgE-triggered local tissue response to worm antigens was likely to limit or even reduce the worm burden, thus identifying the first useful role for IgE. Adjuvants of viral or microbial origin present at the time of exposure to antigen would enhance the production of IgE specific for that antigen, the effect being increased by stress caused by the infectious illness. This degree of knowledge permitted the production of greater amounts of IgE specific for a given artificial (haptenic) antigen, so that binding studies on tissue could be done. Later, production of IgE by hybrido-mas (Milstein et al., 1980), permitted the production of uniform (monoclonal) IgE in lots of many milligrams, so that all work on binding to cells could be strictly quantitative (Katz, 1980; Katz et al., 1983; Kishimoto et al., 1983).

Ishizaka (Ishizaka et al., 1970; Ishizaka K., 1976, 1983) made the crucial observation that mast cells adapt to the level of IgE in their environment, so that the actual number of receptors ($Ig\varepsilon R$) on each mast cell increases markedly when the level of IgE bathing the cell is raised, whereas the number of $Ig\varepsilon R$ decreases when the bathing IgE concentration is lowered. In addition, some of the IgE in plasma was not free to bind to tissue, since it appeared to have its attachment site occupied by a molecule having a structure similar to $Ig\varepsilon R$ which was present in the plasma. In asthmatics the high plasma IgE totally overwhelmed the plasma binding fac-tors in plasma and increased the density of $Ig\varepsilon R$ on mast cell membranes, so that much more IgE was bound per cell. The ability of the mast cell to be triggered by antigen was enhanced even more than this increase in attached IgE would suggest, because triggering involves cross-linking of two IgE molecules by the antigen (see Fig. 6.1). The Ishizakas (Ishizaka, T. et al., 1972, Ishizaka, K. et al., 1983) had shown that monovalent antigens (e.g. linkage of a single hapten molecule to a carrier protein) would prevent subsequent triggering of the mast cell by a polyvalent antigen bearing the same antigenic structures. They had also shown that IgG antibody against the Fc part of the IgE molecule could trigger the mast cell to release and manufacture mediator substances. The latter finding proves that linkage is all that is needed, since the two Fab 'arms' of the IgG antibody can react in no other way than to bridge IgE molecules. If the trigger is subthreshold it will quickly decay. It follows that a raised density of IgE will greatly increase the likelihood of multiple bridging almost immediately on contact with antigen, and hence of exceeding the threshold for triggering. Conversely, any procedure which lessens the chances for bridging will result in a disproportionately great reduction in the likelihood of the mast cell being triggered. Future developments in actually curing asthmatics will utilize this fundamental knowledge.

The factors which lead to the raised synthesis of IgE during helminth infestation in rats and which differentiate high-responder mice from low-responder strains when artificially induced to produce IgE to a specific antigen, have been studied extensively in the laboratories of the Ishizakas and of Katz (K. Ishizaka, 1980; Katz, 1980; Katz et al., 1983). A suppressive factor (SF;SFA) and an enhancing factor (PF;EFA) have been identified as products of T lymphocytes appropriately stimulated. Both substances are of about 16000 daltons and attach to IgE expressed on antigen-committed B cells which are thus either inhibited or induced to mature into IgE-producing plasma cells. The two substances have a closely similar structure, but PF is mannose-rich and shows affinity for lentil lectin and concanavallin A (Con A), whereas SF does not have these sugar-related characteristics. However, both can be produced in vitro from rat T lymphocytes bearing the W3/25 surface marker if activated by Con A for 3 days and then exposed to IgE for 1 day, the only difference is the level of Con A used – 1 μg/ml produces SF and 10 μg/ml gives PF. Furthermore PF production can be switched to SF in this in vitro system at day 3, by the use of the antibiotic tunicamycin which suppresses glycosylation (Ishizaka, K. et al., 1983).

Glucocorticoids influence the balance between PF and SF if given 12 hours before IgE. The increase in SF seen with corticosteroids has been attributed to increased biosynthesis of lipomodulin and resultant inhibition of PLA_2 because mellitin or anti-lipomodulin antibody, both of which lead to increased PLA_2 activity, produce an increase in PF. The well known procedure of producing IgG or IgE selectively by using different adjuvants correlates with the production of SF by complete Freund's adjuvant, and of PF by *B. pertussis* or aluminium hydroxide gel. This is now ascribed to selective mitogenic effects on different sub-sets of T lymphocytes which give either PF, and thus stimulate IgE-committed B cells to mature to IgE-producing lymphocytes, or SF which stimulates activity in suppressor T lymphocytes. (Ishizaka, T., 1983; Katz, 1980). There is also an IgE-binding factor in plasma, which is either deficient or already occupied by IgE in asthmatics. Preliminary findings suggest that it has much in common with the IgE receptor on mast cells and studies on its structure and control are ongoing (Ishizaka, K. et al., 1983).

Much was known about the biochemical reactions of mast cells leading to histamine release and arachidonate metabolism before the details of the trigger were known (Austen, reviews, 1974, 1979; Lewis et al., 1974, 1975) but the sequence of the lipid metabolism in the plasma membrane following the trigger brought all these findings together (Hirata and Axelrod, 1980; Gemsa et al., 1982).

The diversity of the active substances released or synthesized is worthy of special note. Histamine is preformed and released from stores, prostaglandin D_2 is synthesized via the cyclo-oxygenase pathway, leukotrienes C4, D4 and E_4 are synthesized via the 5-lipoxygenase pathway as is the di-HETE leukotriene B_4, PAF is produced by acetylation, ECF-A is a small peptide produced by a serine esterase. The only common features are those preceding the products of PLA2 activity, and all later synthetic or pharmacologic events are so varied that therapeutic measures must employ a battery of drugs to counteract them. Substances currently available are non-specific, or effective in only a few of the above reactions.

The 'late phase' of an asthma attack does not always occur but is frequently severe and often necessitates corticosteroid therapy. It is attributed to an inflammatory condition resulting from the various chemotactic factors, vascular permeability and vasomotor agents, and aggregatory or 'releaser' substances, coming directly from the mast cell or from secondary events in other cells influenced by mast cell products (Casale and Kaliner, 1983; Wasserman, 1983). If the initial phase of the asthma attack is aborted – e.g. by prompt use of a beta adrenergic agent or cromoglycate – the late phase never develops (Howell and Altounyan, 1969; Taylor et al., 1974; Brogden et al., 1974; Morley et al., 1983). At present PGD_2, PAF, LTB_4 and the HETEs seem to be the most important agents. Both PGD_2 and LTB_4 have been shown to set up a local indurated inflammatory response, and PAF has similar properties. All will undoubtedly re-cruit other agents from other types of cell (Ford-Hutchinson et al., 1980; Drazen et al., 1980; Williams and Piper, 1980; Lewis and Austen, 1981; Lefort et al., 1982; Oertel and Kaliner, 1981; Parker et al., 1980; Lewis et al., 1982).

The eosinophilia associated with helminth infections and allergies, and the notable accumulation of eosinophils at the site of an 'immediate-type' allergic reaction remained simply as an observation for many years. It prompted Kay and Austen (1971) to test the possibility that the mast cell released a factor chemotactic for eosinophils at the same time as the other mediators of anaphylaxis, and this they found to be so. They also knew that arylsulphatase (from molluscs) inactivated SRS-A, and that eosinophils contained arylsulphatase, so they set up a study to see if the influx of eosinophils in man might provide a means of terminating the pharmacological activity of SRS-A, (see Wasserman, 1979, review). This process is no longer regarded as a major route of inactivation, but wider roles for the eosinophil have emerged. These include: oxidative deamination of histamine; destruction of PAF by phospholipase D; degradation of many polypeptides and nucleotides (see Goetzl and Austen, 1977), also direct antibody dependent cytotoxicity against parasites involving IgE and the eosinophil in both free radical and basic protein reactions (Capron et al., 1980).

A recent addition to the list of putative mediators of asthma is PAF (1-*O*-alkyl-2-acetylglycerophosphocholine:PAF-acether; AGEPC). The examples most studied are the natural structures with alkyl chains of 16 and 18C at the 1 position, but other lengths and some unsaturated structures are active as is substitution of propionyl for the 'natural' acetyl in position 2. 'PAF' in vivo is thus regarded as a group of active substances related to plasmalogens. It was first reported as a substance released from challenged guinea-pig lung, which was a very potent aggregator of platelets (Benveniste, Henson and Cochrane, 1972). It is now known that it is released in larger amounts from macrophages, and has many pharmacological activities, such as might be expected from a substance able to combine with cell-membranes and having 'detergent' characteristics. These include modest contractile activity on the isolated human parenchymal strip in vitro, which also shows marked tachyphylaxis and very marked increases in local vascular permeability. As its structure would suggest, it is destroyed by phospholipases A, C and D, but additionally, activated macrophages can destroy it by de-acylation in a reversible reaction. In vitro, RBL1 cells and human or rabbit basophils produce and release PAF but rat and human mast cells do not. It is also produced by macrophages, eosinophils and platelets. Bone marrow-derived 'mucosal type' mouse mast cells, passively sensitized and challenged, release both PAF and 5-lipoxygenase projects in about equal amounts in a few minutes. These cells are regarded as equivalent to mast cells of the mucosa of the gut and lung. Platelets release their contents under the influence of PAF, which initiates a dual self-amplifying system in which phospholipase C attacks phosphatidyl inositol to yield diacyl glycerol and phosphatidic acid. These both activate phospholipase A_2, the former via a protein kinase, and the latter by acting as a calcium ionophore, thus generating more PAF and arachidonate products including TxA_2 and 12-HETE. (Benveniste et al., 1972; Pinckard et al., 1983; Arnoux et al., 1982).

In the lung, the release of PAF from sensitized cells when challenged, or by alveolar macrophages when stimulated by phagocytosis, or from other cells in which phospholipases have been activated, will theoretically lead to secondary release or production of autacoids. The platelets are the most sensitive system, and will release thromboxane, 5-HT, ADP and 12-HETE. Macrophages and polymorphs have much higher thresholds for stimulation, but will release 5-lipoxygenase products of the leukotriene and HETE groups. When given intradermally, PAF causes pain and itching and later there is induration with influx of leukocytes typical of immune-based inflammation. It is thus likely that PAF, in conjunction with LTB_4 and other chemotactic factors from arachidonic acid and from polymorphonuclear neutrophils, contributes to the late phase of the asthma attack. There is close similarity between the underlying biochemistry of PAF and the production of SRS-A from sensitized tissue; both require activation of phospholipase and are calcium dependent, and this may encourage attempts to use inhibitors of phospholipases as therapeutic agents.

6.6 The ebb and flow of the 'Humoral theory'

The observation that the symptoms of anaphylactic shock and anaphylatoxin shock produced by i.v. injection were remarkably similar for animals of a given species, whereas the differences between species were striking, formed the basis for the 'humoral theory' of anaphylaxis (Friedberger, 1910). However the early studies with 'anaphylatoxins' generated confusion rather then elucidation, because so little was known about the blood plasma, and by 1920 the humoral theory had given way to the histamine theory (Dale, 1920).

Anaphylatoxin activity can be produced in plasma or serum by shaking it with agar, antigen-antibody precipitate, kaolin, starch, dead bacteria or yeast, or chloroform: these procedures seem to have little in common. The activity decays slowly over several hours. Proteolytic activity increases sharply, and split products of plasma proteins accumulate in the activated serum. Since intravenous injection of saliva (enzymes) or peptone (pepsin digest of fibrin) produced shock syndromes superficially similar to anaphylatoxin given intravenously, the existence of 'anaphylatoxin' as a recognizable substance seemed unlikely. Now that a great deal is known about the complexities of blood chemistry, such as the cascades of enzyme activation in the clotting system, the complement system, and the kinin system, two substances having the properties of 'anaphylatoxin' have emerged. These are C3a and C5a of the complement system. Are they likely to be involved in asthma? (see Vogt, 1974 review; Müller-Eberhard, 1977 and 1980).

The most well known property of complement activation is destruction of 'target' cells to which antibody has been made. When IgG or IgM antibody reacts with its matching antigen on the cell surface either in vitro or in vivo, complement in the extra-cellular fluid is activated and the cascade reaction goes to completion producing a 'lytic complex' of the last 5 complement components. This complex extends right through the cell membrane and forms a pore which destroys the osmotic and ionic gradients across the cell membrane, with rapid swelling and loss of the cell contents. The other classes of immune globulin are not effective activators of complement (see also pp. 608, 609).

Prior to 1970 methods in protein chemistry were not adequate to unravel the closely interrelated proenzymes, enzymes and active fragments of the complement system, much less to perform rational pharmacology. In a remarkably short time all that changed, and many potential roles of complement were apparent (Vogt, 1974). In addition, a non-immune mechanism for activation of complement had been mapped. This was the 'alternative pathway', which Pillemer had called the 'properdin' route, on the basis of non-specific bacterial lysis and zymosan activation of plasma, many years earlier (see Müller-Eberhard, 1977). This system skipped the early reactions of the cascade and activated the system at C3, it was thus less restricted than the 'classical pathway' which required antigen-antibody recognition to activate it. The properdin system could recognize that certain substances, such as the cell walls of bacteria or viruses, were foreign, and attack them without the delay involved in making specific antibody. It could be easily activated artificially, (e.g. by zymosan), to generate 'anaphylatoxin' activity in a relatively simple system, and this activity was located in the C3a and C5a products of the reaction (Cochrane and Müller-Eberhard, 1968). Although these reagents have never seemed likely to play any major role in asthma they may well contribute to the 'late phase' of the attack, especially when the asthma is complicated by infection and IgG reactions as in some bronchitic subjects. The reasons are apparent when the whole picture is considered. First, C3 activation can result from the products of tissue damage, especially the release of proteolytic enzymes, and C3 is present everywhere in substantial amounts. Next, C5a causes release of histamine and a little SRS-A or a similar substance from sliced lung: both C3a and C5a are chemotaxins for polymorphonuclear neutrophils and macrophages and they also increase vascular permeability. Finally the anaphylatoxins are also products of the classical pathway, thus IgG reacting with antigen in mucous membranes or tissue spaces will generate an inflammatory reaction such as is now recognised in 'late-phase' asthma. At present, the dynamics of anaphylatoxin production and catabolism are obscure, and although the very rapid tachyphylaxis seen in the assay on guinea-pig ileum is not evident in vascular permeability reactions, it is very marked when C5a causes mediator release in chopped lung. If this tachyphylaxis is a general phenomemon, the effects of the anaphylatoxins must be extremely brief and much of the pharmacological activity attributed to them must be ascribed to the agents which they release.

Another interesting product of the plasma protein systems which remains enigmatic with respect to asthma, is bradykinin. This substance is a basic peptide comprised of 9 amino acids which is split from a specific precursor by an arginine esterase called kallikrein. The reaction is linked to the clotting system, since the pro-enzyme, prekallikrein is converted to the enzyme by activated Hageman factor and thus as a result of contact between plasma and any cationic charged surface such as glass, kaolin or collagen, or by plasminogen activator. In plasma, Hageman factor is loosely complexed with kininogen from which bradykinin is generated, but this complex is unlikely to leave the bloodstream unless the vessels are unusually permeable as a consequence of an ongoing inflammatory reaction or local production of arachidonate metabolites. Enzymes released from mast cells or lung during anaphylactic reactions in vitro will activate prekallikrein and thus generate bradykinin when added to kininogen (Jonasson and Becker, 1966). The serine protease of the mast cell granules (Austen, 1980) is probably responsible, but many other intracellular or secreted enzymes (e.g. in saliva) are highly active in producing kinin, so the precise identity of the enzyme is irrelevant to its role in asthma.

The pharmacology of bradykinin is extensive. Given intravenously as a bolus it causes vasodilation with a rapid but brief fall in arterial pressure. Very small amounts given intradermally cause increased vascular permeability; therefore, if it is continuously generated in vivo, it could lead to haemoconcentration, and locally it would produce oedema of mucous membranes or of loose connective tissue (as in the orbit). Although it relaxes vascular smooth muscle, it contracts the smooth muscle of the gut, uterus and lung, but human lung gives relatively insignificant responses. When applied to exposed sensory nerve endings (as in skin stripped of the stratum corneum) it causes burning pain. The severity of the pain is greatly amplified if PGE is also present, thus bradykinin is likely to contribute to much of the pain resulting from burns and many other conditions involving inflammation in which both kinins and prostaglandins are produced. In lung it may be important in the initiation of the vagal reflex to irritants and to other agents able to induce ion fluxes across the membrane of nerve-endings. Mucus production in the airways is enhanced by bradykinin, but whether this effect is direct or consequent upon nerve stimulation is not known. The ability of bradykinin, and its close relatives plasma kinins 10 and 11, to contribute to many of the features of the asthma attack is thus beyond question, but the actual contribution is hard to assess. It is difficult to avoid activating the kiningenerating process artificially, when attempting to study it, since any tissue manipulation and even the act of drawing blood will do this. Bradykinin is quickly destroyed in blood and in all organs studied (see Pisano and Austen, 1976; Haberland and McConn, 1979). Kallikrein undoubtedly has a longer half life than bradykinin but it is in a dynamic state and has not yet been adequately studied. However, there is enough kininogen readily accessible to kallikrein in the plasma to generate effective levels of bradykinin in a given organ for several hours at least, and measurable falls in kininogen have been recorded during prolonged systemic anaphylactic reactions. Furthermore the kallikrein inhibitor trasylol (aprotinin) has been shown to diminish those symptoms of anaphylactic shock which resist blockade of all other putative mediators for which inhibitors exist. It therefore seems reasonable to assume that although bradykinin may have little direct effect on the smooth muscle of human lung it does stimulate mucus secretion from goblet cells and increase oedema of the bronchial and upper respiratory tract mucosae, and to postulate that it will amplify vagal reflex activity during asthma. It has recently been cited as the cause of sneezing (Proud et al., 1983). The close association between Hageman factor (HF) and high molecular weight kininogen, and the explosive amplification of kallikrein activity resulting from the reciprocal activation of prekallikrein by active HF and of HF by kallikrein suggests runaway production of bradykinin. Fortunately the system is held in check by an inhibitor of both enzymes: this is the complement-controlling plasma factor 'C1 inhibitor' (Kaplan, 1983).

6.7 Treatment of the asthmatic patient

The widespread and chronic nature of asthma has been a serious medical problem for centuries, but its obscure initiation and the very varied range of agents associated with the onset of dyspnoea has restricted most clinical endeavours to palliative treatment of the 'end-effects' until very recent times. The disease has also provided a fruitful environment for quacks as well as honest but often misguided guesswork, but out of all these trials a few useful agents emerged long before the reasons for the therapeutic effect could be established.

An early example of these fortuitously identified useful agents is stramonium, which was smoked in India to relieve asthma at least 500 years ago. Stramonium contains atropine which blocks the muscarinic receptors for acetylcholine; the reasons for a therapeutic effect are evident from Fig. 6.3. Another example is the herb Ma Huang, used for many ailments by Chinese physicians since antiquity. Its active principle is the alkaloid ephedrine, which is a long lasting and safe sympathomimetic (adrenaline-like drug) introduced into Western medicine about 1920 (Chen and Schmidt, 1926). Fig. 6.3 shows the relevance of such treatment, which was not only to reduce bronchoconstriction but also to reduce the amounts of

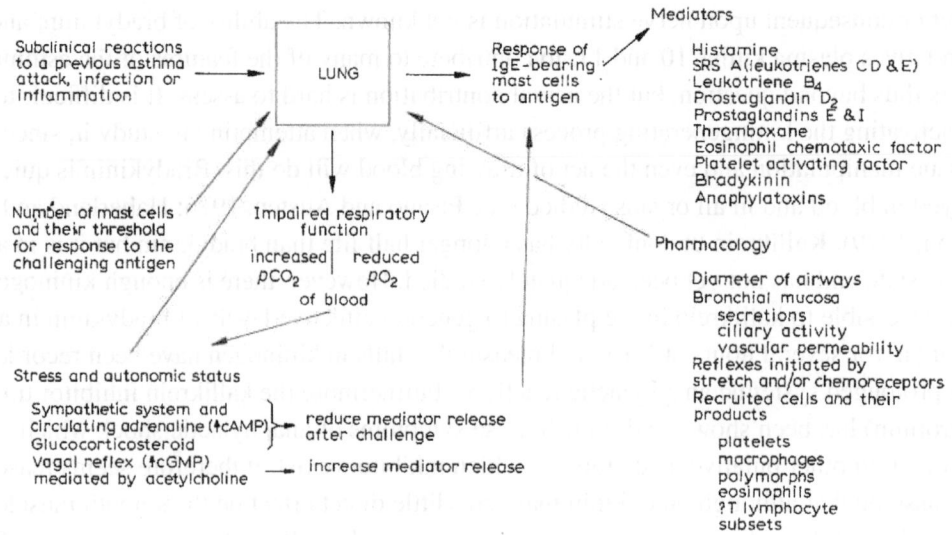

Figure 6.3

Physiological and pharmacological factors mediating or modulating changes in lung function in the asthmatic subject.

mediator produced by a given challenge. Morphine was once popular to allay the anguish of the asthma attack, but when it was realised that it also blunted respiratory drive, the risk of using it in a condition characterized by hypoxia and hypercapnia was unacceptable. A crude adrenal extract was used to reverse status asthmaticus as early as 1900, and it became 'standard treatment' when the active amine adrenaline (epinephrine) was available in crystalline form and could be given parenterally (Bullowa and Kaplan, 1903). Administration by inhalation to relieve or abort asthma attacks of a less serious nature was very widely prescribed when suitable hand-held 'nebulizer' sprays became available (see Graezer and Rowe, 1935). Adrenaline is rapidly destroyed by oxidation in air and light, and has a very short life in vivo, so it has now been replaced by more stable synthetic congeners.

In the absence of any guidance concerning the underlying causes of the dyspnoea during the asthma attack, the clinician could only seek to reverse changes in the airways which were obvious in the clinic or seen post mortem. Many mild bronchodilators of herbal origin were recognized and used over 100 years ago, and their active agents have been the starting point for drug developparent ment in recent times. Two such are tea and khellin. A popular asthma cure in England in the early 1900s consisted of tea and stramonium sprinkled with a solution of potassium nitrate and dried. This was allowed to smoulder and the drug-laden fumes inhaled. The nitrate mainly assisted smooth combustion, but may also have assisted in relaxation of the airways, but the tea provided caffeine which acts indirectly to dilate the airways, and the stramonium contains atropine which prevents any effects of the vagus nerve on the lung, and so reduces the secretion of mucus as well as reversing contraction of the smooth muscle of the bronchial tree. Caffeine (trimethylxanthine) and several related purine alkaloids are inhibitors of the intracellular enzyme phosphodiesterase which inactivates cylic AMP (adenosine monophosphate), the substance which stimulates metabolic activity in the cell. The effect of inhibiting phosphodiesterase will vary with the type of cell in which the cAMP is allowed to rise; thus it will increase the heart rate and stimulate intestinal motility, but will relax the muscle of the lung, and reduce the amounts of mediator substances acting in the lung, by making the mast cell less reactive to challenge (see Fig. 6.3). Theophylline and theobromine are isomeric forms of dimethylxanthine and have effects similar to those of caffeine, but having longer duration of action and somewhat different distribution in the body. Theophylline is currently by far the most widely prescribed treatment for asthma, and has prophylactic as well as therapeutic activity: the reasons will be apparent from Fig. 6.3. Nevertheless it is not an ideal drug, since its actions are far too general, and it is necessary to maintain the tissue concentration within a narrow range to derive adequate benefit without unacceptable unwanted effects.

Whereas the selection of the preferred member of the xanthines has provided no great surprises or excitement, the study of derivatives of khellin had quite unexpected and far reaching significance, and led to the novel drug cromoglycate, and later to the pharmacological 'tool' FPL55712. Khellin is a vasodilator and smooth muscle relaxant substance found in the seeds of an umbelliferous plant and long used medicinally in central Europe. Its unusual chromone structure was taken as the basis for a series of synthetic products to be tested for bronchodilator activity. Since the main bronchodilator application envisaged was in asthma, the tests used included the ability to antagonise the action of SRS-A and to prevent the contraction of isolated sensitized guinea-pig ileum when challenged with antigen. Some of the synthetic products tested showed weak antagonistic activity in these tests, and since no pharmacological antagonist of SRS-A was known at the time (mid 1960s), sufficient interest was generated to extend the series and for a dedicated asthmatic physician (R. Altounyan) to conduct antigen provocation tests on himself. He found that the acidic chromone compound now called disodium cromoglycate had useful antiasthmatic activity, apparently without any unwanted effects, and of a kind quite unlike those of any drugs in use. Although the way(s) in which cromoglycate benefits the 40% of asthmatics who use it are not properly understood even now, this drug has provided a new dimension to the treatment of asthma. It has weak anti SRS-A activity on isolated smooth muscle, and weak ability to inhibit phosphodiesterase, but its most beneficial property is modest ability to 'stabilize' the mast cell membrane. Its structure gives no hint of how this occurs, and other well known membrane stabilisers such as the tricyclic antidepressants and the phenothiazines have not found similar application in asthma. Chromoglycate benefits many asthmatics, by aborting or blunting the attack if taken early, and it has the added advantage of greatly reducing the incidence of late-phase dyspnoea, (Brogden, Speight and Avery, 1974). Perhaps the membrane 'stabilization' includes attenuation of the methylation or phospholipase events which constitute the membrane trigger in IgE-dependent reactions, since the production of PAF and other active lipids is reduced. Considerable advantage must result from rapid availability of the drug in the lung at the onset of an asthma attack, especially when the treatment is aimed at an early stage of the reaction sequence. Cromoglycate is not absorbed orally and is rapidly cleared from the blood by the kidney. The dose is therefore taken by inhalation of suspended minute solid particles. This gives the benefits of speed to the site of action and minimal exposure of other organs, but is regarded as rather cumbersome and variable. A vast amount of effort has failed to discover any substance having comparable activity whilst being acceptable orally, but this work has produced an antagonist of 'SRS-A' (leukotrienes C, D & E) which is now used as a tool to identify activity due to these agents in small impure samples of biological material or within tissues, where other methods of identification are not practicable. Unfortunately this substance (FPL 55712) cannot be used in man (Augstein et al., 1973; Chand review, 1979; Sheard et al., 1977).

A very important advance in the treatment of asthma came with the availability of glucocorticosteroids in the mid 1950s, (Rose and McGarry, 1959). The naturally occurring steroids cortisone and hydrocortisone had been obtained from the suprarenal cortex and shown to be powerful antiinflammatory agents in 'connective tissue' diseases such as arthritis and chronic inflammatory conditions of the intestine or skin, and autoimmune states. An intensive search for a plentiful steroid suitable for synthetic modification was soon successful and produced much more potent drugs including some with a more useful spectrum of activity. Their value in asthma was quickly realised from clinical experience in persons being treated for inflammatory conditions, and they were shown to be life-saving in severe asthmatic attacks in which the sympathomimetic and phosphodiesterase inhibitor drugs were having no effect. However, there were severe limitations to their use which were not immediately recognized. They are hormones, and in normal physiology will be kept in equilibrium with related hormones, and with the requirements of tissues for special function. When supplied in excess by artificial means the benefits of damping down inflammation are offset (depending on the condition and the patient) by such changes as poor electrolyte balance and water retention, reduced tissue growth and repair (especially in tissue requiring rapid renewal or restoration and in young persons), interference in glucose metabolism (diabetogenic), suppression of sex hormones, and reduction of adrenal function. Low dose prophylactic treatment is currently employed in very severe asthmatics, but large doses are strictly reserved for emergencies. The wide range of possible reasons for the striking benefit provided by glucocorticoids in asthma (such as prednisolone given orally or parenterally) provided plenty of speculation concerning their main mode(s) of action, but the delay of 1 hour or more before benefit was seen after i.v. injection suggested a change in cell metabolism, rather than any alteration in the levels of immune globulin which would take longer to be seen, or changes in vascular permeability which take only a short time. Some effects which would be expected after 1 hour would be raised levels of blood glucose and reduced numbers of circulating leukocytes, either of which could attenuate the asthma attack. Present views are based on the recent finding that corticosteroids are potent inhibitors of phospholipase (see Chapt. 10, Part 1), and thus have the ability to attenuate the response of the mast cell to the IgE-antigen trigger at a stage which precedes the appearance of mediators (see Fig. 6.2) and thus approximates the ideal treatment. Latency of at least 1 hour would seem to represent the time taken for the drug to pass from the bloodstream to the mast cell (or other cells involved such as macrophages and polymorphonuclear leucocytes in close proximity to the mast cells) and then be incorporated in the cell membrane. Alternatively the enzymes of the mast cell and macrophage etc. may be partly depleted by the reduction in protein synthesis under the influence of the glucocorticoids. According to T. Ishizaka (1983) activation of PLA_2 causes an increase in the factor potentiating production of IgE (PF) and a corresponding decrease in the suppressing factor (SF). Conversely the inhibition of PLA_2, which would result from an increase of lipomodulin under the influence of glucocorticoid treatment would result in a reduction in the maturation of B cells producing IgE. This indirect and slow effect of the corticosteroids would validate their use prophylactically, but could not account for the effect seen in a few hours. In any case, another major pharmacological parameter has emerged, and new approaches in the search for a steroid with more selective activity in asthma are now indicated. The problem of avoiding systemic effects and shortening the latent period for action was largely overcome by inhalation of a mist of a soluble form of a glucocorticoid (e.g. betamethasone succinate). Unfortunately there are problems of employing the principle of 'delivery to the site of action' in this instance because application of glucocorticoids to mucous membranes suppresses the local inflammatory reaction and thus weakens the ability of the tissue to resist infection and penetration by saphrophytes.

The excessive secretion of tenaceous mucus from the bronchial mucosa during an attack of asthma undoubtedly contributes to the restriction of air flow through the airways. Further-more patients dying after a long period of status asthmaticus often have plugs of firm mucus which can act as valves at the branching points in the bronchial tree, and thus prevent infla-tion of parts of the lung. Although atropine (stramonium, belladonna) reduces the volume of secretions, it tends to make them even more tenaceous and so the balance of advantage is questionable. Potassium iodide given orally increases the volume of bronchial secretion, but makes it more fluid and thus easier for the cilia of the mucosal epithelial cells to move it towards the trachea and then be expectorated or swallowed. Balsams (dried plant exudates) containing volatile aromatic esters such as those of cinnamic and benzoic acids, have been used in lozenges and steam kettles to increase the secretions by their mild irritant action. Enzymes including trypsin, and non-ionic surfactants have been given by inhalation of a spray to make the mucus more fluid or less sticky, but the benefit has not been striking.

Treatments now relegated to history, and often not involving drugs, were legion, but change of job or house, or movement to a different climate were recognised as frequently being effective. Among the more bizarre measures to reduce the frequency or severity of asthma attacks, was a heat-treatment in which the subject spent several hours in a room through which hot moist air was passed. Long after this treatment fell into disuse, the principle was validated by Mongar and Schild (1957) who found that isolated sensitized tissue held at 41°C for 1 hour lost its hypersensitivity. Similarly, sensitized guinea-pigs immersed in a water bath at 41 to 42°C for 1 hour became resistant to challenge with antigen for a period of 2 or 3 days.

The original rationale for injecting minute doses of the known specific allergens in order to diminish the response to natural exposure to these allergens seems to be obscure, but the principle is strongly suggestive of homeopathic medicine. It was introduced in 1903. After the procedure had been 'perfected' as far as a 'trial and error' approach would allow, and with the variations to be expected from a blind approach to therapy, about 50% of cases experienced some benefit with about 20% much improved for periods of up to two years. Typically the injections were given weekly in escalating doses which ideally remain below the response threshold of the subject. The procedure was continued in successful cases until doses of many micrograms of allergen were tolerated. The procedure was called 'hyposensitization' by Cooke (1922) when it was already in wide use, and the main problems were the availability of reliable antigens and correct identification of those responsible for the hypersensitive state. It was believed then, and for over 40 years, that the procedure produced 'blocking' (non-reaginic) antibody and diminished the production of reagin. Nowadays, these beliefs can be tested (see Lichtenstein et al., 1983), furthermore the appropriate sub-threshold dose of antigen at any stage in the course of injections can be estimated by assaying the specific antibody of the IgE (reagin) and IgG (blocking) isotypes in the blood. IgE levels actually show little change and sometimes rise, and the benefit of 'hyposensitization' is now attributed to the great increase of circulating polyvalent IgG and secreted IgA which will combine harmlessly with the antigen in the blood or on the surface of mucous membranes and so prevent significant amounts of it from reaching the IgE fixed to tissues.

Research on asthma has been reminiscent of the battle between Hercules and the Hydra of Lerna. Most of the increases in knowledge have lead to the recognition of a fresh array of problems. In some respects, this provides a happy hunting ground for the professional scientist, but all too often the new challenge takes him into unfamiliar territory where he finds a dearth of both knowledge and technology. In this situation, advances tend to be sporadic with initial painfully slow progress eventually leading to enough data to permit recognition of the basic pattern, and then rapid completion of that part of the jigsaw. The tremendous advances in cell biology, in chemical separation and analysis and in organic and bio-synthesis in the last decade, have permitted a substantial degree of completion of those parts of the jigsaw dealing with the mast cell and the leukotrienes, whilst in other parts, such as the factors controlling IgE synthesis, and the roles of PAF, LTB_4, PGD_2, and the importance of the eosinophil, interesting advances are ongoing. The existence or relevance of other fields is still emerging, e.g. the putative role of IgE in limiting or clearing invasion by parasites and possibly by viruses;

the ability of metabolites of arachidonic acid to amplify or terminate parts of the inflammatory and immune responses and to both attract and activate leucocytes in a variety of clinical conditions. It comes as no surprise that our knowledge of asthma is still incomplete. Perhaps we should be more impressed with what we know, and be expectant that this will become translated into therapeutic benefits in the forseeable future.

References*

Ahlquist, R.P., 1948. Am. J. Physiol. 153, 586–600.

Arnoux, B., Jouvin-Marche, E., Arnoux, A., Benveniste, J., 1982. Agents Actions 12, 713–716.

Augstein, J., Farmer, J.B., Lee, T.B., Sheard, P., Tattersall, M.L., 1973. Nature 245, 215–217.

Austen, K.F. (1974) In: Asthma: Physiology, Pharmacology and Treatment, (Austen, K.F. and Lichtenstein, L., Eds.), Academic Press, New York, NY, pp. 109–121.

Austen, K.F., 1979. Harvey Lectures, 73. Academic Press, New York, NY, pp. 93–161.

Austen, K.F. (1980) In: Advances in Allergology and Immunology (Oehler, A., Ed.), Pergamon, Oxford, pp. 237–247.

Austen, K.F., Brocklehurst, W.E., 1961. J. Exp. Med. 113, 521–528.

Bach, M.K., Brashler, J.R., 1974. J. Immunol. 113, 2040–2044.

Bach, M.K., Brashler, J.R., 1978. J. Immunol. 120, 998–1005.

Bach, M.K., Brashler, J.R., Hammarstrom, S., Samuelsson, B., 1978. Biochem. Biophys. Res. Commun. 93, 1121–1126.

Becker, E.L., Henson, P.M., 1973. Adv. Immunol. 17, 93–193.

Benveniste, J., Henson, P.M., Cochrane, C.G., 1972. J. Exp. Med. 136, 1356–1377.

Brocklehurst, W.E., 1956. A slow reacting substance in anaphylaxis – 'SRS-A. Ciba Symposium on Histamine. Churchill, London, pp. 175–179.

Brocklehurst, W.E., 1960. J. Physiol. 151, 416–435.

Brocklehurst, W.E., 1962. Progr. Allergy 6, 540–560.

Brogden, R.N., Speight, T.M., Avery, G.S., 1974. Drugs 7, 164–282.

Bullowa, G.G.M., Kaplan, D., 1903. Med. New 53, 789–792.

Capron, A., Capron, M., Dessaint, J-P., 1980. Prog. Immunol. 4, 782–793.

Casale, T.B. and Kaliner, M. (1983) ICACI 309–314.

Chand, N., 1979. Agents Actions 9, 133–140.

Chen, K.K., Schmidt, C.F, 1926. J. Am. Med. Assoc. 87, 836–842.

Cochrane, C.G., Muller-Eberhard, H.J., 1968. J. Exp. Med. 127, 371–380.

Cooke, R.A., 1922. J. Immunol. 7, 147–156.

Dale, H.H., 1920. Proc. R. Soc. (B) 91, 126–146.

Dale, H.H., 1950. Ann. N.Y. Acad. Sci. 50, 1017–1028.

Drazen, J.M., Austen, K.F., Lewis, R.A., Clark, D.A., Goto, G., Marfat, A., Corey, E.J., 1980. Proc. Natl. Acad. Sci. U.S.A. 77, 4354–4358.

---

* This chapter is essentially historical narrative covering a wide range of topics and time span. It has proved impractical to quote many of the original references, and since modern science is characterized by interaction and cross-fertilization, selection is often invidious. The references have been compiled as a guide to further reading, with preference for reviews in which original work is cited. The proceedings of two recent international congresses are of special interest: 4th Int. Congress of Immunology: Immunology IV (Fougereau, M. and Dausset, J., Eds.), 1980, Academic Press, New York, NY and XI Int. Congress of Allergy and Clinical Immunology, Proceedings: Invited speakers in Symposia: (Kerr, J.W. and Ganderton, M.A., Eds.), 1983, Macmillan, London (referred to as 'ICACI').

Feldberg, W., 1941. Annu. Rev. Physiol. 3, 671–694.

Feldberg, W., 1954. J. Pharm. Pharmacol. 6, 281.

Feldberg, W., Miles, A.A., 1953. J. Physiol. Lond. 120, 205–213.

Fewtrell, C., Metzger, H., 1981. Biochemistry of the Acute Allergic Reactions. Alan Liss, New York, NY, pp. 295–314.

Foreman, J.C., Mongar, J.L., Gomperts, B.D., 1973. Nature 245, 249–251.

Ford-Hutchinson, A.W., Bray, M.A., Doig, M.V., Shipley, M.E., Smith, M.J.H., 1980. Nature 286, 264–265.

Friedberger, E., 1910. Z. Immunitatsforsch. 4, 636–644.

Gemsa, D., Leser, H.G., Seitz, M., Deimann, W., Barlin, E., 1982. Mol. Immunol. 19, 1287–1296.

Goetzl, E.J., Austen, K.F., 1977. Monogr. Allergy 12, 189–197.

Graezer, J.B., Rowe, A.H., 1935. J. Allergy 6, 415–420.

Griffin, M., Weiss, J.W., Leitch, A.G., McFadden, E.R., Corey, E.J., Austen, K.F., Drazen, J.M., 1983. New Engl. J. Med. 308, 436–439.

Haberland, G., McConn., R., 1979. Fed. Proc. 38, 2760–2767.

Hammarström, S., 1983. Annu. Rev. Biochem. 52, 355–377.

Hirata, F., Axelrod, J., 1980. Science 209, 1082–1090.

Holgate, S.T., Lewis, R.A., Austen, K.F., 1980. Progr. Immunol. 4, 846–859.

Howell, H.B.L., Altounyan, R., 1969. Lancet 2, 1969–1974.

Ishizaka, K., 1976. Adv. Immunol. 23, 1–76.

Ishizaka, K., 1980. Progr. Immunol. 4, 815–828.

Ishizaka, K. (1983) ICACI, 367–370.

Ishizaka, K., Tomioka, H., Ishizaka, T., 1970. J. Immunol. 105, 1459–1467.

Ishizaka, K., Yodoi, J., Suemura, M., Hirashima, M., 1983. Immunol. Today 4, 192–196.

Ishizaka, T. (1983) ICACI, 17–22.

Ishizaka, K., Ishizaka, K., Tomioka, H., 1972. J. Immunol. 108, 513–520.

Jonasson, O., Becker, E.L., 1966. J. Exp. Med. 123, 509–522.

Kahlson, G., Rosengren, E., 1972. Experientia 28, 993–1128.

Kaliner, M., Orange, R.P., Austen, K.F., 1972. J. Exp. Med. 136, 556–567.

Kaplan, A.P. (1983) ICACI, 43–48.

Katz, D.H., 1980. Immunology 41, 1–24.

Katz, D.H., Zuraw, B.L., Chen, P., Cohen, P.A. and O'Hair, C.M. (1983) ICACI, 377–384.

Kay, A.B., Austen, K.F., 1971. J. Immunol. 107, 899–902.

Kellaway, C.H., Trethewie, E.R., 1940. Q.J. Exp. Physiol. 30, 121–145.

Keller, R., 1965. Mast Cells in Immune Reactions. S. Karger, Basel.

Kishimoto, T., Suemura, M., Ishizaka, A., Deguchi, H., Sugimura, K., Maeda, K.,

Kashiwamura, S. and Yamamura, Y. (1983) ICACI, 385–390.

Krilis, S., Lewis, R.A., Corey, E.J. and Austen, K.F. (1983) ICACI, 3–10.

Lefort, J., Wal, F., Chigward, M., Mederios, M.C., Vargaftig, B.B., 1982. Agents Actions 12, 723–725.

Lewis, R.A., Austen, K.F., 1981. Nature 293, 103–108.

Lewis, R.A., Drazen, J.M., Figueiredo, J.C., Corey, E.J., Austen, K.F., 1982. Int. J. Immunopharmacol. 4, 85–90.

Lewis, R.A., Goetzl, E.J., Wasserman, S.I., Valone, F.H., Rubin, R.H., Austen, K.F., 1975. J. Immunol. 114, 87–92.

Lewis, R.A., Wasserman, S.I., Goetzl, E.J., Austen, K.F., 1974. J. Exp. Med. 140, 1133–1146.

Lichtenstein, L.M., 1975. J. Immunol. 114, 1692–1699.

Lichtenstein, L.M., Norman, P.S., Kagey-Sobotka, A., Adkinson, N.F. and Golden, D.B.K. (1983) ICACI, 285–290.

Milstein, C., Clark, M.R., Galfre, G., Cuello, A.C., 1980. Progr. Immunol. 4, 17–33.

Mongar, J.L., Schild, H.O., 1953. Br. J. Pharmacol. Chemother. 8, 103–109.

Mongar, J.L., Schild, H.O., 1957. J. Physiol. Lond. 135, 320–326.

Mongar, J.L., Schild, H.O., 1962. Physiol. Rev. 42, 226–270.

Morley, J., Paul, W. and Basran, G.S. (1983) ICACI, 501–506.

Morris, H.R., Piper, P.J., Taylor, G.W., Tippins, J.R., 1979. Br. J. Pharmacol. 67, 179–184.

Morris, H.R., Taylor, G.W., Piper, P.J., Sirois, R., Tippins, J.R., 1978. Febs. Lett. 87 (2), 203–206.

Mota, I., Humphrey, J.H., 1959. Immunology 2, 31–43.

Muller-Eberhard, H.J., 1977. Hosp. Pract. (Aug.) 33–43.

Muller-Eberhard, H.J., 1980. Progr. Immunol. 4, 1001–1024.

Murphy, R.C., Hammarstrom, S., Samuelsson, B., 1979. Proc. Natl. Sci. U.S.A. 76, 4275–4279.

Oertel, H., Kaliner, M., 1981. J. Immunol. 127, 1398–1402.

Orange, R.P., Murphy, R.C., Karnovsky, M.L., Austen, K.F., 1973. J. Immunol. 110, 760–770.

Ovary, Z., 1958. Progr. Allergy 5, 459–508.

Parker, C.W., Jakschik, B.A., Huber, M.G., Falkenhein, S.F., 1979. Biochem. Biophys. Res. Commun. 89, 1186–1192.

Packer, C.W., Koch, D., Huber, M.M., Falkenhein, S.F., 1980. Biochem. Biophys. Res. Commun. 97, 1038–1046.

Pinckard, R.N., McManus, L.M., Humphreys, D.M. and Hanahan, D.J. (1983) ICACI, 33–38.

Pisano, J.J., Austen, K.F., 1976. Chemistry and Biology of the Kallikrein-Kinin System in Health and Disease. DHEW Publication NIH. U.S. Govt., Washington, D.C, pp. 76–791.

Prausnitz, C., Kustner, N., 1921. Zbl. Bakteriol. (Abt.l Orig.) 86, 161.

Proud, D., Togias, A., Naclerio, R.M., Crush, S.A., Norman, P.S., Lichtenstein, L.M., 1983. J. Clin. Invest. 72, 1678–1685.

Richet, C.R., Portier, P., 1902. C.R. Soc. Biol. Paris 54, 170–180.

Riley, J.F., 1959. The Mast Cells. Livinstone, Edinburgh.

Rose, B. and McGarry, E. (1959) In: International Textbook of Allergy (Jamar, J.M., Ed.), Blackwell, Oxford.

Samuelsson, B., Borgeat, P., Hammarström, S., Murphy, R.C., 1979. Prostaglandins 17, 785–787.

Samuelsson, B., Hammerstrom, S., Murphy, R.C., Borgeat, P., 1980. J. Allergy 35, 375–381.

Schayer, R.W., 1963. Henry Ford Hospital Symposium (on Immunity). Churchill, London, pp. 227–235.

Schayer, R.W., 1959. Physiol. Rev. 39, 116–136.

Schild, H.O., Hawkins, D.F., Mongar, J.L., Herxheimer, H., 1951. Lancet 2, 376–381.

Selye, H., 1950. Br. Med. J. (1) 1383–1392.

Sheard, P., Lee, T.B., Tattersall, M.L., 1977. Monogr. Allergy 12, 145–249.

Taylor, W.A., Francis, D.H., Sheldon, D., Roitt, I.M., 1974. Int. Arch. Allergy Appl. Immun. 47, 175–193.

Uvnäs, B., 1974. Fed. Proc. 33, 2172–2176.

Vogt, W., 1974. Pharmacol. Rev. 26, 125–169.

Walker, J.L., 1973. Adv. Biosci. 9, 235–240.

Wasserman, S.I., 1979. Monogr. Allergy 14, 189–193.

Wasserman, S.I. (1983) ICACI, 29–32.

Williams, T.J., Piper, P.J., 1980. Prostaglandins 19, 779–790.

Commentary on From dyes to drugs by Robert Behnisch

Heinz Moser

Novartis Institutes for Biomedical Research, Emeryville, CA, United States

The article by Behnisch provides a historical insight into early drug discovery that yielded, among other achievements, the first significant class of antibiotics originating from synthetic compounds. Many of the scientists who contributed to this enormous effort participated in World War I, witnessing the impact infections had on wounded soldiers (mainly gas gangrene), indirectly claiming many lives even though with an improving trend compared to earlier wars (Pennington, 2019). 100 years ago, physicians had no therapeutic options to treat such infections that would often end in amputations and/or death. Having witnessed our recent pandemic with Covid-19, we can only imagine the helplessness in those situations and the passionate desire and motivation to find effective therapeutics to treat infections. Below are some observations comparing past and recent approaches to tackle this task:

Chemical matter for screening

Synthetic chemistry was largely driven by a focused effort on dyes, a starting point for many chemical companies along the Rhine. The instinctive belief that some of these dyes could contain antimicrobial activity eventually resulted in the discovery of Prontosil, the first antibiotic within the family of sulfa drugs. Today, the diversity and number of chemicals available to us for screening is larger by roughly three orders of magnitude (Llanos et al., 2019), and our synthetic capabilities have expanded dramatically. Nevertheless, chemists back then were incredibly skilled in the lab, despite the lack of many analytical tools and purification technologies we use today on a routine basis.

Screening and mode of action

Prontosil was identified by directly screening compounds in infected mice, an extreme way of phenotypic screening not practiced nowadays. This molecule would have been missed by minimum inhibitory concentration screening in vitro as it is a prodrug of the active sulfonamide (in vivo cleavage of the $N=N$ double bond). This was discovered only a few years later and

Discoveries in Pharmacology, Volume 3, Hemodynamics and
Immune Defense.
DOI: https://doi.org/10.1016/B978-0-443-18442-0.00009-4

initiated a worldwide effort to expand on this class of compounds. Phenotypic screening in vivo has been abandoned these days and is largely replaced by minimum inhibitory concentration determination in broth or direct screening of essential target proteins. Not only during the period described in the article by Behnisch but also for the following decades, the target was often not known and only discovered years later. In most cases, modern techniques allow rapid target identification, especially if the possibility exists to generate resistant mutants as exemplified by the work of argyrin B (Nyfeler et al., 2012).

Pharmacology and regulation

Compounds were screened for efficacy in different animals, depending on the pathogen of interest. At the same time, animals, organs, and tissues were carefully observed for side effects and thanks to a careful job by pharmacologists, severe toxic effects in clinical trials could largely be avoided. The regulation back then was pretty much non-existent and substantially different compared to the present, with clear guidelines provided by agencies and harmonized globally (https://www.ich.org/page/ich-guidelines).

Pharmacokinetics

The different levels of analytical techniques available during the discovery and optimization period of sulfa drugs limited the insight into pharmacokinetic understanding of a given compound as we know it today. Absorption, distribution, metabolism, and elimination (ADME) is typically determined for compounds of interest in vitro and in vivo, allowing us to understand shortcomings and to figure out how to fix them. Despite the lack of many of these techniques, scientists were able to determine half-lives of drugs, level of absorption, and preferred exposure to organs (e.g., intestine or urine), optimally using specific drugs for a given indication and lowering the dosing frequency by extending half-lives of drugs.

Working culture

As described in the article by Behnisch, it was largely the chemistry community that decided what compounds to make and hand over for screening. The interaction among scientists was minimal and chemists often would not share their plans or ongoing activities with colleagues, almost operating in isolation and fearing ideas might be acquired by others. Across disciplines, the interaction was poor and chemists would complain that they did not receive sufficient information back from pharmacology. This was fundamentally different from how we operate in drug discovery today: Interdisciplinary teams are formed early in the process with frequent meetings, data sharing, and access to all data for everybody involved. Communication skills and the capability to operate efficiently in such an environment are key nowadays for success.

Reporting

It is interesting to read the monthly report by Josef Klarer (November 1932, Figure 7.12, see chapter 7B) that, by today's standards, is minimal and lacks actual data but does include the structures of compounds made. Details of experiments done were typically not reported and eventually were lost over time. Today, it is a standard practice to report such details with the goal to capture critical information—including all analytical data from a given entry—allowing the reproduction of experiments. While lab notebooks were the standard for many decades, chemistry has moved to electronic versions with enhanced features such as substructure search across all existing notebooks within a company or institute.

Patent protection

Sulfa drugs preceded penicillin and were the first functional defense against human infections. The commercial potential was recognized and protecting the rights to inventions was important and practiced by engaged parties. This led in certain areas to complex legal situations that likely only could have been sorted out by lengthy trials in court. This was the case for sulfadiazine and related analogs, and Hoerlein initiated a meeting between interested parties (Ciba, Dehydag, Schering, and IG Farben) and they decided to pool all existing intellectual property together and distribute revenues after a carefully examined formula; an innovative approach to avoid such a complex legal battle and that retrospectively worked out really well.

Scientific recognition

We can hardly imagine how huge the discovery of sulfa drugs was during a time with no reasonable treatment options against bacterial infections. Therefore, it is not surprising that it was recognized internationally, and Domagk was rewarded with the Nobel Prize in 1939. Due to Third Reich politics in Germany, he was not allowed to travel to Sweden and receive the prize in-person. This happened only in 1947 when he was honored but without receiving the prize money. Josef Klarer, who synthesized Prontosil, was not recognized despite his critical contribution; a fact that affected him deeply despite Domagk's repeated recognition of his critical work.

Combination therapy

With the combination of sulfamethoxazole and trimethoprim, another big step was taken early. Both drugs inhibit enzymes in the same pathway, operate in synergy, and reduce the potential for resistance development. The combination, Bactrim or Eusaprim, is still used today and serves as one of the earliest examples of the combination of different drugs to achieve an enhanced effect and slow resistance formation.

References

Llanos, E.J., Leal, W., Luu, D.H., Jost, J., Stadler, P.F., Restrepo, G., 2019. Exploration of the chemical space and its three historical regimes. Proc. Natl. Acad. Sci. 116, 12660–12665.

Nyfeler, B., et al., 2012. Identification of elongation factor G as the conserved cellular target of argyrin B. PLoS One 7, e42657.

Pennington, H., 2019. The impact of infectious disease in war time, a look back at WW1. Future Microbiol. 14, 165–168.

From dyes to drugs

Robert Behnisch

Contents

Disclaimer: The original text that follows is reproduced from the first edition and carries errors and omissions from it. The editors and publisher agreed to retain them and honor the original authors and challenges they had to deal with in publishing back in those times.

Discoveries in Pharmacology, Volume 3, Hemodynamics and
Immune Defense.
DOI: https://doi.org/10.1016/B978-0-443-18442-0.00067-7

7.1 Introduction: A brief history and nomenclature

Paul Ehrlich, 1854–1915, physician, bacteriologist and chemist, was the founder of chemotherapy. During the last ten years of his life, when he was Director of the Institute of Experimental Chemotherapy in Frankfurt/Main, he studied infectious diseases caused by protozoa and together with his coworker Hata, discovered Salvarsan. This agent, which became commercially available in 1910, and its successors afforded a reliable treatment of syphilis and were also effective in trypanosomiasis. This was a sensational discovery and provided an impetus to intensive research in university and industrial laboratories. It had been proved for the first time that synthetic agents for which there were no prototypes in nature could have therapeutic uses. The following 20 years, until about 1930, saw great advances in the fight against malaria, bilharziasis and leishmaniasis, but no agent was found with more than a trace of effectiveness in mice with streptococcal infections. Röhl, Ehrlich's experienced pupil, then working at Elberfeld, also had little hope of discovery in this area since the streptococcus tests he had consistently performed had been negative throughout. His untimely death at the age of 48 denied him success in this field. Only 2 years later he would have come across the first effective compounds. In 1935, exactly 25 years after Ehrlich's famous lecture, Domagk announced to the meeting of the Gesellschaft Deutscher Naturforscher und Ärzte the discovery of streptozone, later named Prontosil, a sulphonamide azo dye, in which he had found a weapon against bacterial infections. This report awakened researchers in the fields of medicine and chemistry all over the world. The search for new, even more effective compounds sparked vehement, often hectic, activities in this area which went on for ten years.

They came to a standstill in 1945 when the efficacy of penicillin discovered by Fleming became general knowledge. Sulphonamides lost their importance and their era seemed to be over. From then on it was chiefly pharmacologists and chemists who systematically studied the wealth of facts then available.

The pharmacokinetics of the sulphonamides, their metabolic reactions, absorption and excretion, the relationship between effect and pK_a value as well as their mechanisms of action were methodically studied. When new findings demonstrated the importance of retention time in the blood a new type of product emerged in the years between 1953 and 1960, the long-acting sulphonamides. This marked the beginning of a new phase of chemical synthesis with the aim of obtaining even better drugs. When this problem too had been solved, research again came to a standstill. Up until 1955 about 1600 papers had been published, several hundred patents granted and some 2500 drugs tested. There are only about 6 active substances that still have some importance today.

However, clinical testing of the sulphonamides provided valuable clues to possible effects in other indications such as diabetes, diuresis, tuberculosis and epilepsy which became the starting point for further research. By 1980 also this work had been largely completed.

The history of these developments up to the time of writing has been described by various authors who quoted a host of supporting literature: Northey (1948), Mietzsch and Behnisch (1955), Krüger-Thiemer (1962). Further summarising accounts have been published by Domagk and Hegler (1944), Behnisch and Horstmann (1965), Ehrhart and Ruschig (1972), Otten and Plempel (1975). No details need therefore be given here. The aim in writing this contribution is rather to show the human aspect of this research, intimating reasons for successes and failures as well as for correct and incorrect working hypotheses. What researchers thought and planned in those days, how they went about their tasks and why they decided the way they did, will be described in the following. The account will also feature the men involved in this work, their different personality traits, their ways of thinking and working. The organisation of research around 1930, the atmosphere which reigned in the laboratories, the relationships between chemists and physicians and interdisciplinary communication also need describing in this context. None of these 'pioneers' is still alive today. The author joined the group of the sulphonamide researchers as a young chemist in 1935 taking an active part in developments until 1958. These notes will therefore be interspersed with personal impressions and experiences. Since up to 1935 research which led from dyes to sulphonamides took place at the Elberfeld plant of what is now Bayer AG, the work done there will be described first followed by that of other research groups.

Almost all of the commercial sulphonamides are derived from sulphanilamide with the exception of mafenidum = Marfanil (25). As suggested by Northey the nitrogen atom of the sulphonamide group is designated N1 while N4 represents the nitrogen atom of the aromatic amine group.

$$H_2\overset{1}{N}-SO_2-\langle\ \rangle-\overset{4}{N}H_2 \qquad \textbf{Sulphanilamide}$$

Apart from the exact names provided according to the rules of the Geneva nomenclature, sulphonamides are known by a number of, often incorrect, names. In addition, there are generic names, free names recommended by the WHO and brand names by which products are often best known.

The correct name for the residue $H_2N\text{-}C_6H_4\text{-}SO_2\text{-}NH$ is 4-aminobenzenesulphonamido- and is often replaced by the abbreviation 'sulpha'. Both forms precede the name of the substituent at the N1 position. The following designations are therefore possible: 4-aminobenzenesulphonamido-2-pyridine or sulpha-2-pyridine. The residue H_2N-C_6H_4-SO_2- is termed aminobenzenesulphonyl- or, briefly sulphanilyl-. This gives rise to the following names: 4-aminobenzenesulphonyl urea or sulphanilyl urea. The number 4- is generally omitted as all sulphonamides with antibacterial effect are derived from 4-sulphanilic acid.

A few names such as sulpha thiourea or sulphaguanidine that have become firmly established in the literature are, however, incorrect and misleading.

The generic names merely designate the class of the heterocycles without clearly indicating the position of the substituents. A key is therefore necessary. The WHO free names, often called INN (International Non-proprietary Names) are generally arbitrarily selected and hardly provide precise information concerning the chemical formula. In the special case of the sulphonamides, however, they are largely synonymous with the generic names. In the following chapters the generic names are given and are marked by asterisks, e.g. *sulphadiazine*.

All brand names mentioned are registered trade marks and thus are protected. Proper reference to proprietary rights having been made herein, the obligatory® sign has been omitted throughout.

The numbers in brackets behind the product names refer to the numbered structures given throughout this chapter.

7.1.1 Successes of chemotherapy: The era of Röhl

The pharmaceutical department of the Farbenfabriken formerly Friedrich Bayer AG of Elberfeld came into being in 1888 on the initiative of C. Duisberg (1861–1935) who was the ruling spirit of the company after the founder's death. He had an unfailing gift for recognising promising new fields of interest and for recruiting qualified staff. The great success Farbwerke Hoechst had had with antipyrine, the antipyretic discovered in 1883, and the favourable reception given to phenacetin which he had developed together with Hinsberg, may have prompted his decision which was a bold one at the time. Suggestions for further new compounds initially came from the universities, however. The job of the chemists working in the new department was mainly formulation development and production control. It was only in 1896 that a pharmaceutical research unit, independent of the production facility and provided with a pharmacological laboratory, was created. Duisberg followed very closely the chemotherapeutic research of Ehrlich of which, however, Farbwerke Hoechst had the exclusive use. He therefore gave generous support to the research of Mesnil at the Institut Pasteur in Paris and of Pflimmer at the Lister Institute, London, whom he supplied with dyes and chemicals. He finally decided to venture into chemotherapy at Elberfeld and when looking for an expert in the field, he found W. Röhl, Ehrlich's assistant. Negotiations took almost a year since Röhl first wanted to qualify as a university lecturer. The employment contract was signed on 1st

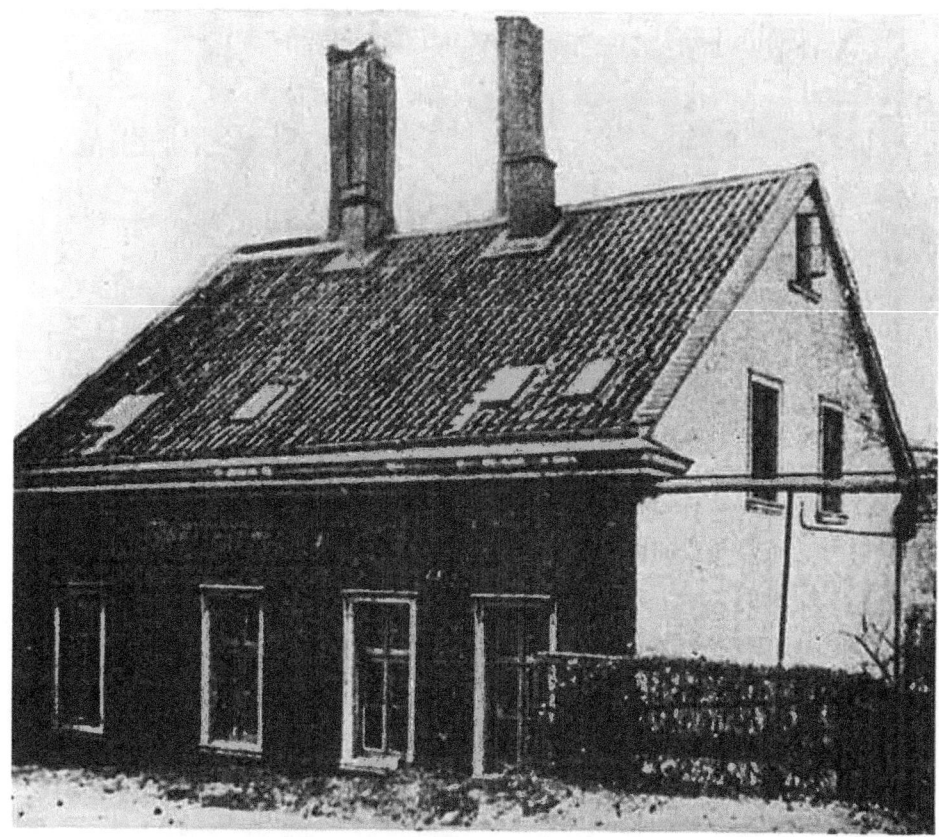

Figure 7.1
First chemotherapeutic laboratory in Elberfeld. Röhl worked here from 1911–1929 and discovered the action of Germanin and Plasmoquine.

April, 1910. Röhl then went to spend a year with Meyer in Vienna to widen his knowledge of pharmacology. In April 1911 he took up work at Elberfeld. This date marks the beginning of the immensely successful phase of chemotherapeutic research at Elberfeld, characterized by such inventions as germanin and plasmoquine.

Who was Röhl? Born in 1881 in Berlin, he came from a family of theologians and mathematicians. He attended secondary school at Naumburg and Halber-Stadt and entered the univerisities of Halle and Heidelberg to study medicine. Röhl took his state examination receiving very high marks and graduated MD with distinction for his thesis on nitrogen metabolism. In the course of his postgraduate training he became an unpaid assistant at the Institutes of Physiology and Pathology at Heidelberg University. Later he became assistant to Ehrlich in Frankfurt, next he joined Moritz at the Medical Clinic in Giessen and finally returned to resume work with Ehrlich. By the age of thirty he had acquired an extensive medical education.

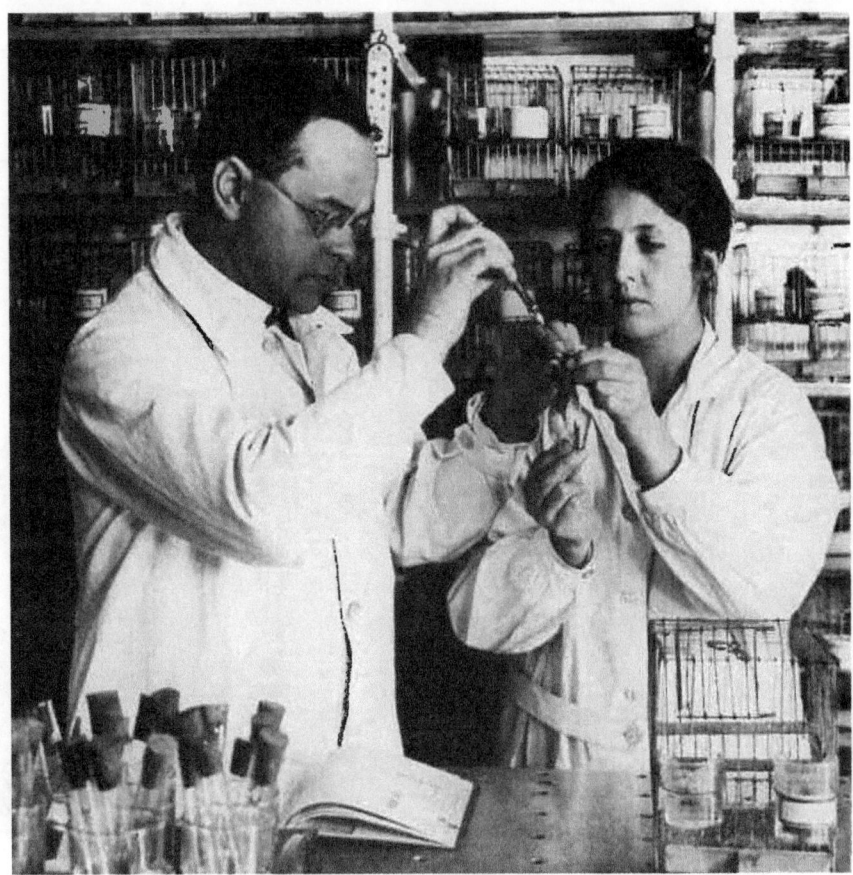

Figure 7.2
Röhl in his laboratory.

At Elberfeld, a small white frame house was placed at his disposal, located near the plant grounds but outside the fence. Whether there was no suitable room in the plant buildings or whether there was fear of infection with pathogens, is uncertain. It was perfectly all right with Röhl. In the modest rooms given him he established his institute and it is rumoured that the only available microscope was his. He first equipped the laboratory in the way he had learnt from Ehrlich and set up animal experiments to test compounds against various strains of trypanosomes, spirochaetae and notably even against bacterial infections, then entirely new territory. A few assistants, laboratory workers they were called, were so thoroughly trained by him as to be able to carry out animal experiments on their own, a method that was to prove very far-sighted during World War I.

It was Röhl who set the tasks. Nobody interfered. Out of consideration for his teacher, Ehrlich, he did not turn to arsenical compounds but picked up the threads of what little else was known. There were a few azo dyes, trypan red, trypan blue, afridol violet and sulphur red acid, which exerted a slight effect on trypanosomes and partly also on spirochaetae. Apart from these classes of substances he studied acridine derivatives and compounds from the oxazine and quinoline series. This marks the appearance of ring systems he selected himself and which were later to form the basic skeletons of the antimalarials Plasmoquine and Atebrine.

The contact between Röhl and the laboratory of science and chemistry at Elberfeld was obviously no more than sporadic since he got his test supplies from the laboratory for azo dyes which had been transferred to Leverkusen in 1911. He told the Director of the Department, Heymann, what he needed and the latter, often rather reluctantly because he did not think anything would come out of it, instructed the chemists Kothe, Dressel and Ossenbeck to synthesize the new dyes. To him, this seemed rather a waste of time. It was uncommon in those days for chemists to send compounds synthesized according to their own ideas to the chemotherapeutic laboratory for testing. This form of cooperation only began 10 years later. As there are only a few colleagues still alive who were able to give information on these three men, a few biographical data should perhaps be added here.

Richard Kothe, born in Leipzig in 1863, studied and took his degree under Wislicenus in Leipzig, became an assistant to his teacher for several years and joined Bayer at Elberfeld in 1891. His field of interest was the synthesis of naphthol and naphthylamine sulphonic acids. He died in 1925 while on holiday in Salzburg, only 62 years old. Kothe is said to have been a quiet, humorous, conciliatory man, at peace with himself, who radiated genuine authority and was admired and respected by his junior colleagues. The same is said of Oskar Dressel, born in 1865 at Sonneberg. He studied chemistry in Heidelberg and Leipzig where he struck up a friendship with Kothe. He took his degree with a thesis on glutaric acid esters and became an assistant to Wislicenus. He joined the company at Elberfeld in 1891, worked chiefly with Kothe and retired in 1929. He died in Bonn in 1941.

Chemists who knew Kothe and Dressel at the height of their activities like to remember the orientation courses the two men organised for junior chemists joining the company who were made to attend these courses for the first 6–8 months from taking up work to be instructed in the plant's processes for the manufacture of intermediate and final products. They were taught quite a few tricks in the process which were not to be found in any of the textbooks, but which a dye chemist had to know nevertheless. Mietzsch (1896–1958), who will feature again later in this chapter, attended these courses in 1922/1923 and kept meticulous notes. He often consulted his carefully preserved notebook later when he was doing research on sulphonamides. The book was found in his estate and attracted great interest. Mietzsch delighted in telling his junior colleagues about these times and passed on many of Dressel's humorous aphorisms which unfortunately defy translation as they are only amusing when told in the original Saxon dialect. The relaxed atmosphere prevailing in those days is reflected by the following authentic dialogue: Dressel calling to Kothe across the hall: 'Richard, we've got to do the melting point of the new compound'. Reply: 'We'll do that tomorrow, it's almost noon now, too late for today'.

The third member of the group was the often forgotten Anton Ossenbeck. Born in 1875, he was some 10 years younger than the two others which made an enormous difference in those days. He came to Elberfeld in 1910 and joined Kothe's group. In 1915 he was appointed provisional head of Röhl's laboratory while the latter was serving as a doctor in the war. Ossenbeck retired in 1935 and died four years later. During his last working years which he spent in the main laboratory, he impressed his young colleagues as a great gentleman who made it clear that he neither appreciated nor sought personal contact with his juniors. He must have been quite a character.

To the collaborative research of Röhl, Dressel, Kothe and Ossenbeck we owe the discovery of germanin. This was synthesized in 1916 and tested in Röhl's laboratory during the latter's war service and is proof of the excellent way in which his staff had been trained by him. The good effect the compound had on various trypanosomes which Röhl was able to verify himself later on, warranted its tentative use against sleeping sickness in humans and animals in Africa. The times prevented the expedition from setting out and it was not until 1921 that it was able to leave. Results of treatment were so convincing as to permit the compound, code name Bayer 205, to be released for general use in the autumn of 1924 under the trade names of Germanin (human sector) and Naganol (veterinary sector). The history of this invention has been described fully by Heymann (1924) and Dünnschede (1971). It is mentioned briefly here for two reasons. For the first time intensive research led to colourless drugs being developed from dyes, an event which was to recur years later, though in a different way, with sulphonamides.

If in the historic understanding of young scientists of today germanin research seems to date back to antiquity, the fact remains that there were a mere three years between the release of germanin and the beginning of sulphonamide research. The experience gained by Röhl and the group around Kothe in eight years automatically led to concepts and working hypotheses that were vividly remembered and passed on for years. Their obvious source was textile chemistry and while they did not stand up to scientific evaluation nevertheless proved a stimulant to later research. It is only from these beginnings that sulphonamide research can be understood.

A therapeutic agent, it was believed, ought to 'fit' the cell of the causative organism in order to disrupt the latter's vital functions. Furthermore, it was said that therapeutically active substituents would be needed to reach the surface or the interior of the cell. The point was to find a suitable molecule into which active groups could be fitted. A beginning was made with acid dyes with a known affinity for fibres. Röhl who was beginning to entertain reservations about having to stain patients red or blue, went to see Heymann about this. 'So you're looking for dyes that do not stain, and we've got them', he said. 'Try diaminobiphenyl urea derivatives.

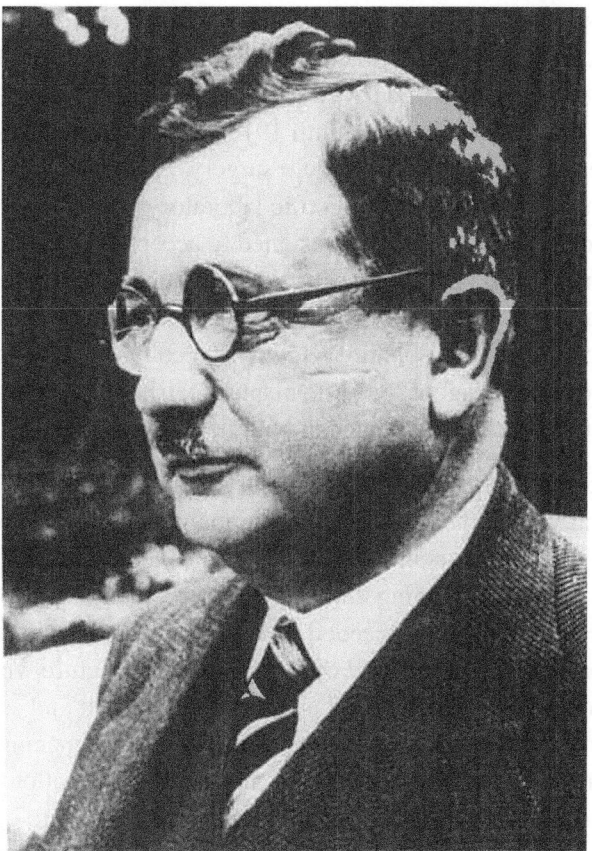

Figure 7.3
Prof. Dr. phil., Dr. Med.h.c., Dr. rer.nat.h.c. Heinrich Hörlein (1882–1954).

They are colourless but will nevertheless be taken up by the fibre'. This was the idea which eventually led to the use of colourless active compounds.

While clinical testing of germanin was still in progress, Hörlein (1882–1954), then Research Director at Elberfeld, was intent on starting a search for synthetic antimalarials. For this project he urgently needed to expand his staff as the research group around Kothe and Dressel could not take additional work. With an unfailing instinct for qualified personnel and aided by recommendations from university professors, he engaged, in 1919, W. Schulemann, in 1921, F. Schönhöfer, and, in 1923, A. Wingler and F. Mietzsch who were to form a successful team in the following years.

Werner Schulemann (1888–1975) was both a physician and a chemist. At the age of 26 he held the degrees of MD and PhD and had already gained some experience as an assistant in surgery, pharmacology, physico-chemistry and internal medicine. His papers on the relationship between structure and vital staining, diffusion rate and distribution of dyes and on aromatic mercury compounds, had attracted Hörlein's attention, notably because this work was closely related to research then underway at Elberfeld. In 1914 Schulemann applied for a job at Elberfeld, but it took several years, until 1919, before he could take up his post after 4 years of war service as a leading doctor in field surgery. At Elberfeld he worked first as a pharmacologist, later as a chemist in the scientific laboratory whose head he became in 1927. He was made a director in 1929. In 1937 he resigned to accept an appointment to a chair in pharmacology in Bonn. He had been a leader in the field of chemical research for 10 years. His leaving the company in a critical phase of sulphonamide research was probably due not so much to his wish to gain a professorship as to internal competence disputes. His ability to guide and inspire young colleagues, to settle disputes fairly, to coordinate chemical and medical research and to give valuable advice in both fields, was sorely missed for many years.

Schulemann too worked first on germanin with the trypan red formula as his starting point. Together with Röhl and Wenker he tried to find a compound against spirochaetae infections that might be able to replace Salvarsan. In 1922 Röhl screened 498 candidate substances for possible application in syphylis, keeping 280 singly-housed rabbits under constant observation for the purpose. He very nearly succeeded. The most effective drug stemming from this research was P 2807, an iodized compound of germanin-like structure which, while showing efficacy comparable to that of Salvarsan, had no advantages over it and so the project was dropped. The group then turned to malaria which had increased menacingly after World War I. Röhl had developed the test on infected canaries to a stage which allowed quantitative conclusions to be drawn about the efficacy of compounds in comparison to quinine. This paved the way for large-scale testing. Schulemann pushed matters from the chemical angle, and for the first time a real team was formed with Schulemann, Schönhöfer, Wingler, Röhl and, later, Mietzsch, as members. Unlike the earlier situation, suggestions now came from the chemists.

The beginning was with the structural formula of quinine. Quinine contains a feebly alkaline quinoline ring attached through a carbon bridge to a quinuclidine ring with higher alkalinity. The quinuclidine ring was hardly susceptible to substitution. This generated the idea of replacing it with alkyl aminoalkyl residues, thus creating a structural principle internally termed 'basic alkylation'. This was tested for many years on any ring systems that were at all accessible. This substitution method also played a considerable part in early work on sulphonamides. Task distribution was on a rational basis. Schulemann prepared the quinoline derivatives, Wingler made the alkaline-substituted alkyl halogenides, a class of substances that was difficult to handle, and Schönhöfer did the compounding. The laborious road to plasmoquine (cf. Schönhöfer, 1965), need not be described here. It should be placed on record, however, that work on antimalarials followed the previous working hypothesis, i.e. combination of a selected ring skeleton with suitable substituents.

7.1.2 Change of generations around 1927: The era of Domagk and Kikuth

The year 1927 opened a new phase of research at Elberfeld. It was a time of radical changes. Röhl's laboratory which was still housed in the old white frame house, no longer met the ever increasing needs. Hörlein therefore decided to have modern facilities built for the medical research division and to carry out a redistribution of assignments. It was an opportune moment for these changes. The last dye plants and the alizarin research laboratories had just recently been moved to Leverkusen. At long last there was sufficient space to rebuild the facility to suit the pharmaceutical department. At the same time some senior positions were falling vacant since the first generation of pharma researchers were due to retire.

The following major decisions were taken: Domagk was appointed head of a new laboratory for bacteriology and experimental pathology. Pending completion of his new rooms he worked in an old, rather modest building. Domagk's assignments were bacterial infections, tuberculosis and cancer while the entire realm of tropical medicine as well as other protozoal infections were to be Röhl's responsibility. The old bacteriological laboratory directed by F. Wesenberg (1871–1958) was dissolved. When the head pharmacologists Impens and Eichholtz left, H. Weese (1897–1954) was engaged. When, in 1929, Röhl died of septicaemia from an insufficiently treated carbuncle of the neck acquired while on a business trip to Africa, W. Kikuth (1896–1968) succeeded to his position. Thus, the years from 1927 to 1929 were a period of great changes. Testing capacity had increased severalfold and the chemists now sent their preparations to 3 or 4 laboratories to be tested. This was the situation when work which was to lead to sulphonamides was begun. Before we go on to the sulphonamides, the external conditions and human relations which had a bearing on work around 1927, need to be described. Without them, the history of research cannot be understood unless this is to be reconstructed merely from strictly factual accounts in the scientific literature.

7.1.3 The laboratory of pharmaceutical science of the IG Farbenindustrie AG Elberfeld around 1927

The research laboratories were outdated. Devised by Duisberg in 1891, they consisted of a system of boxes that were jestingly referred to as 'the stables'. Right and left of the aisle there were six boxes each with furniture painted black and lead-topped tables. For the chemists there were a standing desk and a high chair, with no floor-space wasted. There was no writing room, a deliberate omission, as the chemist was supposed to spend his working hours in the laboratory. With the green-shaded hanging lamps casting their soft light in the afternoons, the room seemed almost cosy. The only modern equipment that had been installed since the beginning of operations consisted of transmissions and holding devices for agitators whose steady drone provided a typical background noise. Workroom 4 was a curiosity. It had been built into the attic as an afterthought. Instead of windows it had skylights on the very low

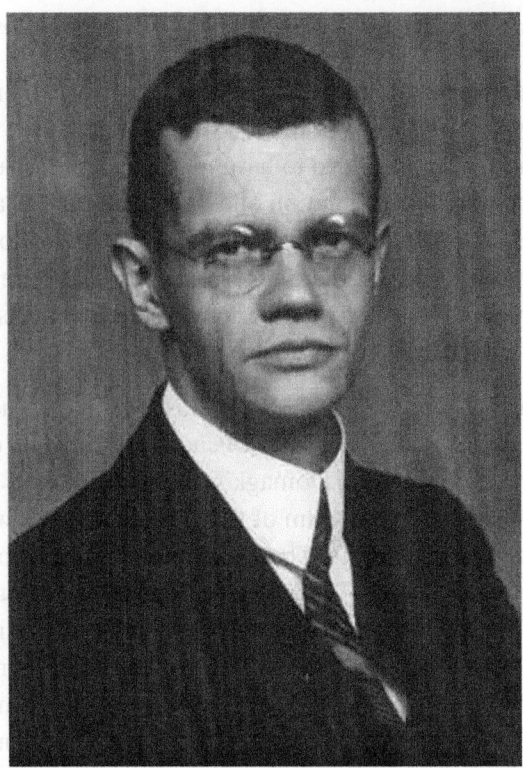

Figure 7.4
Werner Schulemann (1888–1975).

ceiling which also formed the roof. In summer the heat was such that it made the diethyl ether boil in the bottles, but this was accepted uncomplainingly. This particular room saw such inventions as Evipan, Zephirol, Atebrine, Prontosil and many others. The complete freedom which chemists enjoyed with regard to the choice of their themes and methods more than made up for the spartan surroundings. Research was not indication-oriented but focused on chemical reactions and classes of substances. The imagination of the individual was given full scope even in cases where the original theme had long since been abandoned. As a guide beginners were given the motto: 'To make a catch you have to set a large number of traps, the more the better'. The only thing that counted eventually was the commercial product, every chemist's dream. This made them all lone fighters. The team spirit which had been highly successful with plasmoquine, fell into oblivion. While a cheerful, loyal, optimistic and jocular mood reigned in the workrooms, one taboo was rigidly observed. Everyone kept their own work secret. This led to grotesque behaviour, to chemists using codes to mark their bottles and containers. A highly successful colleague had a preference for ingenious abbreviations. Pyrogallol potassium disulphonate became 'Pydisuka' and this was where this particular chemist

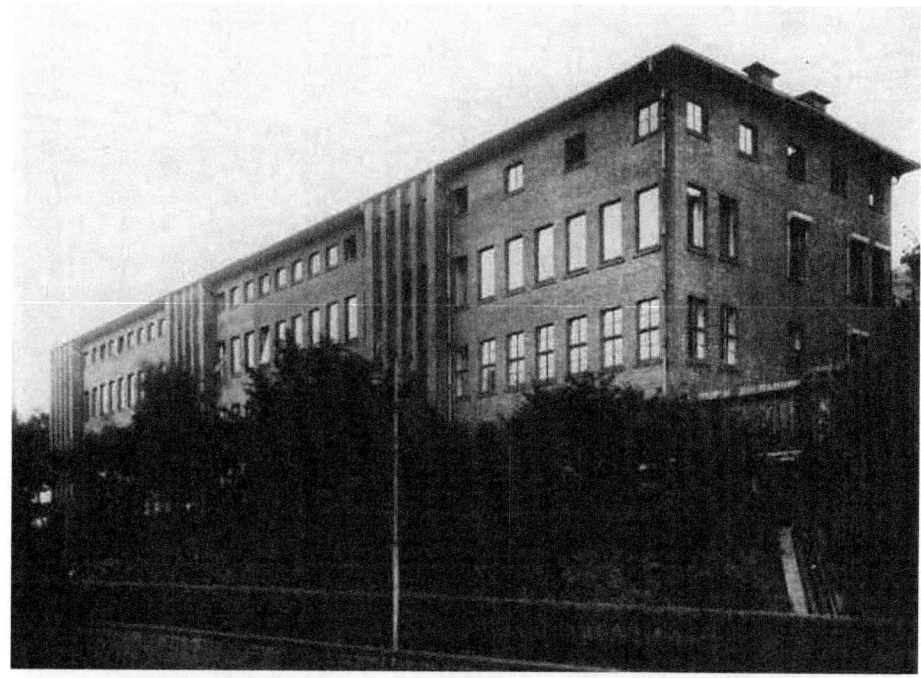

Figure 7.5
The medical laboratories in Elberfeld, 1929. The righthand part of the building was the laboratory of Domagk, in which he worked from 1929–1960. The middle section was Röhl's and was taken over by Kikuth in 1929. The lefthand section, which was later lengthened, housed Biochemical Research.

got his nickname. Work being organised in such a way made duplicate research unavoidable, but such duplication was always discovered and settled when the department head received the monthly reports. Hörlein used to say that four eyes saw more than two and that one would have to see who made the most of it. Permission for publication was only rarely given. It was only the patent application which gave one a general idea of the themes that were being pursued. Projects that were not patentable were shelved and forgotten. There was much less paper work in those days than there is today.

The chemist spent his time in the laboratory doing his own tests. There were no trained technicians then, a workman was trained on the job to give the chemist a hand. The chemical literature had to be studied at weekends. Conferences or group discussions were non-existent. Those were ideal working conditions for whoever was an enthusiastic experimenter with ideas of his own. People today have an indulgent smile for the way in which research was conducted in those days, but what seems to them ineffective now was highly successful 55 years ago.

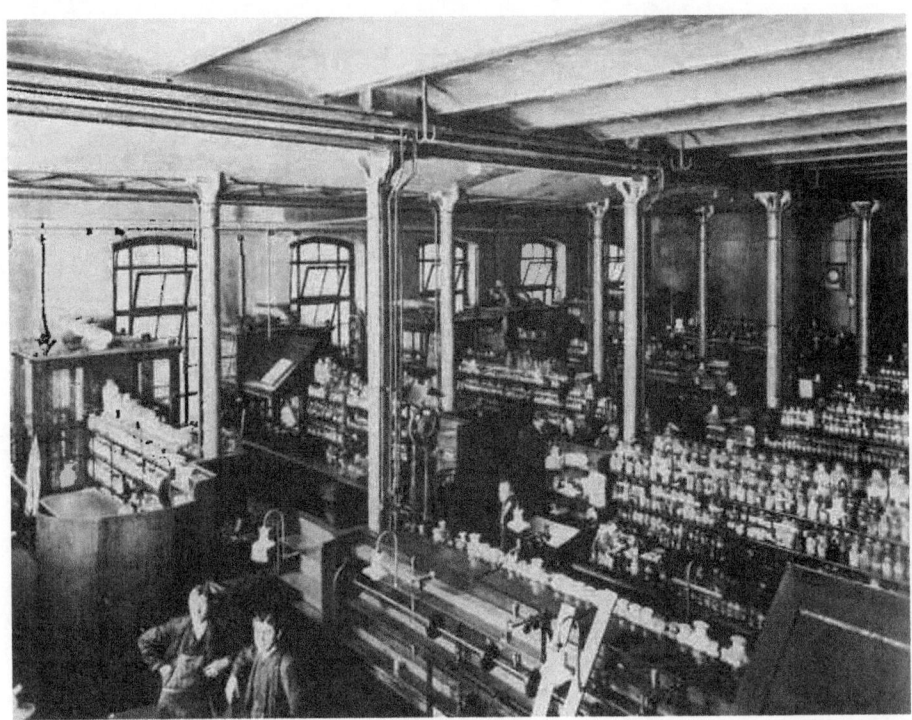

Figure 7.6
The pharmaceutical research laboratory, hall 1 at Elberfeld. Here Schulemann, Schönhöfer and Wingler synthesised Plasmoquine.

7.1.4 The new researchers: Klarer, Mietzsch and Domagk

This was the situation when a new phase of chemotherapeutic research began in 1927. H. Fischer, the Director of the Chemical Institute of the Technical University in Munich, recommended his assistant, Josef Klarer (1898–1953), to IG Farbenindustrie AG at Elberfeld, which he joined in 1927. Klarer was born in Munich, graduated from secondary school in 1916 and served in the first World War. He was severely wounded in action and after his convalescence at home entered Munich University to study mechanical engineering for two years and chemistry for six and a half. He received his doctorate under Fischer, obtaining the highest honours (Summa cum laude) for his sensational thesis on the synthesis of etioporphyrin, etiohaemin and etiophylline which proved to be identical with the breakdown products of blood and leaf pigments. In this way Klarer proved the structure of the dyes. He turned down the professorship he was offered and decided to join industry. At Elberfeld he was given the task of synthesizing compounds that might find application in bacterial infections. It was suggested that he turn to previous IG experiences with azo dyes and subject them to basic alkylation. Klarer was a highly creative, persevering and industrious man. He was an ardent experimenter

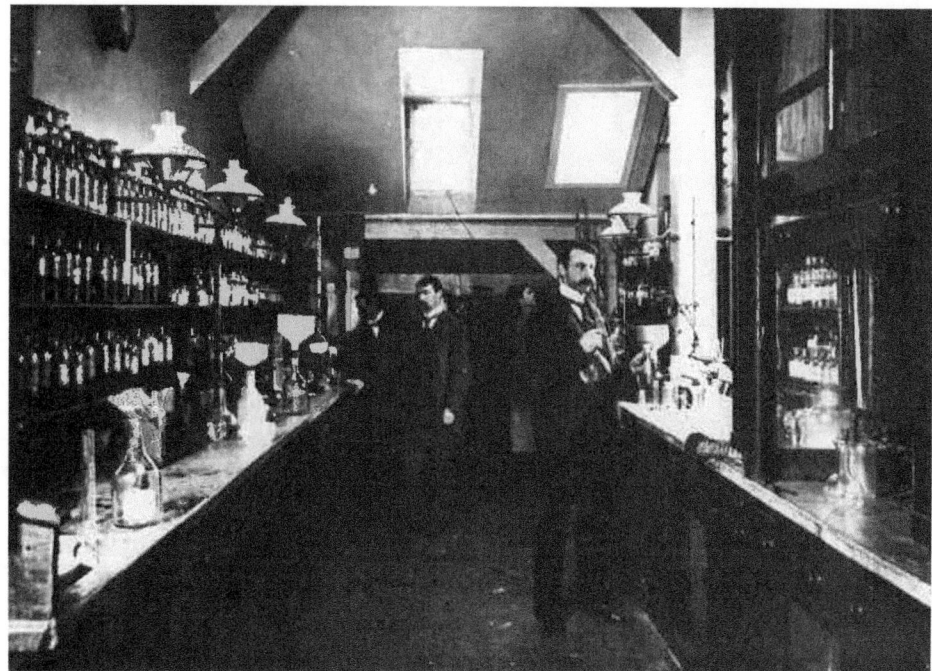

Figure 7.7
The old hall 4. Here preparations such as Luminal, Zephirol, Atebrin and the sulphonamides were discovered. The benches were little changed in 1927.

and had little use for theory. He was rough in his work habits and rather unmindful of his own health. His colleagues received little information about the work he was doing. The only man with whom he slowly made contact was Mietzsch, two years his senior, an experienced dye specialist, who was able to give him a great deal of advice. Beneath his rough surface Klarer was a highly sensitive man who reacted to apparent snubs or lack of recognition with anger turning into depression. During the last years of his life which were marred by ill health, he often had to take long 'rests' from creative thinking. He would retire to his lovely country house at Tegernsee where, under the loving care of his two sisters, he conceived plans for further research in his flower garden. Klarer was the only man to be allowed so much freedom as it was known that he would invariably return with new ideas. His assistant, A. Hirsing, filled in for him while he was away. Klarer worked in such seclusion that even long absences often went unnoticed. His last research project centred on the chemotherapy of carcinoma. He wanted to command success once more, but his untimely death prevented him from pursuing promising clues. Klarer's ideas are no longer reproducible; there is no reference to them in any of the laboratory journals in which he used to jot down his notes on the chemicals he employed. There are a few notes in a now obsolete shorthand, but there is no mention of results.

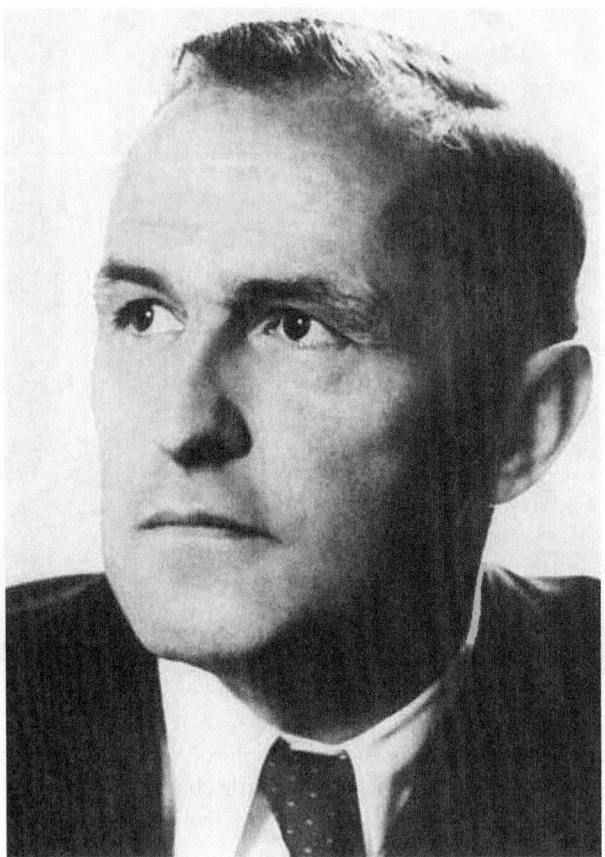

Figure 7.8
Dr. Ing. Dr. med.h.c. Josef Klarer (1889–1953).

Klarer was a self-confident man of original mind who energetically defended his right to do creative research in his own way. In 1937, in recognition of his work, Klarer was accorded the Emil Fischer Memorial Medal and the Gold Medal of the International Art and Technology Exhibition in Paris. In 1945 an honorary doctorate in medicine was conferred on him by the University of Münster. He died in Wuppertal on 21 June 1953.

Fritz Mietzsch (1896–1958) was an entirely different personality. Born in Dresden, he completed his secondary school education taking the 'Abitur' in 1914. In 1915 he was called up and had to interrupt his studies which he was not able to resume until his return in 1919. He took his doctorate in 1922 under König with a thesis on the halochromism of polymethine dyes. After a year as an assistant König recommended him to Farbenfabriken at Leverkusen. He attended Dressel's orientation course and next joined the department handling triphenyl methane dyes. Stimulated by the research Röhl was doing on malaria he wrote a memo

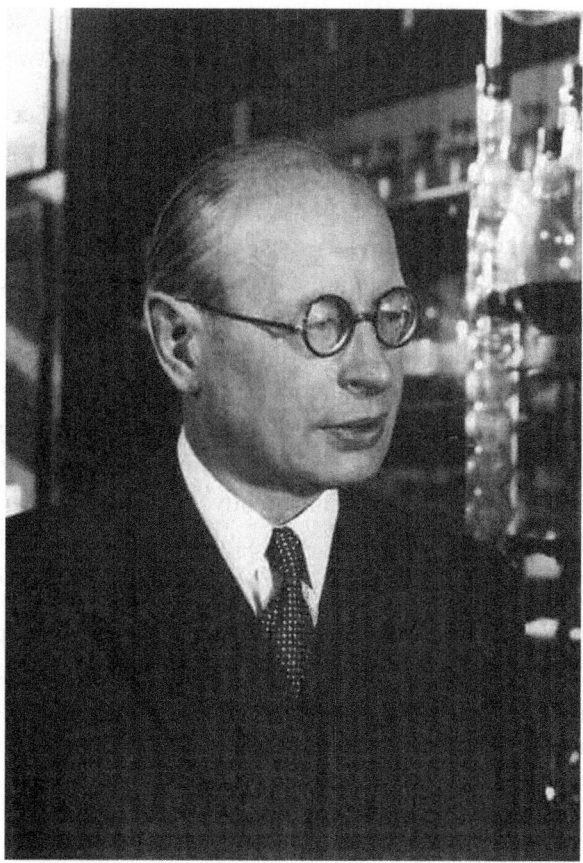

Figure 7.9
Prof. Dr. Ing., Dr. med.h.c. Fritz Mietzsch (1896–1958).

suggesting that compounds be obtained of some structural resemblance to quinine by hydration of 6-methoxylepidine, and to have them tested for antimalarial activity. This attracted the attention of Hörlein who got him transferred to Elberfeld. In the laboratory of pharmaceutical science at Elberfeld he made contact with Schulemann and was able to start work in his own field of interest. Before he was allowed to embark on his own research, however, he was given the assignment of working further on synthetic techniques to get plasmoquine and its intermediary products to the finished-product stage. Apart from this he was already engaged in the pursuit of his own ideas for the development of an antimalarial agent based on acridine. Here again, the procedure was one which had often been used with success, namely selection of a suitable ring system, the right substituents, and discovery of the optimal position in the ring. Five years' screening eventually led Mietzsch and his colleague H. Mauss (1901–1953) to discover the first synthetic agent against schizont parasites, Atebrine. This not only caused a sensation but proved a blessing to friend and foe when used in the combat of malaria during and after World War II. Atebrine was a huge scientific success which received public recognition in 1934 by the award of the Emil Fischer Memorial Medal to the two inventors.

Medical research on the acridine derivatives was initiated by Röhl and continued by Kikuth after the former's death. Kikuth who devised a test on the Java sparrow, was able for the first time to distinguish between gametocides and schizontocides.

Mietzsch was a quiet, distinguished, scholarly man who disliked noisy crowds. He never spoke in a loud voice. When he had reason for criticism his tone became emphatic, but was never brusque. He owed his successes to systematic thinking and diligent effort. He had everything perfectly planned. When he was tackling a problem, he made a statement, analysed the known facts, tested possible variations and worked out a detailed programme. This formed the basis of his weekly test schedules to which, if at all possible, he rigidly adhered. Some of these weekly schedules were found in his estate. One is inclined to think that the two, Mietzsch, a highly organised man and Klarer, an imaginative, spontaneous personality, must have made an ideal team. Nevertheless, while they were complementary to each other, each was too much of an individualist to inform the other fully and in good time of his own progress.

Mietzsch's work in the laboratory ended as early as 1949 when Hörlein appointed him leader of the chemical and pharmaceutical research units and made him a director. In 1953 he received an honorary professorship from the Department of Mathematics and Natural Sciences of the University of Bonn. In 1956 the Technical University Dresden awarded him the honorary degree of Dr. rer. nat. His death marked the end of the second era of chemotherapeutic research at Elberfeld that had lasted about 35 years.

The third member of the study group that created sulphonamide therapy was G. Domagk (1895–1964). He was born the son of a schoolmaster at Lagow (Mark Brandenburg), completed his secondary school education in Liegnitz taking his 'Abitur' at the local Oberrealschule in 1914. He studied medicine in Kiel, volunteered for military service, took part in the battle of Langemark, was wounded in combat on the Eastern front and served as a medical orderly in cholera hospitals. On the Somme and at Verdun he witnessed the helplessness of medicine and the misery of the men suffering from dysentery, hospital gangrene and gas gangrene for which there was no cure.

After the war Domagk returned to university and took his degree under M. Burger, Director of the Schittenhelm Clinic. In 1922 he became a house officer at the Pathological Clinic at Greifswald under W. Gross whom he followed to Münster in 1925. At that time the victims of influenza epidemics and young mothers dying of childbed fever became forever stamped upon his memory. There was no specific therapy for these and other diseases such as pneumonia, tuberculosis, erysipelas, meningitis and many others. Domagk described what was on his mind at the time: 'I thought it would be better to devote my life and knowledge to the search for one single element towards the discovery of a specific treatment rather than give a lifetime service to doing all over again what had been done virtually unsuccessfully for decades'.

In 1923 Domagk was fortunate to escape early death in a train crash. On 31 July 1923, travelling from Greifswald to Southern Germany, he wanted to take the D 88 night train to Munich, but as this was crowded he went on a relief train which left a little earlier. Before Domagk's train reached Kreiensen something was found to be wrong with the engine and the train was kept waiting for a replacement engine at the station. Domagk left his compartment in the rear part of the train to have a drink. At that moment the main train went through the stop sign and hit the relief train at full speed, destroying the rear part completely. Domagk helped to administer emergency treatment to the victims and then continued on his journey.

In 1927 Hörlein offered him the post of head of a Laboratory of Bacteriology and Experimental Pathology which was about to be created. Domagk accepted the offer without hesitation as the funds he expected to need for his research could only be provided by industry. How did Domagk come to be chosen? His work on the destruction of infective agents by the reticuloendothelial system (RES) had aroused the interest of Hörlein who thought this might be a new approach to chemotherapy. While tests to isolate effective compounds from the RES were unsuccessful, it was found that damaged microorganisms are very easily catabolised in the reticuloendothelial cells. This finding suggested that chemical agents be used to damage the microorganisms in order to kill them by phagocytosis. This marked the new approach, i.e. the search for bacteriostatic instead of bactericidal agents, to support bodily defences against bacterial infection. From then on tests in vitro ceased to play a major role and served, at most, as guidelines.

The following is a list of Domagk's spectacular successes:

> 1932: discovery of the chemotherapeutic value of the sulphonamides prepared by Klarer and Mietzsch;
> 1936: successful treatment of gonorrhoea using products prepared by Klarer, Mietzsch and Behnisch;
> 1938: discovery of the effect of chemotherapeutic agents in gaseous infections, using compounds of the Marfanil type made by Klarer;
> 1939: Nobel Prize Award;
> 1941: discovery of the therapeutic effects of the thiosemicarbazones supplied by Behnisch;
> 1945 and after: success in tumour therapy using thymine derivatives found by Westphal, and ethyleneimine quinones discovered by Petersen and Gauss.

Domagk retired in 1960 and died of an infection of the bile ducts at Burgberg (Black Forest) on 24 April 1964, having been dogged by severe rheumatic pain for many years. Domagk was a cheerful man, at peace with himself and modest for all his successes. He devoted his entire

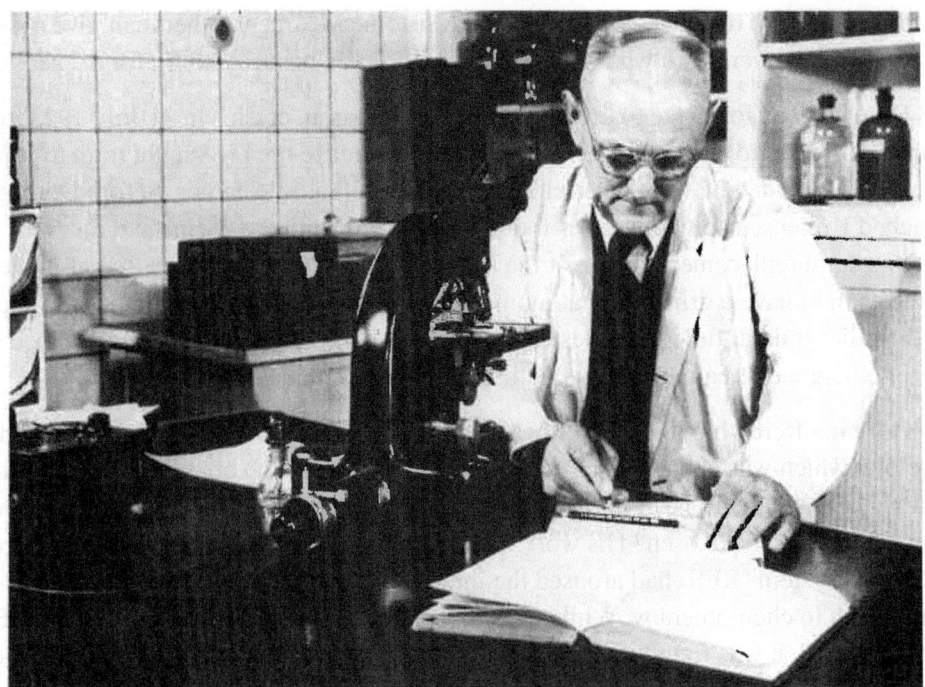

Figure 7.10
Domagk at work.

energy to research and to helping the sick. He loved nature, particularly the lakes and forests of his native region, and the valleys and mountains of Bavaria. Domagk was a connoisseur of the visual arts and a close friend of such eminent painters as Emil Nolde, Christian Rohlfs and Otto Dix. He was an amusing raconteur who held his audience captive with stories of his travels or meetings with well-known politicians, artists and scientists. Once a year he would invite his collaborators and assistants to dinner and a social gathering at his ever open home. These were the highlights of everyday life in those days and are still talked about today. Averse to noisy crowds, Domagk particularly loved brilliant conversation with a small circle of friends. One may wonder what made his life's work so immensely successful. The answer lies primarily in diligent effort, courage to tackle even apparently hopeless problems and perseverance refusing to be discouraged by failures. But there is more to it than that; Domagk had an unfailing gift for recognising even the slightest effects of a given test substance and could distinguish off-hand between compounds that held promise and those that did not. In his studies he observed and followed up even the slightest deviation from the norm. He did his own postmortem dissections and microscopic examinations of animal organ sections. When carrying out his weekly postmortem examinations he was accessible to no one, took no telephone calls and received no visitors. On this part of his work Domagk commented as follows: 'We dissected until we could no longer stand on our feet and looked through microscopes until we could no longer see'. This was his habit till his last working day.

If it also takes luck for a researcher to be successful, Domagk was lucky to meet at Elberfeld junior chemists who did research with the same optimism and intensity as he did and never tired in supplying him with new compounds. In contrast to the widely held view these collaborative projects had no leader. Domagk did not bother about chemistry and the chemists left medicine to him. Successes were founded on mutual trust between equals working in partnership.

7.2 Research 1927–1935

7.2.1 The discovery of Prontosil

When, in 1927, Klarer started his search for effective compounds against bacterial infections, he had very little to go on. Apart from verbal inter-office reports on experiences from germanin, plasmoquine and atebrine research, the only reference in the literature was to some azo dyes used in urinary tract infections such as azohel, azo toluene, pyridium and neotropine (1–4), and to a few quaternary acridine derivatives.

1 Azohel

2 Azo toluene

3 Pyridium

4 Neotropine

Klarer logically combined the basic structure of azobenzene with the principle of basic alkylation and the introduction of further substituents. By the end of 1931 he had prepared some 300 new compounds which he submitted for testing in bacterial and protozoal infections. Having taken possession of the laboratory facility especially equipped for him in 1929, Domagk had substantially expanded testing facilities. In addition to the streptococcal test introduced by Röhl and later improved, there was now routine testing involving staphylococci, pneumococci, meningococci, coli bacteria, gonococci, *Clostridium septicum,* gas gangrene, parathyphoid fever, tubercle bacilli and carcinoma. Domagk managed to carry out this comprehensive test programme with 6 women technicians and a few workers for animal care. All compounds he received were subjected to the complete series of tests. During the first

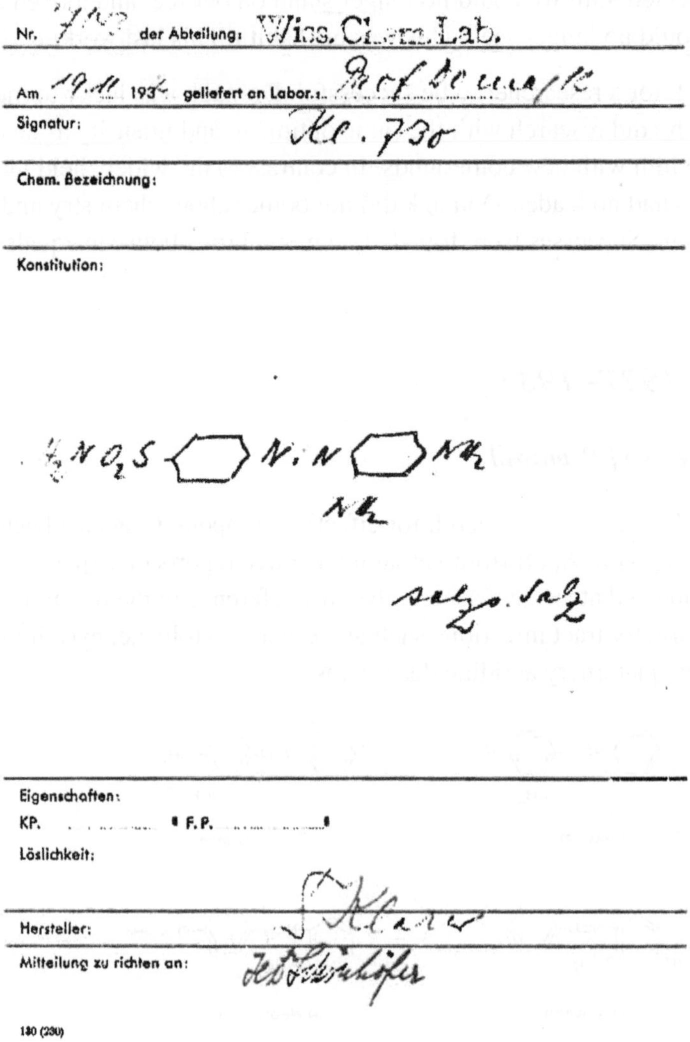

Nr. *7..?* der Abteilung: Wiss. Chem. Lab.

Am *19.11* 193*2* geliefert an Labor.: *Prof Domagk*

Signatur: *Kl. 730*

Chem. Bezeichnung:

Konstitution:

H₂NO₂S ⬡ *N:N* ⬡ *NH₂*

NH₂

salzs. Salz

Eigenschaften:

KP. . . . . F.P. . . . .

Löslichkeit:

Hersteller: *Klarer*

Mitteilung zu richten an: *Hörlein*

180 (230)

Figure 7.11
With this delivery note, Klarer first sent Domagk, on 19th November, 1932, preparation Kl 730,
later called Prontosil.

4 years results were not particularly encouraging, but Domagk remained optimistic. There
were only five compounds that seemed to have merit. When tested by Röhl, (5) showed an
effect in bird malaria, (6) cured mice infected with *Trypanosoma gambiense* in Kikuth's
experiments and (7) attracted Kikuth's interest in view of its effect in rat leprosy. In 1931
Wesenberg noticed that (8) and (9) were moderately effective in destroying streptococci,
staphylococci and coli bacteria in vitro, an effect Domagk was unable to confirm in animals.

Modification of molecules failed to lead to any useful drugs being developed from these compounds.

This inspired the search for new substituents that had not so far been tested. At this juncture the major question occurs as to who first brought up the words 'sulphonamide group'. There is no definite answer to this question. According to Mietzsch, the suggestion came from Hörlein who himself never so much as claimed authorship. Klarer stated that, in conversation, Hörlein had referred to the patent processes for the manufacture of substantive cotton dyes he had filed together with Kothe and Dressel and suggested that they should be studied for suitable substituents. Thereupon he, Klarer, had first selected the sulphonamide group as it was easy to isolate. However it came about that the sulphonamide group achieved the first breakthrough. When Domagk tested the dye K1695 (10) prepared by Klarer, he found that its effect in mice with streptococcal infections was superior to anything that had been investigated before. From then on the molecule was systematically manipulated and reduced until, in 1932, the drug Kl 730 (11) was finally born and Domagk suggested that it be tested in patients. In a few months' time Klarer had prepared 35 new compounds and the necessary intermediate products, the result of enormous diligence! After careful pharmacological and toxicological testing, the product (11) named streptozone was sent to a few specially selected hospitals for clinical evaluation in patients.

As there was general scepticism, the study had a very slow start, but in the months that followed it yielded surprisingly good results in such diseases as puerperal sepsis and erysipelas as well as in mild cases of pneumonia. Results after two years were sufficiently conclusive to warrant the launching of streptozone. At first the decision team showed reluctance and was highly sceptical of the results, and it was only thanks to Domagk's passionate pleading and convincing arguments that it was eventually decided to market the drug under the brand name of Prontosil.

10   H_2N-SO_2—⟨benzene⟩—N=N—⟨benzene⟩—$\underset{C_2H_5}{N}-CH_2-\overset{OH}{CH}-CH_2-NH_2$

11   H_2N-SO_2—⟨benzene⟩—N=N—⟨benzene, $\underset{NH_2}{}$⟩—NH_2 Prontosil

11a H_2N-SO_2—⟨benzene⟩—NH_2 Sulphanilamide

12   H_2N-SO_2—⟨benzene⟩—N=N—⟨naphthalene, OH, NaO_3S, SO_3Na⟩—$NH-CO-CH_3$ Prontosil soluble

The drug could only be administered as tablets. For injection, an azo dye, M783 (12), pre-pared by Mietzsch, was chosen. This dye, obtained from diazotized sulphanilamide with acetyl niobic acid, formed a sodium salt easily soluble in water at neutral pH, which could be injected without causing irritation. This was named Prontosil S, often termed Prontosil solubile. Both products soon came into their own. Domagk's first publication (1935) created a sensation and requests for supplies started flowing in from everywhere. Apart from many positive reactions there were disappointments and drawbacks. Endocarditis proved not to be amenable to Prontosil therapy and results in urinary tract infections failed to come up to ex-pectations. Fourneau attacked Hörlein for having kept this major invention secret for so many years. Hörlein emphatically rejected the attack contending that a new class of compounds such as the above called for particular caution with regard to safety before permitting its un-restricted use. There were frequent reports of spectacular successes. As early as 1933 Domagk used Prontosil successfully in his 4-year-old daughter whose arm was to be amputated as she had acquired septicaemia from a phlegmon. The author is able to report a similar instance involving his then sixty-year old mother in Breslau whose case is an example of Domagk's great kindness. Mrs. B. had had a fall and broken her metacarpal bone. A large wood splinter that had penetrated deeply into her hand had been overlooked and amputation was required for septicaemia affecting the entire limb. When telephoned to give his permission for surgery, her son immediately got in touch with Domagk who directly contacted the head of the Breslau pharma office. The latter immediately set out to the clinic with a hospital pack of Prontosil. Doctors there had not yet had occasion to test the drug that had only recently been launched. With great hesitation they agreed to try chemotherapeutic treatment since they felt the patient had little chance of surviving the amputation because of her poor general condition. Intensive treatment cured the septicaemia, the splinter could be removed and the fracture treated. The patient made an uneventful recovery and was discharged from hospital after five weeks. Cases such as this brought the product great recognition. Prontosil was thought a wonder drug by the mothers cured of the dreaded childbed fever. A wonder drug it certainly was not, but put to the right use in the hands of the physician it could be of the greatest value. Domagk received many letters from grateful patients; Klarer never got one.

Dr. Klarer.

Monatsbericht für November 1932.

In Fortsetzung der Arbeit basischer Azofarbstoffe wurde, da
sich der im September-Bericht bereits beschriebene Körper von
der Formel :

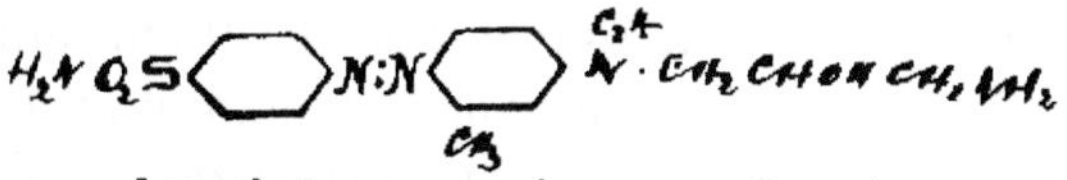

gegen Strept. Seps. als wirksam erwies, wurde eine grössere An-
zahl mit der Sulfamidgruppe substituierterDerivate hergestellt.

Es ist bekannt dass Chrisoidin eine gewisse bakterizide Wirkung
aufweist. Um den Einfluss der Sulfamidgruppe auf diesen Körper zu
studieren und ferner die Patentlage zu erweitern, gewann ich fol-
gende Körper :

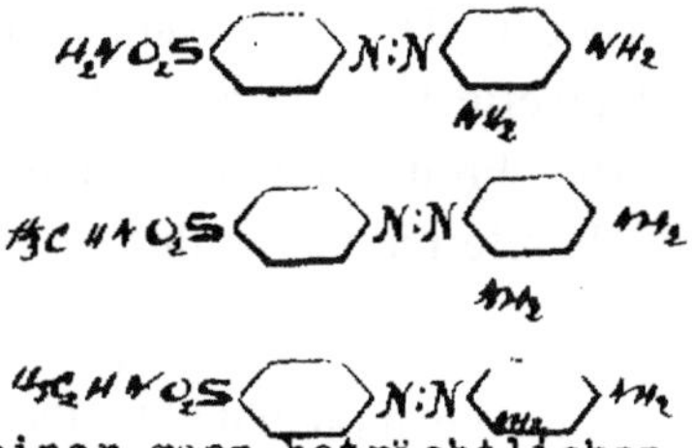

mit dem Erfolg einer ganz beträchtlichen Steigerung der Wirkung
gegen Streptococcen.

Wuppertal-Elberfeld, den 5. Dezember 1932.

Figure 7.12
Extract from Klarer's monthly report for November 1932, in which the structure of Prontosil was
written for the first time.

7.2.2 The turning point: Advent of colourless products, Trefouel and Fourneau

Soon after the clinical results became known, industrial and research laboratories all over the world began intensive work on the sulphonamides. Here again, research was concerned mainly with azo dyes. Of the many new compounds from diazotized sulphanilamide only two attained temporary importance. The drug (13) described by Goissedet et al. in 1936 was used in Egyptian eye disease under the name of Salosept, but its effects were not convincing. Authors of the introductory paper were Burnet et al. (1939); the drug became also known by the names of Lutazol, Azoique 33, Jodosil and Chromosulfol. The drug (14) described by Levaditi and Vaisman (1935) and Gley and Girard (1936) was commercially available as Rubiazol, a competitor product of Prontosil. Prontosil was so popular with doctors mainly because of its excellent tolerance that it was not withdrawn from the market until 1966, after 30 years of use. The injectable solution was on sale until 1958.

When Klarer and Mietzsch were still busy completing the patents, the famous publication of Tréfouel et al. (1935) appeared and had the effect of a bombshell. In summary, the article read that the active principle was not the azo dye, Prontosil, but the other part of the molecule, the simple sulphanilic acid amide (11a) briefly referred to as sulphanilamide and described by Gelmo in 1908.

The excitement caused by this paper can only be appreciated by those who witnessed it. Many chemists had been working on this product, but nobody had had it tested. At Elberfeld, where it had been manufactured by the ton, nobody thought it possible that Domagk should not have tested it. But all enquiries were fruitless. A large number of sulphanilic acid alkyl- and dialkylamides had been tested and found ineffective. Only the parent substance had been forgotten. Everybody thought they could fall back on the other; lack of communication, too, had had a negative effect. Fourneau again raised accusations against Hörlein for withholding the truth about sulphanilamide the better to sell the patented product, Prontosil. In Hörlein's honour it must be said that he was indeed unaware of the effectiveness of sulphanilamide, improbable as this may sound. This dispute, too, was resolved.

Intensive research on sulphanilamide derivatives now began worldwide with the objective of finding more potent drugs. At Elberfeld steps were also taken to regain lost ground. A further chemist, R. Behnisch, born 1909, joined the group of the sulphonamide researchers. The question keeps recurring why it was not possible in this critical situation to expand the study group for the sake of making rapid headway. The answer is simple. Domagk's research laboratories were working to capacity even then and while it would have been quite possible to recruit additional staff, provide the money and find the space, animal supplies presented an insurmountable problem.

Mietzsch immediately set about assigning tasks. Klarer was to handle N1 substitution, Behnisch N4 substitution and Mietzsch substitution in the ring. To him, the field of substitution in the ring seemed to hold great promise as experience with plasmoquine and atabrine had taught him the great role that type and position of substituents could play in increasing effectiveness. Efforts in this direction were unsuccessful as it became clear that substituents in the aromatic ring diminish or abolish potency.

N4 substitution, that is, substitution at the group of the aromatic amines, was studied by many research groups both domestic and foreign. A host of drugs were tested, but only a few gained temporary importance on the market such as the condensation products with formaldehyde sulphoxylate, formaldehyde bisulphite, acetaldehyde and cinnamaldehyde bisulphite. The latter compound (15) prepared by Rhône-Poulenc in 1936, was commercially available for many years under the name of Soluseptazine. As a sodium salt it had the advantage of being readily soluble in water at a neutral pH. It was very well tolerated. Its effect was based on gradual hydrolysis whose equilibrium was measured by Barber and Wilkinson in 1946.

Conversion of a slightly soluble sulphonamide to a readily soluble form without loss of effectiveness, a principle first employed with Soluseptazine, was often used with success in the years that followed. Another condensation product based on sulphanilamide, glucose, formaldehyde and sodium hydrogen sulphite prepared by Boehringer Mannheim in 1949, proved its value in paediatric practice when given as a high-per cent aqueous solution (Ladogal).

Of the N4-alkyl and aralkyl derivatives only N4 benzyl sulphanilamide was on the market for a few years under the names of Septazine (16) (manufacturers Rhône-Poulenc) and Proseptazine (May and Baker). According to James and Fuller (1940) the effect of this product was also based on the slow separation of sulphanilamide.

15   $H_2N-SO_2-\langle\ \rangle-NH-CH-CH_2-CH-\langle\ \rangle$ Soluseptazine
                              | |
                            SO_3Na   SO_3Na

16   $H_2N-SO_2-\langle\ \rangle-NH-CH_2-\langle\ \rangle$ Septazine

The N4 acetyl compounds were very thoroughly studied. Effective products containing the residues of isovaleric acid, oleic acid and mandelic acid, had no appreciable advantages over the parent compound. *n*-butylaminoacetyl-N4-sulphanilamide (17) was clinically tested against angina for several years as Be 365 or Angonal. Despite the promising results the drug eventually failed to gain wide acceptance in view of the bitter taste characteristic of many sulphonamides which could not be masked without loss of efficacy. With the importance of N1 substitution becoming known, this research direction was soon abandoned.

7.2.3 Start of worldwide sulphonamide research: The first antigonorrheal agents

Linkage of two sulphanilamide molecules by a sulphonamide bridge yields compounds of the diseptale type (18–20) which bear a structural resemblance to the N1 or N4 derivatives. This class was investigated by Mietzsch, Klarer and Behnisch in 1936 and was found by Domagk (1937) to have a specific effect in gonococcal infections and to be increasingly effective in staphylococcal and gas gangrene infections. With oral administration alone both male and female patients could be cured of acute and chronic gonorrhoea. On account of the clinical results obtained by Felke (1937), Fischer (1937) and Schreus (1937), Uliron (18) was launched in 1937. Two years later the slightly more potent Neo-Uliron (19) emerged with Grütz (1937). Uliron C (20) was the most potent drug of this series, but as it frequently produced cyanosis it was unsuitable for practical application.

When the ulirones were given for prolonged periods and in excessive doses they were associated with side effects such as exanthema and nervous lesions. Reputed German clinicians, Felke in particular, worked out a dosage scheme for sulphonamides involving the short-term use of massive doses spaced sufficiently far apart to avoid the above lesions. The concept of massive-dose therapy was applied to all subsequent sulphonamides. After many years of successful application efficacy began to decline due to the formation of ulirone-resistant bacterial strains remaining unaffected by further treatment.

17	H_2N-SO_2—⟨ ⟩—$NH-CO-CH_2-NH-C_4H_9$	Angonal
18	$(CH_3)_2N-SO_2$—⟨ ⟩—$NH-SO_2$—⟨ ⟩—NH_2	Uliron (diseptal)
19	$CH_3-NH-SO_2$—⟨ ⟩—$NH-SO_2$—⟨ ⟩—NH_2	Neo Uliron (diseptal B)
20	H_2N-SO_2—⟨ ⟩—$NH-SO_2$—⟨ ⟩—NH_2	Uliron C (diseptal C)

When sufficient penicillin became available for the treatment of gonorrhoea, therapy with Neo-Uliron experienced a drastic decline but did not fade into disuse until 1966. Research on N1 derivatives of sulphanilamide was taken up with great intensity by researchers all over the world in 1936. Discoveries occurred in quick succession and research activities became hectic. At this stage differences of opinion arose occasionally between Domagk and the chemists about the evaluation of test results. For the sake of continued research planning the chemists wanted quantified results to be able to quickly distinguish effective from less effective drugs. They met with a friendly, but categorical, refusal from Domagk who explained his attitude roughly as follows: 'it is impossible to compare findings of this week with those of the next. When I say: effect, some effect, no effect, this applies to one series only. I look at each series personally and can tell you with certainty if there is something we can use. I shall be glad to run any comparative test you want if you tell me what's to be compared'. An agreement was invariably reached on this basis. In the light of present-day knowledge Domagk was right. In point of fact, he never overlooked an effective compound, and apart from this the available animal material did not permit him to be more precise. The mice had to be bought in large or even very small lots from a variety of suppliers from far and wide. The animals were of different strains and quality, some of them suffering from infections, just as they happened to be available, for there were never enough of them. There was neither time nor room for placing them in quarantine. Domagk took it all in his stride but under circumstances which no department head would accept today, he was unable to produce comparable data.

There was also a need for many new ideas from the chemical world as conventional methods had often failed with the N1 series. The first launch came as a surprise from Schering, namely N1-acetylsulphanilamide (21) *Sulphacetamide*, prepared by Dohrn and Diedrich in 1938, brand name Albucid. This compound, of simple chemical structure, was very effective against gonococci, the sodium salt being readily soluble in water and neutral in solution. The drug was very well tolerated and proved its value as a concentrated injectable solution in gonorrhoea, meningitis, trachoma and urinary infections. Spiethoff (1938), Vonkennel and Korth (1938) were the authors of the clinical papers.

Geigy developed N1 dimethylacroylsulphanilamide (22), commercially available since 1941 under the brand name of Irgamid. It was used for the treatment of bacterial infections of the eyelid, conjunctiva, and cornea. Author of the introductory paper was Högger (1941). The drug is still currently being employed in a small way as Irgamid eye drops. Two further compounds of this series, also stemming from Geigy research, were N1-3,4-dimethylbenzoyl sulphanilamide (23), brand name Irgaphen, launched in 1943. It was a broad-spectrum drug for use in infections caused by streptococci, pneumococci and coli bacteria, but was withdrawn a few years later because of occasional instances of cyanosis. A further compound was N1-4-isopropoxy benzoyl sulphanilamide (24) *Sulphaproxylinum*. Combined with *Sulphamerazin* this drug continues to occupy a place on the market down to the present day (brand name Dosulfin syrup), although it may cause side effects that require medical supervision. Moreover, the series of N1 acetyl compounds which offers unlimited scope for variation, has been thoroughly tested in all directions. Nothing new or superior to the compounds described above has been discovered.

21–24 Derivatives of the general formula: H₂N—⟨benzene⟩—SO₂–NH–R

	R=	*Generic name*	Brand name(s)
21	–CO–CH₃	*Sulphacetamide*	Albucid, Urosulfon
22	–CO–CH=C(CH₃)(CH₃)	*Sulphadicrymidium*	Irgamid
23	–CO–⟨C₆H₃(CH₃)(CH₃)⟩		Irgaphen
24	–CO–⟨C₆H₄⟩–O–CH(CH₃)(CH₃)	*Sulphaproxylinum*	Component of Dosulfin

7.3 Dramatic changes 1937–1945

In the minds of those directly concerned with sulphonamide research, the years between 1938 and 1941 represented a period of dramatic tension and exciting discoveries. Articles in chemical and medical journals appeared in such profusion as to make critical appraisal almost impossible. Four new classes of substances with surprising effects were discovered. These were 4-aminomethyl benzole sulphonic acid amide with a specific effect against anaerobic bacteria (Section 7.3.1.), 4,4'-diaminodiphenyl sulphone and its derivatives (Section 7.3.2.), the sulphanilyl ureas (Section 7.3.3.), and the sulphonamides substituted in the heterocycle that were studied for nearly 20 years and will be dealt with in a separate section (4.). The award of the Nobel Prize to Domagk in 1939 is described in Section 7.3.4.

The four fields were investigated simultaneously and results coincided in such a manner that it would be confusing to give the chronological history. Instead, developments are herein described on the basis of chemical relationships.

7.3.1 First agents effective against anaerobic infections

Klarer was one of the few researchers who would not be influenced by the general excitement. He innovated research in his own way and avoided handling the heterocyclic sulphonamides as long as he possibly could. In 1938 he synthesized 4-aminomethyl benzole sulphonic acid amide (25), later to become known as Marfanil. Domagk's investigations (1942) revealed that the drug, when administered topically, was highly effective against streptococci, microorganisms causing gas gangrene and *Clostridium septicum.* It had, however, only little effect when given orally. Mitchell et al. (1944) confirmed that the drug had penicillin-like activity. The action of Marfanil, unlike that of the other sulphonamides, was not nullified by 4-aminobenzoic acid; it remained effective even in the presence of PAB. Marfanil proved a blessing in the treatment of wound infections in World War II and saved the lives of thousands of wounded soldiers and civilians. The first publication came from Klarer and so did the IG patent (1939). In order to achieve a dispersing cone covering as large a surface as possible, Marfanil was used mainly in combination with sulphanilamide as an MP powder (Marfanil-Prontalbin). Packed in convenient small sifter-top containers, it was to be found not only in every soldier's kitbag but also in the medicine chests of many homes and was very popular as an emergency treatment of wounds in danger of infection. It was not until 1981 that sales of the product were discontinued. Haferland (1941) provided a review of the application of the powder. Marbadal, prepared by Klarer in 1944, a further development, consisted of a stable salt from the strongly alkaline Marfanil and the acid sulphanilyl thiourea. It is said to possess increased potency due to synergistic action and is still employed as a pharmaceutical chemical today.

Author of the first publication was Klarer (1947). Many laboratories worked on this class of substances, but a better product never emerged.

25   H_2N-SO_2-⟨benzene ring⟩-CH_2-NH_2 *Mafenidum*   Marfanil

7.3.2 Discovery of sulphones with bacteriostatic effects

While the discovery of 4,4′-diaminodiphenylsulphone (DADPS) (26) dates back to 1908, nothing was known about its antibacterial effects. Two independent research groups, Buttle et al. (1937) and Fourneau et al. (1937) discovered that the compound was about ten times as effective as sulphanilamide and also exerted slight activity in leprosy and tuberculosis. An alarming report! A compound containing no sulphonamide group but having a similar spectrum of action did not agree with any of the theories then existing on the mechanism of action of the sulphonamides. Domagk was able to confirm these findings but also observed tenfold higher toxicity. Thus the problem was to use substituents to achieve a tenfold decrease in toxicity without loss of efficacy. Fourneau et al. (1937) found that the 4,4′-diacetyl compound, launched by Rhône-Poulenc under the name of Rodilone (27), largely met these requirements. The product did not make headway; its effects failed to come up to expectations and there were instances of cyanosis. Domagk made the interesting observation that the drug was highly toxic only when given by the oral route. When the extremely poorly soluble compound (27) was administered parenterally as a very finely dispersed suspension, its effect and tolerance improved considerably. Such preparations were not, however, suitable for use in human patients.

In order to tackle the large field of the sulphones systematically, new ways of synthesising the starting material (26) had to be found. Eight newly synthesized compounds patented in quick succession are an indication of the interest the subject had attracted in many places. At Elberfeld, Behnisch and Pöhls (1906–1975) were instructed to undertake efforts in this area.

They found that coal slurry, a waste product of sulphonamide manufacture containing the byproduct (27), seemed to be a suitable source of the starting material they were looking for. The idea was to find readily soluble injectable derivatives gradually releasing DADPS into the circulation. Only two out of some 200 compounds tested met these requirements. The 4,4'-diaminodiphenyl sulphone digalactoside (28) prepared by Behnisch was launched in 1941 under the brand name of Tibatin. Among the glycosides prepared it was the only one whose isolation in crystallized form presented no technical problem. Tibatin was very well tolerated when given in daily doses of up to 10 g by the intramuscular, intravenous and intralumbar routes. It proved its value in severe septicaemia, particularly in puerperal sepsis and otogenic sepsis where it was clearly superior to previous therapy with Prontosil S. For the veterinary sector Behnisch prepared the condensation product with 2 moles of acetaldehyde hydrogen sulphite sodium (29), brand name Baludon, which was effective in the same indications. Tibatin remained on the market for about 14 and Baludon for 34 years until both products were displaced by antibiotics. All attempts to create from this series effective agents against leprosy and tuberculosis were eventually unsuccessful despite promising beginnings. After 1950, selective research in this area was abandoned.

26	$H_2N-\langle\rangle-SO_2-\langle\rangle-NH_2$	*Diphenylsulphone*	DADPS
27	$CH_3-CO-NH-\langle\rangle-SO_2-\langle\rangle-NH-CO-CH_3$		Rodilone
28	$C_6H_{11}O_5-NH-\langle\rangle-SO_2-\langle\rangle-NH-C_6H_{11}O_5$		Tibatin
29	$CH_3-CH(SO_3Na)-NH-\langle\rangle-SO_2-\langle\rangle-NH-CH(SO_3Na)-CH_3$		Baludon

7.3.3 Carbonic acid derivatives of sulphanilamide

Apart from combination drugs, the sulphanilyl compounds of urea, thiourea and guanidine, did not gain importance as chemotherapeutic agents except in special indications. Considering their simple structure it is surprising that they were not investigated until 1939, when sulphapyridine and sulphathiazole were already known. The reason is that urea and thiourea do not react with sulphochlorides while guanidine does so only under strictly limited conditions. As long as there were more important things to do, the search for new ways of product synthesis was put off to a future time.

7.3.3.1 Sulphanilyl ureas

Sulphanilyl urea (30), mostly incorrectly referred to in the literature as sulpha urea, was intensively studied by the Heyden company at Radebeul, later Munich, and by Geigy who discovered and patented the major new manufacturing processes. The drug is very rapidly absorbed and 90% is excreted in the urine. It is therefore particularly suited to the treatment of urinary tract infections, but supplemental doses must be given at short intervals to maintain adequate blood levels. It is the sulphonamide with the shortest elimination half-life, viz. 2–3 hours. Domagk's judgement was cautious as his tests had shown the drug to be markedly inferior to the standard sulphonamides. This finding was undoubtedly test-related as no provision had been made in the design for supplemental doses to be given at short intervals, all the more so as the significance of elimination half-lives was unknown then. The product (Euvernil, Heyden) has remained on the market to this day. The same suppliers prepared an ingenious variant of Euvernil. Conversion by means of phthalic acid anhydride and formaldehyde yielded the compound (31) Intestin-Euvernil (Heyden). This drug presents the readily absorbable Euvernil in a form of which 90% is excreted in the intestine and which is therefore used with success in intestinal infections.

The author of the introductory paper was Hartenbach (1954). Both products, though now superseded by more effective drugs, count among the oldest sulphonamides in the therapeutic armamentarium. The work of Haack on sulphanilyl urea marked the opening of the era of the oral antidiabetics which are briefly described in Section 7.6.1.

30	$H_2N-C(=O)-NH-SO_2-C_6H_4-NH_2$	*Sulphanilyl urea*	Euvernil
31	$HO-CH_2-NH-C(=O)-NH-SO_2-C_6H_4-NH-CO-C_6H_4-COOH$		Intestin-Euvernil
32	$H_2N-C(=S)-NH-SO_2-C_6H_4-NH_2$	*Sulphanilylthiourea*	Badional, Fontamide
33	$H_2N-C(=NH)-NH-SO_2-C_6H_4-NH_2$	*Sulphanilyl guanidine*	Resulfon

7.3.3.2 Sulphanilyl thioureas

Sulphanilyl thiourea (32), first described as an intermediate product by the Chinoin company, was tested for bacteriostatic effect in France and Germany. Apart from its efficacy in the known sulphonamide indications, it was found to be effective in mycosis and skin tuberculosis by Mayer in 1941, and in leg ulcers by Heinrichs in 1944. Its advantage over the other sulphonamides lay in its strongly acid reaction which made it possible to prepare neutral salts, of which Marbadal (cf. Section 7.3.1.) was probably the most important. To prepare Marbadal, large amounts of sulphanilyl thiourea were required that were not at all easy to come by. Within a few years eight new processes were patented, all of them posing considerable problems with regard to technology and equipment. They involved the use of substances that are among the most foul-smelling in chemistry and also toxic, such as hydrogen sulphide, thioacetic acid or mercaptane. It was only in 1946 that mass production could be started. The pure substance, sold under the brand name of Badional (Bayer) and Fontamide (Rhône-Poulenc) played no great role in oral therapy. Conversely, drugs for external application retained their place in practice for more than 10 years. Badional Gel for the treatment of burns, scaldings, skin lesions and wound infections remained a household remedy for decades. In the literature, sulphanilyl thiourea is mostly referred to incorrectly as sulpha thiourea. The generic name 'Sulphathiourea' is also a rather unfortunate choice.

7.3.3.3 Sulphanilyl guanidine

Sulphanilyl guanidine (33), mostly incorrectly termed sulphaguanidine, occupies a special place among the sulphonamides. It is insoluble in alkali and, according to the theory of the relationship between pK_a value and effect, ought to be ineffective. In spite of this, it was very thoroughly studied. Only 40% is absorbed and excreted mainly in the intestine. It proved its value in the treatment of chronic and acute intestinal infections. Although the product was initially offered by many manufacturers, it was only Resulfon (manufacturer Nordmark) that remained on the market until the early 1980's. Synthesis offered a wide range of activities in chemistry. Approximately 12 new syntheses were patented within a few years' time. The major importance of sulphanilyl guanidine is as an intermediary product in sulphapyrimidine synthesis.

7.3.4 The Nobel Prize

As early as 1938 there had been plans to award Domagk the Nobel Prize, but he was not nominated by the Nobel Committee until one year later. Since it was known that the Third Reich forbade Germans to accept the Nobel prize, Folke Henschen, the Deputy Chairman of the Nobel Committee, tried to obtain an exemption for Domagk and wrote a personal letter to Goring, to which he received no reply. A few days before the decision was to be taken, another telegram was sent to the Foreign Office in Berlin. The reply was: 'Nobel prize award to a German national absolutely undesirable'. The next day Domagk was awarded the prize unanimously. He was delighted to be the recipient of this award. Although he was not allowed to accept it, he wanted at least to travel to Stockholm to express his thanks. However, the Gestapo arrested him, searched his home, his correspondence and refused to let him leave the country. One of the things he said 'it is easier to destroy a thousand lives than to save one' is supposed to have made the Gestapo furious. Domagk was released from prison after one week and was allowed to go back to his work. He rarely spoke about his time in prison, it was only one particular incident he related from time to time. When asked by a prison warder what he had done, Domagk answered: 'I got the Nobel Prize' to which the warder replied: 'We've got a madman here'. Even in the years that followed Domagk never showed a moment's hesitation in making brilliant comments on the political situation, which certainly did not make him a favourite with the big shots of the Third Reich, but he was spared further persecution.

Despite the great honour the award represented for Domagk, the company and all those who had taken part in the sulphonamide project, the study group was not spared tensions. Mietzsch and Klarer were especially involved. Although the prize had perfectly correctly been awarded for 'the discovery of the effects of the sulphonamides' and not for their preparation, Klarer held that the effects could not have been discovered without someone having pioneered the isolation of the sulphonamides and submitted them for testing. While Domagk invariably made it clear both verbally and in writing that a major part of the discovery was due to the chemists, it was eventually the Nobel Prize winner who received all the credit. Klarer was very disappointed and embittered at what he felt was a disregard of his own achievement. He lost all interest in the sulphonamides and Marbadal was his last major success. He took only very little part in the development of the sulphonamides substituted in the heterocycle. Mietzsch took things more philosophically or in his reticent way put on a good face. It was only eight years after he had been awarded the prize, namely in 1947, that Domagk was able to go to Stockholm to accept his award, but the prize money was forfeit. Henschen reported that Domagk had lost a lot of weight, looked much older than he was and carried the traces of the privations of the war years.

7.4 Sulphonamides substituted in the heterocyclic ring system

Whitby's report (1938) on the striking effects of sulphapyridine (34) in pneumococcal infections that was to win fame precipitated an avalanche of patent applications. All experts had a feeling that the N1-substituted sulphonamides might be a source of highly effective compounds. They were not mistaken. Yet nobody wanted to wait until such time as the best compounds had been selected from the vast number of candidates, a process that would have taken years of chemical synthesizing and clinical testing. Patent claims thus covered nearly all the known heterocycles, but failed to cite sufficient examples of their preparation and effectiveness. From the wealth of scientific literature it gradually emerged that the interest in this phase of development focused mainly on the sulpha derivatives of pyridine (Section 7.4.1.), thiazole (Section 7.4.2.), thiodiazole (Section 7.4.3.) and pyrimidine (Section 7.4.4.).

Combining the N1 nitrogen atom with heterocyclic rings was not altogether a new theory. A few years previously Mietzsch had prepared sulpha derivatives with the quinoline, acridine and carbazole ring systems which seemed particularly promising to him from his experience in plasmoquine and atebrine research, but this time his hopes were not realised. The compounds showed little or no effect.

7.4.1 Sulphapyridine

Even before Whitby's paper appeared, Ciba and, later, Rhône-Poulenc and May & Baker had sought patents for the preparation of sulphapyridine (34). Further applicants claiming special manufacturing processes followed; of these, the process developed by Loop and Lührs of the Nordmark company in 1939 had the greatest technical merit. Among the commercial products appearing on the market soon afterwards Dagenan (Rhône-Poulenc) and Eubasin (Nordmark) were the most widely known. The effect in pneumonia came up to expectations, but side effects such as vomiting and anuria called for caution. The N4-acetylated metabolic derivative formed in the body led to crystalluria; this resulted in renal tubule obstruction and, in some cases, even in uraemia. These incidents showed that it would be necessary in future to give the greatest attention to the solubility of the acetyl compounds. Many tests were made to improve tolerance by substitution at the N4 nitrogen atom, and promising results were obtained. Before they could be put into practice, however, sulphapyridine had become outdated and disappeared from the market.

Only one derivative, after being forgotten for almost 40 years, has found renewed interest. This compound, an azo-dye synthesised by Svartz in 1942 from diazotized sulphapyridine and salicylic acid, was tested at that time under the names salazopyrine and sulphasalazine in rheumatoid arthritis and ulcerative colitis. The trials were broken off because of toxic side-effects. Two British research groups have recently reported new trials with this compound (Neumann et al., 1983; Pullar et al., 1983). They come to the conclusion that sulphasalazine is an effective and safe drug capable of producing remissions in active rheumatoid arthritis. Their results, they suggest, also lend confidence to the use of preliminary open trials as a means of screening for remission inducing drugs in rheumatoid arthritis.

34	$\langle N \rangle$—NH–SO$_2$—$\langle \rangle$—NH$_2$	*Sulphapyridine*	Eubasin, Dagenan
35	$\langle S,N \rangle$—NH–SO$_2$—$\langle \rangle$—NH$_2$	*Sulphathiazole*	Eleudron, Cibazol

7.4.2 Sulphathiazole

Sulphathiazole (35) which is also the generic name, soon displaced sulphapyridine. It is much better tolerated, undergoes far less acetylation in the body and is just as effective. While sulphathiazole is slower in producing afebrility in pneumonia, healing rates are the same with the two compounds. Furthermore, its action against staphylococci and gonococci compares favourably with that of other sulphonamides. Sulphathiazole was the first compound found by Domagk to have pronounced activity in tuberculosis of the guinea pig. Ciba has undisputed priority to this drug. Subsequent patent applications were filed in quick succcession by Rhône-Poulenc, May & Baker, Winthrop, Gedeon Richter, Chinoin and others. Later, applications were also filed claiming special manufacturing processes. However, the scope of Ciba's pioneer patent was such that the analogous British patent was revoked by precedent of court of last resort in a spectacular patent suit. In the opinion of the court the patent contained claims for a host of ineffective compounds such that the inventive idea was not clear. This decision was unprecedented in the practice of patent law. The product dominated the sulphonamide market for a few years under the names of Cibazol (Ciba) and Eleudron (Bayer).

36   [structure] —NH–SO₂—⟨benzene⟩—NH–CO–CH₂–CH₂–COOH   Sulphasuxidine

37   [structure] —NH–SO₂—⟨benzene⟩—NH–CO—⟨benzene⟩   Taleudron
                                                            COOH

Among the large number of known derivatives only three gained importance as therapeutic agents. A polycondensation product of sulphathiazole with formaldehyde, Formo-Cibazol (Ciba) was used with success in intestinal infections such as enteritis, colitis, bacterial dysentery and summer diarrhoea. Sulphasuxidine (36) (Sharp & Dohme) N4-halbamide of succinic acid and Taleudron (37) the N4-halbamide of phthalic acid (Bayer), were effective in the same indications.

7.4.3 Sulphathiodiazole

To Dohrn and Diedrich of the Schering company and the publications by Vonkennel et al. (1940/41) we owe our knowledge of the sulpha-1,3,4-thiodiazoles. Although these compounds had already appeared in earlier patent applications, they had not been investigated. 5-Ethyl-sulphathiodiazole (38) *Sulphaethidolum* became widely known under the brand name of Globucid (Schering). It is very well tolerated, does not cause irritation when injected and is effective in pneumonia, meningitis, dysentery, pyelitis and, particularly, in gonorrhoea. Next to Albucid and Neo-Uliron it was the third drug fully effective in this disease.

A comparison of the 5-alkyl sulphathiodiazoles is particularly interesting because of the differing properties within this homologous series. The 5-methyl compound *Sulphamethizolum* is a typical short-acting sulphonamide. 95% of it is excreted in the urine within 5–6 hours and because of its low pK_a value it is optimally effective at pH 5.5. It is therefore beneficial only in infections of the urinary tract. Well-known commercial products were Lucosil (Lundbeck & Co.) and Urolukosil (Warner & Co.).

5-Isopropylsulphathiodiazole *Glyprothiazolum* exerted a pronounced effect against the organisms of gas gangrene, but as it had strong hypoglycaemic activity it had no value as a chemotherapeutic agent. 5-*tert*-butylsulphathiodiazole *Glybuthiazolum* had such hypo-glycaemic potency that it could be used as an oral antidiabetic agent, brand name Glipasol (Rhône-Poulenc). However, antidiabetics with additional antibacterial activity are not used anymore.

7.4.4 Sulphapyrimidine and sulphaisoxazole

This development phase which continued to the end of World War II reached its climax with the synthesis of the sulphapyrimidines. Dohrn & Diedrich of the Schering company undoubtedly pioneered the preparation of non-substituted sulphapyrimidine in 1939, as the patent application proves. While the Dehydag company was able to cite a prior claim on the basis of an application filed a few months earlier, there was reason for doubt, in view of the insufficiency of the experimental data, that the compound had been available at the time of the application. Sharp & Dohme, Cyanamid, Ciba and others had filed patent applications, but these were still under examination and therefore as yet unpublished. Public attention was first drawn to this class by the report of Roblin et al. (1940 and 1942) who were associated with the American Cyanamid Corporation. Further scientific publications appeared in quick succession: Caldwell and Kime (1940), Caldwell et al. (1941), Sprague et al. (1941), Raiziss and Freifelder (1942), Backer and Grevenstuk (1942), Jensen et al. (1942). In Germany, publications did not appear until later. Studies centred on three compounds:

(i)   sulphapyrimidine (39) *Sulphadiazine*; (ii) sulpha-4-methylpyrimidine (40) *Sulphamerazine*; (iii) sulpha-4,6-dimethylpyrimidine (41) *Sulphadimidine*.
All investigations showed sulphadiazine to be the most effective compound against streptococci, pneumococci and *Klebsiella*.

38–53   Derivatives of the general formula: H_2N—〈 〉—SO_2–NH–R

No.	R =	*Generic name*	Brand name(s)
38	(structure) C₂H₅	* Sulphaethidolum *	Globucid, Sulfaperlongit
39	(structure)	* Sulphadiazine *	Debenal, Pyrimal
40	(structure) CH₃	* Sulphamerazine *	Debenal M Component of many combination drugs
41	(structure) CH₃	* Sulphadimidine *	Diazil

The careful comparative studies performed by Lehr (1953) in infected mice given identical doses of the three compounds yielded the following results:

Streptococci	100	64	50
Pneumococci	100	93	82
Klebsiella	100	79	26
Sulpha-	diazine	merazine	dimidine

Domagk fully corroborated these findings and told the chemists jestingly: 'I really ought to advise you to stop looking for further drugs. As I am able to cure 100% of my infected mice with minimal doses, I cannot see anything better. Sulphadiazine is the king of the sulphonamides'.

While this statement was correct in relation to efficacy, the position was different as far as solubility at pH 5.5 and tolerance were concerned. At this pH, the solubility of sulphadimidine was about 4 times that of sulphadiazine. The hazard of crystal formation by the free compound and the acetyl derivatives was therefore lowest with sulphadimidine. Surprisingly in this series, the acetyl compounds were more readily soluble than the free amines and therefore constituted no added risk.

Though sulphadimidine had inferior absolute efficacy to the other compounds it proved its therapeutic value over many years of practical clinical application. Tolerance increased in the following order: 39 < 40 < 41 (sulphadiazine < sulphamerazine < sulphadimidine) and was thus in inverse ratio to efficacy. Nevertheless, the decision as to which product was best suited to practical application was based chiefly on chemical considerations.

Testing of the compounds in Germany began in 1941, but it was not clear from the patent situation who was entitled to produce which product. Dehydag's patent was weak, Ciba's patent too broad and Schering's patent was subsequent to that of the Dehydag company. Time-consuming and expensive lawsuits seemed to be the only way to clarify the intricate legal situation. It was then that Hörlein took the initiative and asked the responsible men at Ciba, Dehydag, Schering and IG Farben to join him at the conference table, just as Duisberg had done successfully decades ago in disputes relating to dyes. An agreement was soon reached not to object to the 38 patent applications of the participant companies and to settle the matter without a court case. It was decided to pool all patents except sulphathiodiazole for free exploitation by the parties. The royalties were first to be transferred to the pool and later to be allocated to the parties according to a carefully worked out formula. Initially, there was a controversy as to the extent to which IG was to participate. IG had, or so it appeared, no further applications for the manufacture of heterocyclic substituted sulphonamides and only appeared to have a moral claim as pioneers in the field. A nominal fee was probably what the meeting had in mind. Then Hörlein, to the surprise of those present, produced from his pocket a patent application and probably said something like this: 'I've got a patent here that will enable us to make all heterocyclic substituted sulphonamides without having to fall back on your processes. We would thus be legally free; nevertheless we are prepared to contribute the parent to the pool'. (These events were recounted to the author by Mietzsch who had the information from Hörlein himself). An awkward silence fell after these remarks, everybody showed polite interest, examined the patent and agreed to the proposal. It was indeed a hitherto unknown method for the synthesis of these sulphonamides. Formula and procedure were quickly decided upon, and a four-party contract was concluded in November 1942 which opened the path for productive research and functioned extremely well until the patents ran out.

The secret of this patent was oxidation of sulphene, a process that had been developed at the IG by Lorenz (1910–1976) and Behnisch in 1940. The first step of this process yielded sulphenamides of the R-S-NH-heterocycle that could be converted to sulphonamides by mild oxidation. Surprisingly, the heterocycle was not broken up in this reaction step. This work had been started with an entirely different objective. Lorenz whose chief line of activity was plant protection, had experience with chlorides of sulphenic acids while Behnisch wanted to prepare and test sulphenamides of analogous structure to the sulphonamides. So the two men joined forces. The sulphenamides proved to be ineffective. However, in an effort to find some use for them they were subjected to oxidation and thus converted to the known sulphonamides. No one had the slightest idea then that this reaction would become as important as it eventually did.

In order to be able to fully understand the history of the sulphapyrimidines it is necesssary to look at the chemical problems they carried. Sulphamerazine and sulphadimidine were easy to make, sulphadiazine was not. There was no workable synthesizing technique for the necessary intermediate product, 2-aminopyrimidine. The patent literature of the following years shows more than ten processes relating to the synthesis of this product. But there was always the difficulty of isolating the water-free amine, a substance that is most readily soluble in water. Entirely new processes were therefore developed that were able to do without aminopyrimidines. In laboratory jargon these processes were called 'further ring closure reactions'. N4-acetylated sulphanilyl guanidine was condensed with β-dicarbonyl compounds or their equivalents such as propinal diacetal or β-dimethylaminoacroleine, thus closing the pyrimidine ring. These processes are still being used today.

There was a war on and the best processes were useless at a time when raw materials were unobtainable. Unlike the United States, Germany was no longer able to maintain regular production. It was only in 1947/48 that this was slowly resumed, but then interest in the sulphonamides was already dwindling. In 1948, sulphadiazine was launched in Germany by Schering (Pyrimal) and Bayer (Debenal).

In the meantime Domagk had been busy working intensively on combinations of various sulphonamides and was enthusiastic over the properties of a mixture of the sulphonamides 39, 40 and 41 which he used as reference standards in all his tests. While this triple sulphonamide had some advantages over sulphadiazine, it had no wider spectrum of action and was therefore held in abeyance to be used a few years later in combination with orally effective penicillins. Instead, a combination of sulphamerazine and Marbadal was chosen, which covered not only the typical sulphonamide indications but anaerobic infections as well. This drug, brand name Supronal (Bayer) remained a top-selling product for 20 years. It was supplemented in 1952 by Solusupronal, a neutral injectable solution prepared by Behnisch that was used up to 1971. Combination drugs were manufactured all over the world.

Around 1955, 46 combination drugs containing two, three or four sulphonamides and 10 combining sulphonamides with penicillin, were commercially available in the United States. During the period ending 1945 another two sulphonamides of major importance were found. These were: (i) 4-sulpha-2,6-dimethylpyrimidine (42) *Sulphisomidine*; and (ii) 5-sulpha-3,4-dimethylisoxazole (43) *Sulphafurazole*. Sulphisomidine was first investigated by Schering (1939), by Geigy (1940) and by Ciba and Nordmark in 1941. The latter two companies in particular tested this preparation very thoroughly and launched it after prolonged clinical testing under the brand names of Elkosin (Ciba) and Aristamid (Nordmark).

R=	*Generic name*	Brand name(s)
42	*Sulphisomidine*	Aristamid, Elkosin
43	*Sulphafurazole*	Gantrisin, Entrusul

Loop and Lührs (1953) of the Nordmark laboratories developed an interesting new technique for the manufacture of the substance by dispensing with pure pyridine that was both costly and in short supply. Sulphisomidine is a typical short-acting sulphonamide with an elimination half-life from human serum of 7.4 hours. It is very well tolerated. Although its efficacy in mice with streptococcal and pneumococcal infections was only one third of that of sulphadiazine, it proved its value in medical practice and is still being used on a small scale in 1983. The authors of the introductory papers were Gsell (1944) and Meier et al. (1944).

The sulpha derivatives of oxazole and isoxazole were developed at Hoffmann-La Roche by Wuest and Hoffer. 5-Sulpha-3,4-dimethylisoxazole was launched in 1944 under the brand name of Gantrisin (43). The generic name *Sulphisoxazole* and the WHO free name Sulphafurazole are not identical and are used concurrently. Gantrisin is a short-acting sulphonamide with an elimination half-life of 6 hours and a pK_a value of 4.72. Both values suggest its use chiefly in biliary, urinary and eye infections, but the product also proved its value in the combat of other sulphonamide-sensitive organisms. Experimental results in animals were reported by White et al. (1952) while Randall et al. (1954) described blood levels and excretion.

As the drug had an extremely bitter taste, Gantrisin syrup for use in the treatment of children was prepared from the largely tasteless N1-acetylated derivative. Sulphisoxazole is good evidence of the fact that, as distinct from the early days of the sulphonamides, it was pharmacokinetic considerations that now played a decisive part in product assessment. In the usual animal tests sulphisoxazole was clearly inferior to the reference drugs sulphadiazine and triple sulphonamide and would not have been given a chance of success in the early days. However, considering its solubility in urine at pH 6.4 which is 25 times that of sulphadiazine, one recognizes the advantages of the drug which have later been confirmed in medical practice.

7.5 Standstill and renewal of research: Long-acting sulphonamides

The triumph of the antibiotics that began in 1948 (see Chapter 9B) gradually brought research aimed at sulphonamide synthesis to a halt. Although there were still gaps to fill and hitherto unexplored heterocyclic ring systems to test, no fresh impulses of any significance arose from this work; it appeared that research had achieved its utmost. The available material was so extensive that the time seemed ripe for critical re-appraisal and re-evaluation in the light of the latest scientific advances. The rapid development of chemical analysis, the changeover from the old wet processes to modern physical techniques facilitated pharmacokinetic studies on the behaviour of the sulphonamides in the body, their distribution, acetylation, binding to serum, excretion and mechanism of action. It became clear why some highly effective compounds did not come up to expectations in practical application and why less effective drugs forged ahead of them.

More detailed knowledge of the metabolic processes following sulphonamide administration also allayed the fears of using compounds with long retention times in serum. Initially, pharmacologists entertained serious reservations about sulphonamides that were not rapidly excreted. There was fear of cumulation in organ tissues, and in view of initial side effects following high doses everybody felt it their duty to exercise particular caution. It was therefore a courageous decision of the Lederle company to launch, in 1957, a new sulphonamide that had an elimination half-life of about 40 hours. This product, 3-sulpha-6-methoxypyridazine (44) *Sulphamethoxypyridazine*, which became known by many brand names such as Kynex, Lederkyn, Davosin and Myasul Sultirene, marked a new phase in sulphonamide research. The terms long-, short- and medium-acting sulphonamides were coined.

R =	*Generic name*	Brand name(s)
44 (structure with —OCH3)	*Sulphamethoxy-pyridazine*	Kynex, Davosin, Lederkyn, Midicel

The convincing results obtained with sulphapyridazine sparked an entirely unexpected interest in the sulphonamides. A distinction was now made between old and new sulphonamides, 'new' meaning simply that they were launched after 1957 and not that they were hitherto unknown compounds (Table 7.1).

How did Domagk feel about this new development? He noted the therapeutic success of the antibiotics with satisfaction. On the other hand he did not fail to see the disadvantages associated with their uncritical and exaggerated use such as gastrointestinal upsets, staphylococci-induced diarrhoea, moniliasis and colitis pseudomembranacea. He therefore regretted the waning interest in the sulphonamides and maintained that such drugs as sulphadiazine and supronal were supreme achievements. As from 1948, his work centred on the treatment of tuberculosis and carcinoma, sulphonamides being pursued merely as a sideline. The chemical laboratories barely offered him any new sulphonamides now. The old study group was no longer in existence. Klarer had died in 1953, Mietzsch had given up his

Table 7.1: List of important sulphonamides arranged according to elimination half-lives.

Number of drug listed in this chapter	Generic name	Elimination half-life (h)	Known brand names
30	Sulphacarbamide	2–3	Euvernil
	Sulphamethizol	2–3	Lucosil, Urolucosil
32	Sulphathiourea	3–6	Badional, Fontamid
35	Sulphathiazole	3.6–4	Cibazol, Eleudron
43	Sulphafurazole	6	Gantrisin, Entrosul
42	Sulphasomidine	6–7	Aristamid, Elkosin
34	Sulphapyridine	6.5–9.4	Dagenan, Eubasin
46	Sulphachlorpyridazin	7	Sonilyn, Nefrosulfin
38	Sulphaethidol	7–8	Globucid, Sulfaperlongit
11a	Sulphanilamide	8.8	Prontalbin
53	Sulphamethoxazole	10–11	Gantanol, Sinomin
51	Sulphamoxole	10.6	Sulfuno, Tardamid
52	Sulphaphemazole	10.7	Orisul, Sulfabid
21	Sulphacetamide	12–14	Albucid, Urosulfon
24	Sulphaproxylinum	12	Dosulfin
41	Sulphadimidine	14	Diazil
39	Sulphadiazine	16.7	Debenal, Pyrimal
40	Sulphamerazine	17	Debenal M, Constituent of many combinations
49	Sulphaperine	35–40	Pallidin
44	Sulphamethoxypyridazine	37.7	Kynex, Lederkyn, Davosin
47	Sulphadimethoxine	37.9	Madribon, Madriquid
45	Sulphameter	38.2	Durenat, Kiron, Bayrena
50	Sulphalen	65	Kelfizina
48	Sulphormethoxine	156	Fanasil, Fanzil

laboratory in 1949 to become Director of Chemical Research and, as he died in 1958, did not live to witness the comeback of the sulphonamides. Behnisch was engaged in developing new anti-tuberculosis agents from thiosemicarbazones and took care of the sulphonamides as some kind of general executor until 1958. With Domagk retiring in 1960 there were none of the inventors of the sulphonamides left.

7.5.1 Sulphapyrimidines, sulphapyridazines and sulphapyrazines

Mietzsch with his habit of exploring research areas systematically had noticed that sulphapyrimidines with substituents in the 5-position had not been investigated. His suggestion that this class be thoroughly studied inspired research developments culminating in the synthesis of 2-sulpha-5-methoxypyrimidine (45) *Sulphameter* which became known by the name of Durenat. The road to success was laborious. It was one of Mietzsch's last far-sighted decisions shortly before his illness to create yet again a study group to tackle this task. The group was headed by Behnisch and members were, successively, U. Wörffel (born 1924), R. Lorenz (born 1919) and H. Horstmann (born 1933). It took three years to solve the problem and to find the synthesis. Almost simultaneously Schering had attained the goal via a similar route and it was decided by mutual consent between Bayer and Schering to market the product jointly under one name, Durenat.

Therapeutic and pharmacological studies were performed very thoroughly by the two companies. Bünger and Koch (1961), Hecht et al. (1961), Horstmann et al. (1961), Kimbel and Garn (1961), Knott et al. (1961), Scholtan (1961). The findings justified the hope that Durenat might achieve a prominent position among the long-acting sulphonamides. It was superior in efficacy to sulphadiazine, well tolerated and characterized by such features as low acetylation, low protein-binding, rapid absorption and an elimination half-life of about 38 hours, thus allowing for an ideal dosage interval of 24 hours. The product eventually had the success anticipated at the time of its introduction in 1961.

In addition to the two compounds (44) and (45) mentioned earlier, another eight belonging to the 'new generation' gained some importance as therapeutic agents. Of these, 3-sulpha-6-chloropyridazine (46) *Sulphachlorpyridazine* is of particular interest. Chemically, it is a precursor of compound (44) and carries a chlorine atom in place of the methoxy group. It is a typical short-acting sulphonamide with an elimination half-life of 7 hours. The process patent had been issued to the American Cyanamid Company as early as 1953, Druey et al. had been working on it in Switzerland in 1954. It is recommended for use in infections of the urinary tract. Goldammer (1961) reported on clinical experiences with the drug. It is sold under the names of Consulid (Ciba), Sonilyn (Mallinckrodt) and Vetisulid (Ciba) for use in veterinary medicine.

4-Sulpha-2,6-dimethoxypyrimidine (47) *Sulphadimethoxine* gained wide usage. It is similar in chemical structure to sulphisomidine (42) but unlike the latter it is a long-acting sulphonamide with an elimination half-life of 35–53 hours. The compound first appeared in a patent of the Österreichische Stickstoffwerke in 1951 but was not methodically tested until about 1957. It was introduced into therapy by Hoffmann-La Roche under the brand name of Madribon in 1959. The compound has excellent tolerability and can be used in all infections caused by sulphonamide-sensitive bacteria. For clinical findings see Schütze (1959).

4-Sulpha-5,6-dimethoxypyrimidine (48) *Sulphormethoxine* is an isomer of (47) with an extremely long elimination half-life (156 hours). For maintenance of effective blood levels no more than an initial dose of 1 g and maintenance doses totalling 1 g in 7 days are needed. Hoffmann-La Roche introduced this product under the name of Fanasil in 1961, but it failed to make headway. 2-Sulpha-5-methylpyrimidine (49) *Sulphaperine*, an isomer of sulphamerazine (40) and hence sometimes called isosulphamerazine, was described by Sprague et al. as early as 1941, but it was not before 1960 that it was recommended for use as a chemotherapeutic agent by Hepding et al. It has a broad spectrum of action, is well tolerated and has achieved a firm position in therapy as a long-acting sulphonamide under the names of Pallidin (Merck) and Sulfene (Sharp & Dohme).

R =	*Generic name*	Brand name(s)
45	*Sulphameter*	Durenat
46	*Sulphachlor-pyridazine*	Sonilyn, Nefrosulfin
47	*Sulphadimethoxine*	Madribon, Madriquid
48	*Sulphormethoxine*	Fanasil, Fanzil
49	*Sulphaperine*	Pallidin

The sulphapyrazines lay almost forgotten for about 20 years. Recent studies carried out in Italy showed that 2-sulpha-3-methoxypyrazine (50) *Sulphalene* has uses as an ultra long-acting sulphonamide with an elimination half-life of 65 hours. The drug was launched by Farmitalia under the name of Kelfizina in 1962 but did not attain a position outside Italy. Apparently the ultra long-acting sulphonamides were only reluctantly accepted by the medical profession.

In contrast, two medium-acting sulphonamides from the 'new generation' came into their own and have retained a position in the therapeutic armamentarium ever since:

(i) 2-sulpha-4,5-dimethyloxazole (51) *Sulphamoxol* originated with the Nordmark company. The literature cites two different elimination half-lives, namely 10.8 and 24 hours, the lower value being the more likely of the two. This compound is characterized by rapid absorption, fairly rapid excretion, good tolerability and a broad spectrum of action. The compound has been on the market since 1955 under the names of Sulfuno (Nordmark), Tardamid (Grünenthal) and Nuprin (Upjohn). (ii) 5-Sulpha-1-phenylpyrazole (52) *Sulfaphenazole* originated with the Ciba laboratories. It was introduced in 1957 under the name of Orisul (Ciba), its properties are largely similar to those of (51) and it has proved its value to this day.

7.5.2 Sulphoxazole and Trimethoprim

The end of the 'sixties' saw the advent of a new combination drug whose enormous success all over the world is attributable to the ingenious idea of combining *Sulphamethoxazole* from Hoffmann-La Roche research with *Trimethoprim*, a product of Wellcome. 3-Sulpha-5-methylisoxazole *Sulphamethoxazole* (53) has been known since 1960 as a medium-acting sulphonamide with an elimination half-life of 10.7 hours, brand names Gantanol (Hoffmann-La Roche) and Sinomin (Shionogi). Like all sulphonamides it blocks folic acid synthesis by antimetabolic interference with 4-aminobenzoic acid. 2,4-Diamino-5-(3′,4′,5′-trimethoxybenzyl)-pyrimidine *Trimethoprim* (54), often abbreviated TMP, has a broad spectrum of action against many Gram-positive and Gram-negative bacteria. It inhibits the reduction of folic acid to dihydrofolate and tetrahydrofolate, a subsequent step to that inhibited by the sulphonamides. Double blockage eventually inhibits the formation of protein and ribonucleic acid. When given in high doses trimethoprim produced haemotoxic effects and haematopoiesis which prevented it use in therapy at the time. However, when mixed with sulphamethoxazole in the proportion of 1:10–1:5 the side effects were largely suppressed and a synergistic effect was obtained.

	R =	* Generic name *	Brand name(s)
50		* Sulphalene *	Kelfizina
51		* Sulphamoxol *	Sulfuno, Tardamid
52		* Sulphaphenazole *	Orisul, Sulfabid

The combination drug is used with success in the treatment of urinary infections. The healing rate is 70–95% in acute infections and 60–80% in chronic cases not associated with obstruction. While bronchitis and gonorrhoea are aslo possible indications these are not commonly treated with the drug because of the risk of growing resistance to TMP. The drug has found worldwide acceptance under the brand names of Bactrim (Hoffmann-La Roche) and Eusaprim (Wellcome) and is now being marketed under different names by many companies.

Attempts were made to use *Tetroxoprim* (65) instead of TMP. Products containing sulphadiazine (39) as their sulphonamide component in the proportion of 1:2.5 are Tibirox (Hoffmann-La Roche) and Sterinor (Heumann).

	R =	* Generic name *	Brand name(s)
53		* Sulphamethoxazole *	Gantanol, Sinomin
54	H_2N ... CH_2 ... OCH_3	*Trimethoprim *	
55	$C_4H_9-NH-C-NH-SO_2$—NH$_2$	* Carbutamide *	Nadisan, Invenol
56	$C_4H_9-NH-C-NH-SO_2$—CH$_3$	* Tolbutamide *	Rastinon, Artosin

7.6 Fields of study directly stemming from sulphonamide research

To complete this account, another four areas need to be described briefly as they are based on observations stemming from sulphonamide research and have gained great importance. These four areas are 6.1. Hypoglycaemic agents, 6.2. Diuretics, 6.3. Anti-tuberculosis agents and 6.4. Antiepileptic agents and will be described only in the light of their relationship to the sulphonamides.

7.6.1 Hypoglycaemic agents

The oral hypoglycaemic agents stem from an invention made by Haack at the Heyden company, Radebeul. When doing research on sulphanilyl ureas he prepared, among other compounds, sulphanilyl-*n*-butyl urea (55) *Carbutamide*, BZ 55. It was to be submitted for clinical testing as it had proved to have good antibacterial activity. It is not known whether the trial was actually started in the last years of the war, but there were obviously no confirmed results. When Haack moved to Mannheim to join Boehringer he initiated clinical testing there. In these clinical trials a number of patients were found to collapse following treatment with the drug. Franke and Fuchs (1955) interpreted this phenomenon correctly as being due to a substantial fall in blood sugar. After thoroughly checking these findings Boehringer launched the compound (55) under the name of Nadisan, thus creating the first potent oral hypoglycaemic agent.

A team led by H. Ruschig (born 1906) was also working at the same time at Hoechst A.G. on oral antidiabetics. In order to rule out bacteriostatic activity, which was undesired in an antidiabetic agent, this group removed the N4-aromatic amino-moiety completely. The first great success with this approach was the compound 4-toluolsulphonyl butyl urea (56), *Tolbutamide*, which was more potent than Nadisan and had no bacteriostatic activity. In view of the structural similarities between the two compounds, Hoechst and Boehringer came to an exemplary agreement whereby both firms would work together in this area in the future and market both drugs from both companies. Thus, Nadisan also became known under the tradename Invenol (Hoechst) and *Tolbutamide* was marketed as Rastinon (Hoechst) and Artosin (Boehringer). References to the worldwide development of this field which began soon afterwards can be omitted here.

The activity of today's top-ranking products is about 300 times that of Rastinon. In spite of their complex structure the relationship with the ancient sulphanilyl urea (30) is still apparent in such drugs as Euglukon (57) (Hoechst and Boehringer), *Glibenclamide* and Pro-Diaban (58) (Bayer and Schering), *Glisoxepide*.

7.6.2 Diuretics

The invention of new, non-mercurial diuretics also stems from sulphonamide research. When administering sulphanilamide, commercially available since 1936, it was noted that high doses were frequently followed by a fall in serum pH below the norm of 7.35. Mann and Keilin (1940) interpreted this effect as being due to the inhibition of the enzyme carbonic anhydrase which catalyzes hydration of carbon dioxide. Eight years later Krebs (1948) published a table presenting data of carbonic anhydrase inhibition by numerous sulphonamides, but made no use of the therapeutic potential that lay in these observations. It was not until 1950 that Roblin and Clapp began to study this field systematically. The major product originating from this research was *Acetazolamide* which has been known since 1953 under the brand name of Diamox (59). It is a typical carbonic anhydrase inhibitor and a natriuretic agent. Primarily it promotes the excretion of the sodium ions, increased excretion of water being a secondary process. The importance of this compound diminished when new, much better agents, the saluretics and the high-ceiling diuretics, were discovered in 1957 and later. With a few exceptions, they are structural analogues of the sulphonamides.

59	$CH_3-CO-NH-\overset{N-N}{\underset{S}{\parallel}}-SO_2-NH_2$	*Acetazolamide*	Diamox
60	Cl—⟨⟩—SO_2-N-CH_2... CH_3 CH_3, SO_2-NH_2	*Mefruside*	Baycaron
61	H_2N-SO_2... Cl ... *Hydrochlorothiazide*	*Hydrochlorothiazide*	Esidrix
62	H_2N-SO_2... COOH ... $NH-CH_2$ ... Cl	*Furosemide*	Lasix
63	$CO-NH-NH_2$ ... pyridine ... N	*Isoniazide*	Neoteben

Without elaborating on this development the author would like to cite three typical representatives of these new diuretics whose formulae indicate the relationship with the sulphonamides. These are (i) *Mefruside* (60); (ii) *Hydrochlorothiazide* (61); and (iii) *Furosemide* (62).

7.6.3 Antituberculosis agents

Domagk tested all sulphonamides submitted to him, namely more than two thousand, for anti-tubercular activity in guinea-pigs and rabbits. He intimated that only two drugs,

Sulphathiazole (35) and *Sulphethidole* (38), had been slightly effective, but no notice was taken of his suggestion for a few years. When, in 1941, Behnisch took up this problem, he reasoned that, of the many sulphonamides studied only two having shown a trace of effectiveness, the sulphonamide group could not very well be the part of the molecule that mattered. The fragments 2-aminothiazole, 2-amino-5-ethyl-1,3,4-thiodiazole and sulphanilic acid were ineffective. Perhaps the molecular arrangement of the elements nitrogen and sulphur was important. On splitting the ring of the 2-amino-5-ethylthiodiazole the arrangement of the atoms was that present in the thiosemicarbazides and thiosemicarbazones, namely:

Domagk found that benzaldehyde thiosemicarbazone had considerable activity in tuberculosis. This finding provided an incentive to planned research in this field in which Mietzsch and Schmidt (1886–1959) collaborated. Of the eight drugs clinically tested three were put on the market: (i) Tb I, Conteben (4-acetylamino-benzaldehyde thiosemicarbazone); (ii) Tb VI, Solvoteben (benzaldehyde thiosemicarbazone-4-carbonic acid and (iii), Nikoteben (pyridine-3-aldehyde thiosemicarbazone).

In the fight against tuberculosis that had spread rapidly after World War II, these drugs did a world of good. In 1946 Domagk acquainted the medical profession with this new class. The status of chemical research was reviewed by Behnish et al. (1948 and 1950).

The results of medical research were summarised in a monograph of which Domagk was the author (1950). The thiosemicarbazones were gradually replaced by isonicotinic acid hydrazide in 1954 or so. Offe (born 1912), working at Elberfeld, shortened the thiosemicarbazone chain by another two links and obtained the structure of the acid hydrazides of which the hydrazide of isonicotinic acid proved to be the most effective anti-tuberculosis agent.

Although nothing in the structure of isonicotinic acid hydrazide (63) *Isoniazide*, Neoteben (Bayer), INH, is reminiscent of sulphethidole (38), it was a logical development that led from sulphethidole to Conteben to Neoteben.

7.6.4 Antiepileptic agents

B. Helferich (1887–1982) during the last years of his tenure as Director of the Chemical Institute of Bonn University had been engaged in research on sultamens, cyclic sulphonamides. The pharmacologist Schulemann, also of Bonn University, found that a compound of the structure of (64) exerted a suppressive effect on psychomotor epilepsy. As the project could not be pursued further in Bonn the two researchers turned it over to Bayer subject to their priority rights. Bayer gave the assignment to Behnisch.

W. Wirth (born 1898) did the pharmacological testing. It emerged that changes at the sulthame ring did not improve efficacy while substituents at the aromatic ring did. 4-Tetrahydro-2-H-1,2-thiazine-2-yl-benzolsulphonamide-S,S-dioxide (64) *Sultiam*, a drug that carried a sulphonamide group in the 4-position, came out best as regards efficacy and tolerability and after prolonged clinical testing was brought onto the market under the brand name of Ospolot. It proved its value in temporal lobe epilepsy, Jackson epilepsy and grand mal. The structural relationship with the sulphonamides is undeniable. The history of the compound has been reviewed by Behnisch et al. (1963).

7.6.5 Disappointments

This account has so far been concerned with cases where clues pointing to effects outside the typical sulphonamide indications were pursued with success. The number of cases where such efforts failed is, however, far greater. Suffice it to cite three instances.

Ch. Hackmann, a collaborator of Domagk, had found a significant anti-geriatric effect in old rats he had treated over long periods with subtherapeutic doses of sulphadiazine. The symptoms of arthrosis, stiff legs, bent back and difficult movement of limbs disappeared. The ruffled fur with bald patches began to grow again and looked like that of young animals. Senile cataract improved and the animals recovered their agility and appetite. Similar results were obtained in old dogs. Colleagues with heavy loss of hair volunteered for trials in humans and took 0.1 g of Debenal daily. Because of unwanted substantial weight gain which had also occurred in the animals the tests were discontinued. A scientifically monitored, statistically confirmed clinical trial in old people's homes proved to be impracticable so that the hope to obtain an anti-geriatric drug had to be abandoned. Sulphadiazine has found successful application only in veterinary medicine where it is used in combination with vitamins and restoratives in the treatment of dogs.

W. Kikuth and L. Mudrow-Reichenow tested sulphonamides in malaria. They were seeking a causal therapy capable of preventing the outbreak of the disease by attacking the E forms. Sulphanilyl-3,5-dibromanilide, Be 768, also called Bemural, that had been prepared by Behnisch in 1938, attracted their attention. It was able to cure monkeys infected with *Plasmodium knowlesi* without relapse. It was also effective against *Plasmodium relictum* and exerted pronounced prophylactic activity. Could it be that this was the causal therapy they had been looking for all this time? The clinical trial started with high hopes ended in disappointment. The findings in animals were only insufficiently confirmed in man.

W. Kikuth and R. Gönnert did intensive research on the effects of sulphonamides in viral infections. They investigated an azo dye Behnisch had prepared in 1938 by coupling diazotized sulphapyridine with acetyl niobic acid. This azo dye, closely related in structure to Prontosil S, was tested in mice with lymphogranuloma inguinale and bronchopneumonia and proved to be many times superior in efficacy to the fragment, sulphapyridine. At long last a drug against viral infection had been found, or so it was thought. The sodium salt (Be 1034) and the diethanolamine salt (Be 1115) were clinically tested in typhoid fever and trachoma some time in 1941/42. Because of the war the trial that had just got underway had to be stopped and was never resumed after the war. Another disappointment had to be faced.

The era of the sulphonamides as far as their use in bacterial infections is concerned, is slowly coming to its close. Attempts to synthesise hitherto unknown sulphonamides have been given up in nearly all research laboratories. But for the antibiotics, the sulphonamides would still be among the most valuable medicines. Interest in this class, with the exception of sulphamethoxazole, is steadily declining and their economic importance has also dwindled. Notwithstanding pessimistic forecasts some of them have retained a position on the market and have even outlived a great many antibiotics. 35 years of research have not been in vain. As Fleming put it: without sulphonamides no antibiotics.

Acknowledgement

I would like to thank Bayer A.G. Leverkusen for permission to use photographs from their archives.

References

Backer, H.J., Grevenstuk, A.B., 1942. Rec. Trav. Chim. Pays Bas 61, 291–298.
Barber, H.J., Wilkinson, J.H., 1946. Pharmacol. J. 157, 105.
Behnisch, R., Mietzsch, F., Schmidt, H., 1948. Angew. Chem. 60, 113–115.
Behnisch, R., Mietzsch, F., Schmidt, H., 1950. Am. Rev. Tuberc. 61, 1–7.
Behnisch, R., Hoffmeister, F., Horstmann, H., Schraufstätter, E., Wirth, W., 1963. Sulfonamide mit anticonvulsiver Wirkung. Med. Chem. (Leverkusen) VII, 296–314 Chemie G.m.b.H. Weinheim.
Behnisch, R., Horstmann, H., 1965, 2nd Edn. Ullmanns Encyclopädie der technischen Chemie, 16. Urban und Schwarzenberg, München und Berlin, pp. 491–528.
Boehringer, C.F., Söhne, Rabald, E., Hagedorn, A., 1949. Verfahren zum Wasserlöslichmachen von Sulfonamiden. Dtsch. R. P. 838050 K130h, angem. 25.3.49 /ausgeg. 5.5.52.
Bünger, P., Koch, G., 1961. Arzneimittleforschung 11, 726–736.

Burnet, E., Cuénod, E., Nataf, R., 1939. Bull. Acad. Nat. Med. (Paris) 122, 317–324.

Buttle, G.A.H., Stephenson, D., Smith, S., Dewing, T., Foster, G.E., 1937. Lancet 232, 1331–1334 *I*.

Caldwell, W.T., Kime, H.B., 1940. J. Am. Chem. Soc. 62, 2365.

Caldwell, W.T., Kornfeld, E.C., Donnel, C.K., 1941. J. Am. Chem. Soc. 63, 2188–2190.

Dohrn, M., Diedrich, P., 1938. Muench. Med. Wochenschr. 85, 2017–2018.

Domagk, G., 1935. Dtsch. Med. Wochenschr. 61, 250–253.

Domagk, G., 1937. Klin. Wochenschr. 16, 1412–1418.

Domagk, G., 1942. Klin. Wochenschr. 21, 448–455.

Domagk, G., Hegler, C. (1944) Chemotherapie bakterieller Infektionen. 3nd Edn., Hirzel S., Leipzig.

Domagk, G., Behnisch, R., Mietzsch, F., Schmidt, H., 1946. Naturwissenschaften 33, 315.

Druey, J., Meier, K., Eichenberger, K., 1954. Helv. Chim. Acta 37, 121–140.

Dünnschede, H.B., 1971. Tropenmedizinische Forschung bei Bayer. Düsseldorfer Arbeiten zur Geschichte der Medizin. Triltsch, Düsseldorf, pp. 15–55.

Ehrhart, G., Ruschig, H., 1972, 2nd Edn. Arzneimittel, 4. Verlag Chemie, Weinheim, pp. 86–142.

Felke, H., 1937. Dtsch. Med. Wochenschr. 63, 1393–1395.

Fischer, C., 1937. Fortschr. Ther. 13, 553–559.

Fourneau, E., Tréfouel, J., Nitti, F., Bovet, D., Tréfouel, J., 1937. C.R. Hebd. Seances Acad. Sci. 204, 1763–1766.

Franke, H., Fuchs, J., 1955. Dtsch. Med. Wochenschr. 80, 1449–1452.

Gelmo, P., 1908. J. Prakt. Chem. 77, 369–382.

Gley, P., Girard, A., 1936. Presse Med 44, 1775–1777.

Goissedet, P., Despois, R., Gailliot, P., Mayer, R., 1936. C.R.Hebd. Seances Soc. Biol. 121, 1082–1084.

Goldhammer, H., 1961. Arzneimittelforschung 11, 131–132.

Grütz, O., 1937. Muench. Med. Wochenschr. 84, 1201–1205.

Gsell, O., 1943. Schweiz. Med. Wochenschr. 73, 692–699.

Gsell, O., 1944. Schweiz. Med. Wochenschr. 74, 1095–1103.

Haferland, H., 1941. Arch. Klin. Chir. 202, 580–610.

Hartenbach, W., 1954. Med. Klin. 49, 2071–2074.

Hecht, G., Junkmann, K., Langecker, H., Gloxhuber, Ch., Harwarth, A., Wirtz, S., 1961. Arzneimittelforschung 11, 695–700.

Heinrichs, A., 1944. Dtsch. Med. Wochenschr. 70, 561–562.

Hepding, L., Hoffmann, A., Wahlig, H., 1960. Arzneimittelforschung 10, 440–448.

Heymann, B., 1924. Angew. Chem. 37, 585–589.

Högger, D., 1941. Schweiz. Med. Wochenschr. 71, 901–904.

Horstmann, H., Knott, Th., Scholtan, W., Schraufstätter, E., Walter, A., Wörffel, U., 1961. Arzneimittelforschung 11, 682–684.

Farbenindustrie A.G., I.G., Klarer, J., 1941. Verfahren zur Herstellung von 4-Aminoalkyl-benzolsulfonamiden. Dtsch. R. Pat. 853444 9.8.40/23.10.52 KI 120.

James, G.V., Fuller, A.T., 1940. Biochem. J. 34, 648–656.

Jensen, K.A., Falkenberg, P., Thornsteinsson, Th., Lauridsen, M., 1942. Dansk. Tidsskr. Farmakol. 16, 141–153.

Kimbel, K.H., Garn, F.W., 1961. Arzneimittelforschung 11, 721–726.

Klarer, J., 1941. Klin. Wochenschr. 20, 1250.

Klarer, J., 1947. Dtsch. Med. Wochenschr. 72, 670–671.

Knott, Th., Kutzsche, A., Walter, A., 1961. Arzneimittelforschung 11, 684–694.

Krebs, H.A., 1948. Biochem. J. 43, 525–528.

Krüger-Thiemer, E., 1962. Handbuch der Haut- und Geschlechtskrankheiten, 5. Springer, Berlin und Heidelberg, pp. 962–1122 Teil 1.

Lehr, D., 1953. Antibiot. Chemother. 3, 71–93.

Levaditi, C., Vaisman, A., 1935. C.R.Hebd. Seances Acad. Sci. 200, 1694–1696.

Loop, W., Lührs, E., 1953. Liebigs Ann. Chem. 580, 225–236.

Mann, T., Keilin, D., 1940. Nature 146, 164–165.

Mayer, R.L., 1941. Rev. Med. Fr. 1941, 3–19.

Meier, R., Allemann, O., v. Meyenburg, H., 1944. Schweiz. Med. Wochenschr. 74, 1091–1095.

Mietzsch, F., Behnisch, R., 1955. Therapeutisch verwendbare Sulfonamid- und Sulfonverbin-dungen, 2nd Edn Verlag Chemie, Weinheim/Bergstrasse.

Mitchell, G.A.G., Rees, W.S., Robinson, C.N., 1944. Lancet 246, 627–629.

Neumann, V.C., Grindulis, K.A., Hubbal, S., McConkey, B., Wright, V., 1983. Leeds-Birmingham trial. Br. Med. J. 287, 1099–1102.

Nordmarkwerke, G.m.b.H., Loop, W., 1939. Verfahren zur Herstellung von Sulfanilsaüreamidopyridinen. Dtsch. R.P. 749794 KI 12q, angem. 28.3.39 /ausgeg. 6.12.44.

Northey, E.H., 1948. The Sulfonamides and Allied Compounds. Reinhold Publ. Corp., New York.

Otten, H., Plempel, M., 1975. Antibiotica und Chemotherapeutica. Antibiotica Fibel. 110–146 G. Thieme, Stuttgart.

Pullar, T., Hunter, J.A., Capell, H.A., 1983. Br. Med. J. 287, 1102–1104.

Raiziss, G.W., Freifelder, M., 1942. J. Am. Chem. Soc. 64, 2340–2342.

Randall, L.O., Engelberg, R., Iliev, V., Rose, M., Haar, H., Mc Gavack, T.H., 1954. Antibiot. Chemother. 4, 877–885.

Rhône-Poulenc, 1936. Herstellung von wasserlöslichen Produkten des 4-Aminobenzolsulfonamids. Dtsch. R. P. 704447 angem. 14.5.37/ausgeg. 31.3.41 Fr. Prior. 1936.

Roblin, R.O., Williams, J.H., Winnek, P.S., English, J.P., 1940. J. Am. Chem. Soc. 62 2002–2005.

Roblin, R.O., Winnek, P.S., English, J.P., 1942. J. Am. Chem. Soc. 64, 567–570.

Roblin, R.O., Clapp, J.W., 1950. J. Am. Chem. Soc. 72, 4890–4892.

Schönhöfer, F., 1965. Arzneimittelforschung 15, 1256–1258.

Scholtan, W., 1961. Arzneimittelforschung 11, 707–720.

Schreus, H.Th, 1937. Dermatol. Z. 76, 253–262.

Schütze, E., 1959. Med. Klin. 54, 2339–2341.

Spiethoff, B., 1938. Dtsch. Med. Wochenschr. 64, 1097–1102.

Sprague, J.M., Kissinger, L.W., Lincoln, R.M., 1941. J. Am. Chem. Soc. 63, 3028–3030.

Svartz, N., 1942. Acta Med. Scand. 110, 577–598.

Tréfouel, J., Tréfouel, J., Nitti, F., Bovet, D., 1935. C.R.Hebd. Seances Soc. Biol. 120, 756–758.

Vonkennel, J., Korth, B., 1938. Muench. Med. Wochenschr. 85, 2018–2021.

Vonkennel, J., Kimmig, J., Korth, B., 1940. Z. Klin. Med. 138, 695–743.

Vonkennel, J., Kimmig, J., 1941. Klin. Wochenschr. 20, 2–8.

Whitby, L.E.H., 1938. Lancet 234, 1210–1212 *I*.

White, H.J., Wadsworth, B.C., Redin, G.S., Gentile, A.J., 1952. Antibiot. Chemother. 2, 659–688.

Development of β-lactams since 1986. Commentary on The discovery of penicillin and cephalosporins by Sydney Selwyn

Søren Brøgger Christensen

Department of Drug Design and Pharmacology, University of Copenhagen, Copenhagen, Denmark

Penicillins

The pathogenicity of some bacteria is a feature that is mentioned very seldom during discussion on the importance of antibiotics. Even though this statement seems trivial today, it was not addressed before the end of the 19th century (Christensen, 2021). Subsequently, a hunt for antibiotics was rationalized. In his review from 1986, Selwyn describes the discovery of penicillin (Selwyn, 1986).

Ethnopharmacological use by the Aztecs of extracts of mold for treatment of infected wound infections inspired Lister and Tyndall to scientific studies on the broth of cultures. In some cases, a bactericidal effect was found. However, when Fleming in 1928 observed inhibition zones on a plate of *Staphylococcus* variants accidentally contaminated with a *Penicillium* species, he was not aware of these studies. The development of a drug based on Fleming's observation was hindered by two obstacles: the structure of the active agent was unknown and the active principle could not be produced on an industrial scale. The production problem was solved by Florey, Chain, and Heatly and the structure was elucidated by Hodgkins (Christensen, 2021). Large scale production of penicillin was prioritized by the American Army during the Second World War and huge amounts of penicillin were brought with the soldiers for the invasion of Normandy in 1944. The unique features of penicillin are the presence of a reactive β-lactam ring (Fig. 8.1) and the structural similarities to the residue D-Ala-D-Ala involved in cross coupling of the cell walls in bacteria (the Tipper–Strominger hypothesis). The four-membered ring makes the amide a strong acylating reagent. The penicillin binds to and acylates serine residues in penicillin-binding proteins and consequently prevents cell wall formation (Christensen, 2021). The first penicillin isolated from the broth of

Discoveries in Pharmacology, Volume 3, Hemodynamics and
Immune Defense.
DOI: https://doi.org/10.1016/B978-0-443-18442-0.00004-5

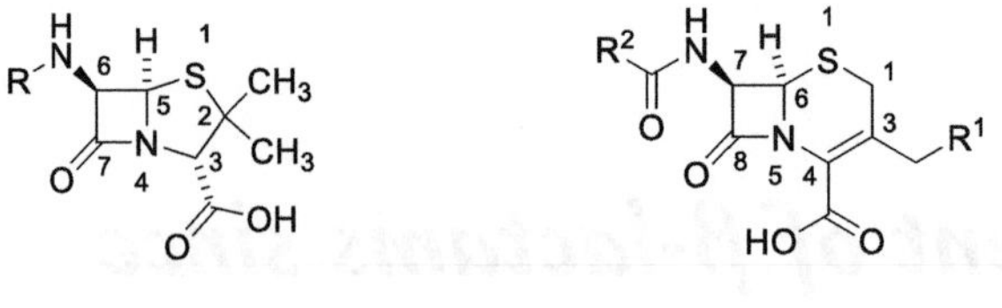

Figure 8.1
The scaffolds of penicillin (*left*) and cephalosporin (*right*).

Penicillium was cleaved in the acidic environment in the stomach, ruling out oral administration. Replacing the β-methylene group with an oxygen atom in the acid-acylating N-6 stabilizes the compound enabling oral use. In the second penicillin generation, an amino group was introduced at the α-carbon of the side chain (ampicillin, epicillin, amoxicillin, and ciclacillin). Ampicillin penetrates the cell wall of gram-negative bacteria. Protonation in acidic media of the amino group stabilizes the β-lactam ring. Another tool for decreasing acid lability was the introduction of a carboxylic group in the acyl side. Carbenicillin, sulbenicillin, ticarcillin, piperacillin, and mezlocillin are examples of such drugs.

Early on, Fleming observed the existence of penicillin resistance. The resistance is caused by either expression of β-lactamases, modifying the penicillin-binding protein (as is seen in *Staphylococcus aureus*) or in the case of gram-negative bacteria by expressing pumps that remove the drug from the bacteria. β-lactamases inactivate the penicillin by opening the lactam ring. To meet the challenge of β-lactamases, voluminous acids like benzoic acid with two substituents in the two ortho positions have been acylated at N-6 to give third-generation penicillins like methicillin, oxacillin, and nafcillin. β-lactamase inhibitors like clavulanic acid and sulbactam tazobactam are used in combination with penicllins to treat otherwise resistant infections.

Prodrugs such as ampicillin, in which the carboxylic acid of the penicillin nucleus has been masked, have been introduced to improve the oral absorption.

Cephalosporins

The first cephalosporin-producing mold, *Cephalosporium acremonium* (*C. acremonium*) was found in Sardinian sewage. Injection of an extract of the broth cured patients suffering from typhoid and other infectious diseases. Again, an advantage of the discovery was not obtained before Dr. Florey at Oxford was involved. During the isolation of antibiotic compounds from the broth of *C. acremonium*, the first true cephalosporin C (Fig. 8.1, $R_1 = OOCCH_3$, $R_2 = -OCCH_2-CH_2-CH_2-CH(NH_2)COOH$) was isolated in addition to penicillin N, fusidic acid, and penicillic acid (Newton and Abraham, 1955). The first-generation cephalosporins (narrow spectrum) have activity against gram-positive bacteria like *Staphylococcus* species, even though they express β-lactamases, and a few gram-negative bacteria, e.g., *Escherichia coli*,

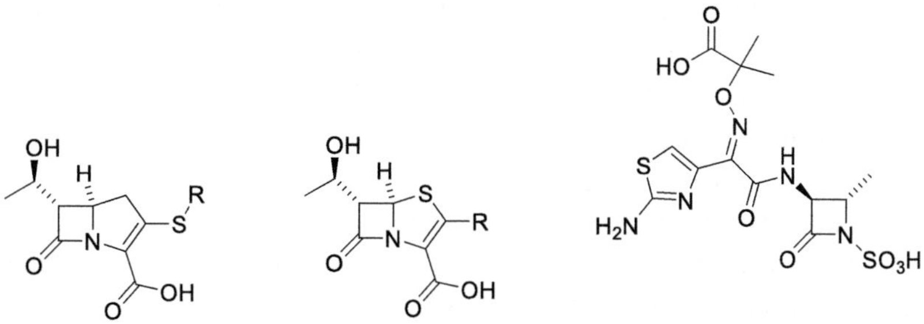

Figure 8.2
The scaffolds of carbapenems (*left*), thiophenes (*middle*), and the monobactam aztreonam.

Haemophilus influenza, and *Klebsiella* species. Examples of first-generation cephalosporins are cephalexin, cefradrine, and cefadroxil. Second-generation agents include cefaclor and cefuroxime. These possess activity against aerobic gram-negative bacteria like *Moraxella*, *Salmonella*, and *Shigella* species. Clinically, they are used against upper and lower respiratory tract infections. Third-generation, broad-spectrum cephalosporins include cefotaxime, ceftazidime, and ceftizoxime. They have activity against gram-negative bacteria and are more resistant toward β-lactamases. Fourth-generation cephalosporins include cefepime, cefpirome, and cefquinome. With the introduction of an ammonium group, they more efficiently penetrate the cell wall of gram-negative bacteria. They can be used against bacteria like gram-positive cocci, including methicillin-resistant *Staphylococcus epidermis*, penicillin-resistant *Staphylococcus pneumonia*, and *Enterococcus faecalis*. In addition, they are used for the treatment of infections with many gram-negative bacilli including *Escherichia coli* and *Pseudomonas aeruginosa* both producing β-lactamase.

Other β-lactams

Besides penicillins and cephalosporins, some other antibiotics possessing a β-lactam ring have been discovered (Fig. 8.2). These include carbapenems, thiophenes, and monobactams. The monobactams and carbapenems were found by the screening of molds for antibacterial effects, whereas the thiophenes are of synthetic origin (Lima et al., 2020). Some carbapenems like imipenem, panipenem, meropenem, and doripenem are used against infections with gram-positive bacteria, and aztreonam is used in the clinic. No thiophenes have been introduced to the market. Meropenem, in combination with the β-lactamase inhibitor clavulanic acid, is used against infections of resistant *Mycobacterium tuberculosis*.

Development of antibiotics for the present and future society

Despite the appearance of drug-resistant bacteria, the development of new antibiotics is an orphan discipline. This might be considered a positive statement since it could mean that few resistant bacteria are threatening the general health of the world. Consequently, only a poor profit can be expected, even though a brilliant drug could be developed. Cephalosporins, quinolines, macrolides, and β-lactamase inhibitors are the drug types among which new revolutionary drugs primarily are expected to be found. In the period 2000–2019, only 24 new antibacterial drugs were approved. The market value of five of these agents has fallen to a value of zero (Rex and Outterson, 2021). As an example, a registered product (meropenem-vaborbactam) sold for only $21 million in the first 2 years and the sponsor, Melinta Therapeutics, declared bankruptcy in 2019 (Rex and Outterson, 2021). The poor expected profit has discouraged large companies from the field.

World Health Organization (WHO) and increasingly medical experts continuously warn against the development of resistant pathogenic bacteria. In 2019, the WHO published a list of 12 pathogenic bacteria that pose the greatest public health threat. Among these, carbapenem-resistant *Acinetobacter baumannii*, carbapenem-resistant *Pseudomonas aeruginosa*, and carbapenem-resistant *Enterobacteriaceae*, also resistant to third-generation cephalosporin, were considered the most dangerous (Weiss, 2019). Among the 25 antibiotics in clinical trials in 2020, eight were expected to have activity against the mentioned pathogens (Dheman et al., 2021). Initiatives like Transatlantic Taskforce on Antimicrobial Resistance (an EU–US collaboration), ND4BB (an EU multidisciplinary initiative) the Generating Antibiotics Incentives Now (GAIN) program passed by the U.S. Congress are governmental and international bodies created to generate new efficient antibiotics.

References

Christensen, S.B., 2021. Drugs that changed society: history and current status of the early antibiotics: salvarsan, sulfonamides, and β-lactams. Molecules 26, 6057.

Dheman, N., Mahoney, N., Cox, E.M., Farley, J.J., Amini, T., Lanthier, M.L., 2021. An analysis of antibacterial drug development trends in the United States, 1980-2019. Clin. Infect. Dis. 73, e4444–e4450.

Lima, L.M., da Silva, B.N.M, Barbosa, G., Barreiro, E.J., 2020. β-lactam antibiotics: an overview from a medicinal chemistry perspective. Eur. J. Med. Chem. 208, 112829.

Newton, G.G.F., Abraham, E.P., 1955. Cephalosporin C, a new antibiotic containing sulfur and D-α-aminoadipic acid. Nature 175, 548.

Rex, J.H., Outterson, K., 2021. Antibacterial R&D at a crossroads: we've pushed as hard as we can … now we need to start pulling! Clin. Infect. Dis. 73, e4451–e4453.

Selwyn, S., 1986. The discovery of penicillin and cephalosporins. In: Parnham, M.J., Bruinvels, J. (Eds.), Pharmacological Methods, Receptor & Chemotherapy (Discoveries in Pharmacology). Elsevier, pp. 284–301.

Weiss, G., 2019. 2019 Antibacterial Agents in Clinical Development. An Analysis of the Antibacterial Clinical Development Pipeline. WHO. https://apps.who.int/iris/bitstream/handle/10665/330420/9789240000193-eng.pdf.

The discovery of penicillin and cephalosporins

Sydney Selwyn

Contents

The history of penicillin is logically divided into four phases. The first is the pre-scientific use of mould preparations. This phase ended with the observations of John Burdon Sanderson, Joseph Lister and others in the early 1870s. The second phase continued for 60 years until the 1940 publication by Howard Florey's Oxford group of their first paper on the chemotherapeutic use of penicillin. Only 20 years were to elapse before the start of the present era of semi-synthetic penicillins was heralded by the report in 1959 from the Beecham group on the preparation and modification of the penicillin nucleus.

8.1 Pre-scientific applications of 'penicillin'

The use of fungi, particularly moulds, in the prevention and treatment of superficial infections has been a feature of folk medicine throughout the world since earliest times (Selwyn, 1980). Fig. 8.1 depicts, in pre-Columbian Central America, damp bread as the source of mould, an extract of which is being administered orally. Far more commonly, however, such preparations

Discoveries in Pharmacology, Volume 3, Hemodynamics and Immune Defense.
DOI: https://doi.org/10.1016/B978-0-443-18442-0.00068-9

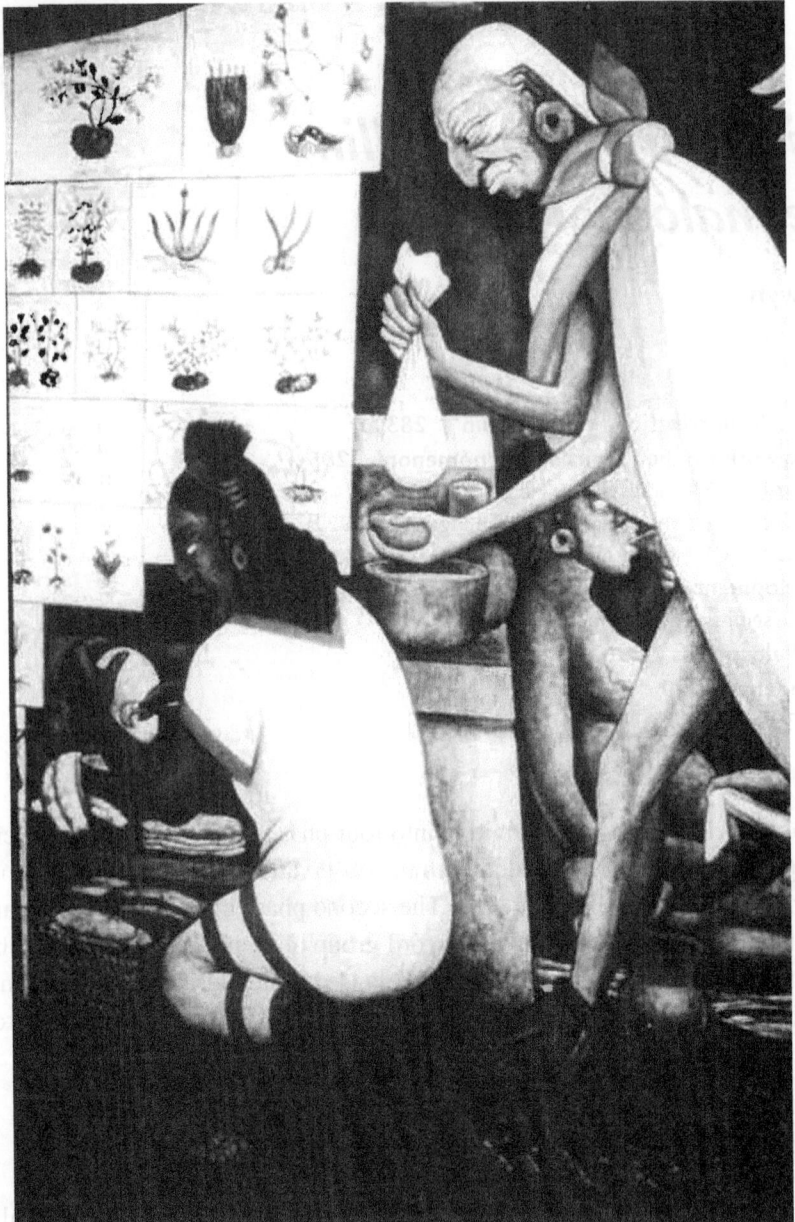

Figure 8.1
Representation of ancient Aztecs cultivating *Penicillium* mould on bread, extracting crude penicillin and swallowing it for therapeutic purposes. (A coloured mural by Diego Rivera in Centro Medico 'La Raza' del Instituto Mexicano del Seguro Social, Mexico City).

were applied topically in the form of salves and poultices. Several typical examples of such applications are described by Florey (1949).

The following account quoted by Townend (1943) is representative of many such uses:

> ['I have received the following note from Mr. H.L. Watkinson, headmaster of Mexborough Grammar School, Yorkshire]:
> 'During my undergraduate days at Cambridge, within the period 1911–13, I called at the Botany Laboratory to do a little extra work. We were studying fungi and the activities of the class were centred at the time on *Penicillium glaucum*. It was the custom in the class to be provided with a growth of the fungus which had been previously grown on old pieces of shoe leather. Only a portion of the growth was used and on the occasion of my calling the old laboratory attendant was collecting the stuff left on the students' benches. I was somewhat curious and asked why he was so carefully scraping off the fungus into a jar. He told me that he used it for a salve which had been used in his family for a very long time. It was used for what he called gatherings. I presume by this he meant septic wounds.' [Perhaps we have not yet made a serious enough attempt to investigate such home remedies.']

These therapeutic procedures would, nevertheless, have been very unreliable due to the great variability in the antibiotic productivity of *Penicillium* and related moulds, as well as the instability of penicillin solutions.

8.2 Scientific work on the 'penicillin phenomenon'

8.2.1 1870–1927: Studies before Fleming

Between 1869 and 1876 there were several fascinating British reports of observations on the antibacterial activity of *Penicillium* species (Selwyn, 1979). The first of these, described a study carried out in 1870 by John Burdon Sanderson (1871), who was at that time 'Medical Officer of Health' for the London Borough of Paddington – the district where Fleming also carried out his work nearly 60 years later. Like penicillin itself in the 1930s, Sanderson subsequently moved to Oxford where he became Professor of Physiology and eventually of Medicine.

Sanderson's findings were made during the course of pioneer bacteriological work in which he established that bacteria were entirely distinct from microscopic fungi, and were not stages in a complex life cycle, as had been claimed by Hallier. In one of Sanderson's experiments he placed two heat-sterilized glasses:

> 'on a shelf under a glass shade, one of which marked a. contained unboiled Pasteur's solution [simple culture fluid], the other, marked b., boiled solution. On October 10 glass

a. was turbid, and was found on microscopical examination to be teeming with bacteria – a thick whitish scum had formed on its surface. Glass b. was perfectly clear; there were, however, great numbers of torula cells on its surface, but no bacteria. On October 12b. exhibited numerous tufts of penicillium, but the liquid still remained limpid and free from bacteria; five days later similar tufts appeared on the surface of a.'

Later, after five glasses of media had been prepared,

'all the glasses showed tufts of penicillium, those on 3 and 5 were more advanced than the rest, and had become greenish from the development of heads of spores. At this time, and on all subsequent occasions, the liquid in 5 was found to be perfectly limpid and free from microzymes'. [Béchamp's term for bacteria.]

Sanderson also noted that the presence of mould in animal tissues inhibited bacterial growth. After exposing excised guinea pig thigh muscle to air, it 'shortly became covered with a crust of penicillium . . . On removing the crust and cutting into the muscle it was found to be . . . of natural appearance. There was a musty but no putrefactive smell'. However, bacterial overgrowth and rapid putrefaction occurred in muscle that had been moistened with non-sterile water.

Sanderson misinterpreted his observations to indicate that while fungi were airborne, bacteria were not, and they could be transmitted only in contaminated water.

Five years earlier, Joseph Lister had introduced his Antiseptic System of surgery based on a belief that the bacteria which infected wounds were carried in the air as well as on hands and various inanimate objects. Sanderson's report therefore threatened to undermine Lister's recommendations, consequently, in his Edinburgh residence, he undertook a detailed series of investigations to evaluate and extend Sanderson's work.

Starting on 16 th November 1871, Lister used as the main culture medium his own urine, which he collected after disinfecting the glans penis with carbolic acid. He was able to refute Sanderson's conclusions by showing that bacteria as well as fungi were indeed almost constantly present in the air. However, he also observed that cultures containing 'beautiful branching and jointed filaments' of mould showed either no bacteria or only degenerate forms. Interpreting this correctly, Lister continued his studies 'with the view of ascertaining whether the growth of fungi renders the liquid a less favourable nidus for bacteria'. He examined two subcultures microscopically:

'. . . both exhibited bacteria in abundance, but there was a very marked difference between them as regards their activity. Those from [tube] 2' [which had but a slight growth of *Penicillium*] exhibited the most amazing energy, not only as individuals but in the dense groups which were frequently seen, and in which the intense jostlings going on among the individuals were really surprising. Those from [tube] 5' [which had developed a heavy

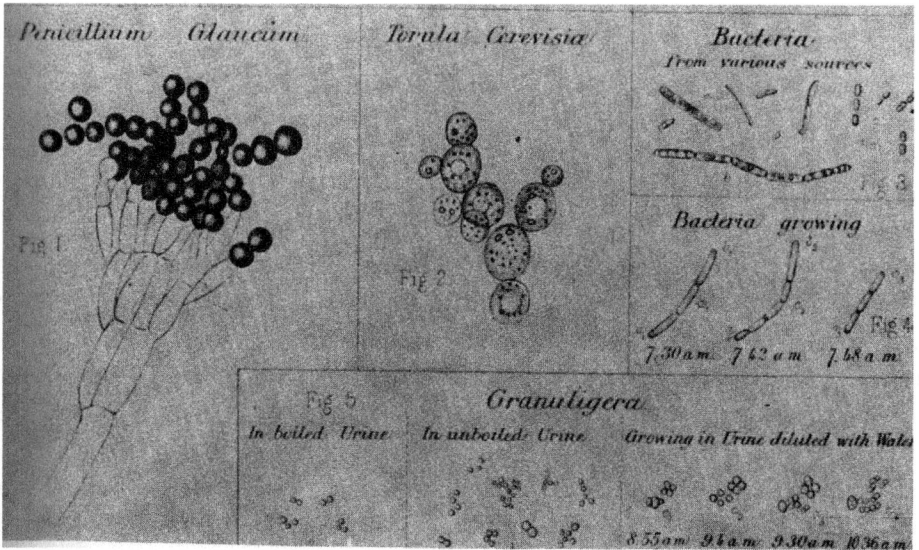

Figure 8.2
Engraving of a *Penicillium* species and other micro-organisms from a publication by Joseph Lister in 1875 (*Transactions of the Royal Society of Edinburgh,* 27: 313–344).

growth of *Penicillium*] were comparatively languid, multitudes were entirely motionless and there was not the same appearance of dense groups.'

Lister identified the fungus as *Penicillium glaucum* and he prepared excellent illustrations of it (Fig. 8.2). This species name was used uncritically by subsequent workers, and had originally been applied by Link in 1809, to the type species of that group of Hyphomycete fungi which produce 'conidial fructifications' in the form of a brush (penicillus in Latin).

The clinical possibilities of applying the antibacterial effect of *Penicillium* were clear to Lister, who sought an antiseptic that would be less toxic than carbolic acid. He wrote in 1872 while still performing his experiments, 'should a suitable case present I shall endeavour to employ *Penicillium glaucum* and observe if the growth of the [infecting] organisms be inhibited in the human tissues'.

Lister remained interested in applying *Penicillium,* and there is a report of his clinical use of a culture extract in the local treatment of a gluteal abscess in 1884 at King's College Hospital, London, to where he had moved seven years earlier (Selwyn, 1979). Unfortunately Lister did not publish the results of his clinical work with *Penicillium,* and we must assume that they were very inconsistent.

Three other British scientists carried out relevant studies of the antibacterial action of *Penicillium* shortly after Lister. The first of these was William Roberts, Professor of Medicine in Manchester, who in 1874 confirmed Lister's results (Roberts, 1874). Roberts wrote:

'the growth of fungi appeared to me to be antagonistic to that of bacteria, and vice versa. I have repeatedly observed that liquid, in which the *Penicilium* [sic] *glaucum* was growing luxuriantly could with difficulty be artificially infected with bacteria.'

Two years later in 1876 the distinguished physicist John Tyndall reported his experiments which helped to disprove the time-honoured concept of spontaneous generation (Tyndall, 1876). As an incidental observation he noticed, like Lister and Roberts, that where cultures were 'crowned by beautiful tufts of mould . . . the *Bacteria* lost their translatory power, fell to the bottom, and left the liquid between them and the superficial layer clear'. Tyndall, however, incorrectly supposed that 'the thick tough layer' of mould which covered the culture surface 'must have seriously intercepted the oxygen said to be necessary to Bacterial life'. Nevertheless he made the fascinating observation that in a culture containing 'a bright yellow-green pigment . . . no trace of mould was to be seen . . . it cannot be doubted that the mould-spores fell into this tube also, but in the fight for existence the colour-producing *Bacteria* has the upper hand'. This was to be very prophetic of the problems posed in the antibiotic treatment of *Pseudomonas* infections a century later.

The great biologist Thomas Henry Huxley attempted to dissuade his friend Tyndall from the false concept of oxygen lack as the mechanism by which *Penicillium* produced its antibacterial effect. Huxley also independently studied this phenomenon in 1875, but he described the results only in his private correspondence.

Between 1896 and the summer of 1928 the inhibitory effect of *Penicillium* on bacteria was rediscovered several times by Gosio, Duchesne, Sturli, Gratia and others (Selwyn, 1980). Although these investigators carried out interesting in vitro and even, occasionally, in vivo experiments, their results had minimal impact. The same cannot be said (ultimately) of the work of Alexander Fleming in the autumn of 1928.

8.2.2 The observations of Alexander Fleming (1928–1929)

The well known and romantic story of Alexander Fleming's origins, his discovery of penicillin and the drug's subsequent development may be summarised as follows. He had a poverty stricken childhood in the Scottish countryside, and had to struggle against every kind of difficulty in order to qualify as a doctor with a steadfast interest in conquering infection. Then in 1928 Fleming (Fig. 8.3) noticed that one of his cultures of *Staphylococcus aureus* had become contaminated with a *Penicillium* spore which had blown in through his laboratory window in St. Mary's Hospital, London. In the vicinity of the resulting mould growth the staphylococcal colonies had been dissolved to an extent inversely proportional to their distance from the mould. Fleming tried in vain to purify the penicillin antibiotic responsible for the bacterial lysis, in order to use it for the treatment of human infections. He encountered indifference and active opposition, even from his own colleagues. Only after the outbreak of

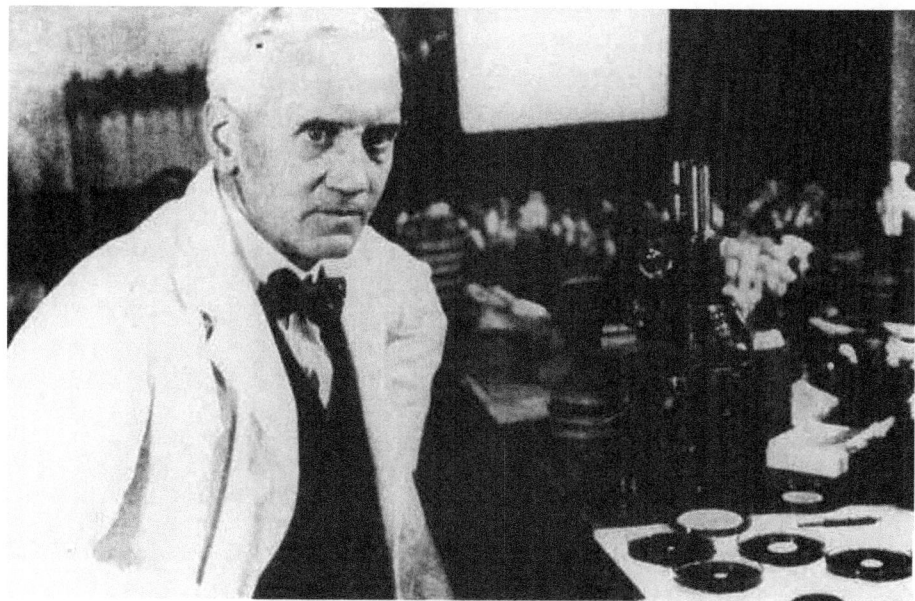

Figure 8.3
Alexander Fleming in his laboratory at St. Mary's Hospital, London (about 1944).

World War II eleven years later, with its enormous problems of infected wounds, was Fleming able to persuade some research workers in Oxford to produce enough penicillin for clinical use.

Almost every detail of this story is now known to be incorrect. A comprehensive recent biography (Macfarlane, 1984) confirms that Fleming was the son of a relatively prosperous farmer, and his medical education was facilitated by a family legacy. He had intended to be a surgeon, but turned to bacteriology because, by chance, he was offered a grant in that subject.

The circumstances of Fleming's observations on penicillin are based on his own published account and his comments more than 13 years later. His original paper (Fleming, 1929a) was significantly entitled *On the antibacterial action of cultures of a Penicillium, with special reference to their use in the isolation of B. influenzae.* It begins:

> 'While working with staphylococcus variants a number of culture-plates were set aside on the laboratory bench and examined from time to time. In the examinations these plates were necessarily exposed to the air and they became contaminated with various microorganisms. It was noticed that around a large colony of a contaminating mould the staphylococcus colonies became transparent and were obviously undergoing lysis'

Fleming was apparently unaware of earlier observations on the antibacterial effect of some (but by no means all) strains of *Penicillium* species. Hare (1970) who was a colleague of

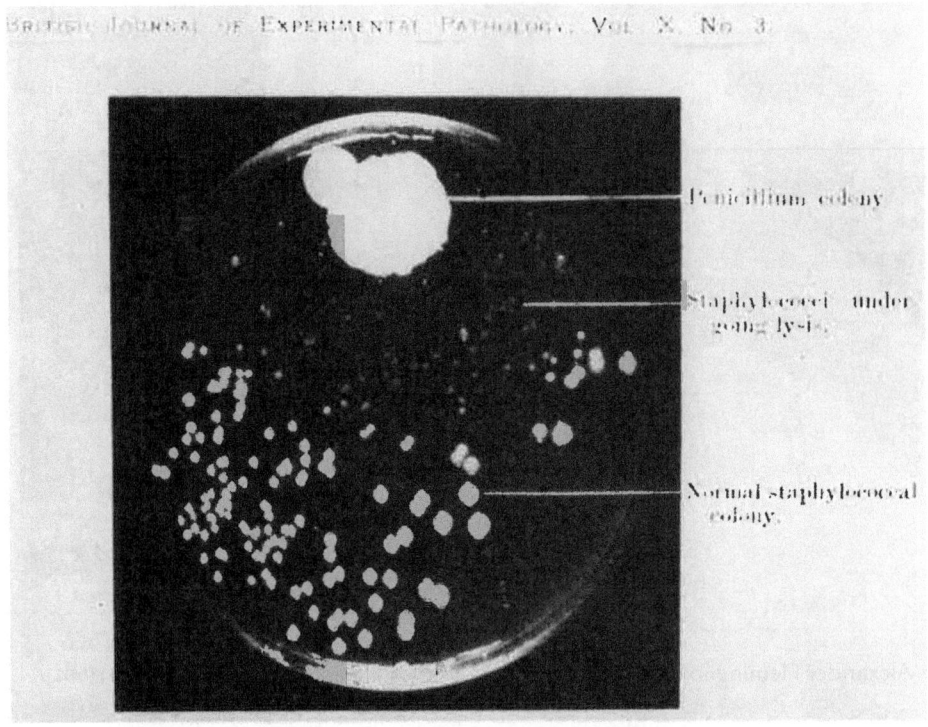

BRITISH JOURNAL OF EXPERIMENTAL PATHOLOGY. VOL. X. No 3.

Penicillium colony

Staphylococci undergoing lysis.

Normal staphylococcal colony.

Figure 8.4
The original culture of *Staphylococcus aureus* growing in the presence of *Penicillium notatum* (Fig. 81 of Fleming's 1929 paper).

Fleming in 1928 clearly showed that the celebrated culture had been misinterpreted by Fleming. Even enormous amounts of penicillin cannot lyse mature staphylococcal colonies, but can only produce lysis of the actively growing bacteria in 'young' colonies. Indeed Fleming's own published illustration shows that only small colonies were affected by lysis and showed premature cessation of growth (Fig. 8.4). The lysis is in fact the secondary result of defective cell wall synthesis.

Hare (1970) has reconstructed the details of the original discovery with the help of meteorological records and practical experiments. The original fungal spore (or possibly two spores, judging by the resulting double mould colony, shown in Fig. 8.4) probably did not blow through Fleming's window since this was apparently always kept shut. The mould is likely to have originated in the nearby mycological laboratory of C. J. La Touche, who was studying a wide range of fungi as allergens.

Fleming had almost certainly not incubated his culture plate after he had originally inoculated it with *Staphylococcus aureus* – which he was studying in great detail in 1928 while preparing a chapter on this species for a major textbook (Fleming, 1929b). The fungal contaminant landed on the culture medium either before the bacteria were inoculated or certainly before visible bacterial growth had occurred. After leaving the culture plate on his laboratory bench, Fleming went on a short vacation at the end of July.

While he was away, the summer temperature was at first (from 27th July to 6th August) unusually low, fluctuating between 12°C and 20°C. This permitted good growth of the *Penicillium* but not the staphylococci. The ambient temperature then rose and ranged from 21°C to 26°C for several days, allowing adequate growth of the staphylococci – except in the vicinity of the penicillin-producing mould.

After returning at the beginning of September, Fleming discarded his accumulated cultures into a shallow tray containing the disinfectant lysol. Fortunately the disinfectant did not penetrate into the mould-contaminated culture; and on about 3rd September when Fleming was finally examining the discarded cultures in the presence of one of his junior colleagues, D. M. Pryce, he remarked 'That's funny', and he immediately sub-cultured the mould. Fleming's eye and mind were prepared for such microbial inhibitions ever since 6 earlier when he had observed that his nasal mucus, which was being cultured, had caused the dissolution of a contaminating bacterium (*'Micrococcus lysodeikticus'*). He thus discovered lysozyme (Fleming, 1922).

In the last four months of 1928 and the first four of 1929, Fleming carried out very thorough in vitro tests into the antibacterial effects of his *Penicillium* strain. He showed that very high dilutions of the filtrate from the mould cultures inhibited most Gram-positive bacteria including staphylococci, haemolytic streptococci, pneumococci and diphtheria bacilli. The important anaerobic bacilli, the *Clostridia,* were, however, omitted. He found that most Gram-negative bacteria were resistant, except the *Neisseria* group of cocci.

Fleming also showed that his crude penicillin was harmless to polymorph leucocytes and to whole animals and man, reporting that:

> 'the toxicity to animals of powerfully antibacterial mould broth filtrates appears to be very low. Twenty c.c. injected intravenously into a rabbit were not more toxic than the same quantity of broth. Half a c.c. injected intraperitoneally into a mouse weighing about 20 gm. induced no toxic symptoms. Constant irrigation of large infected surfaces in man was not accompanied by any toxic symptoms, while irrigation of the human conjunctiva every hour for a day had no irritant effect.
> *In vitro* penicillin which completely inhibits the growth of staphylococci in a dilution of 1:600 does not interfere with leucocytic function to a greater extent than does ordinary broth.'

Perhaps surprisingly, however, Fleming did not assess the activity of his antibiotic preparation against systemic infections in laboratory animals. This may partly have been due to his observation that penicillin is eliminated rapidly from the animal body, whereas he believed that the agent had a very slow antibacterial effect.

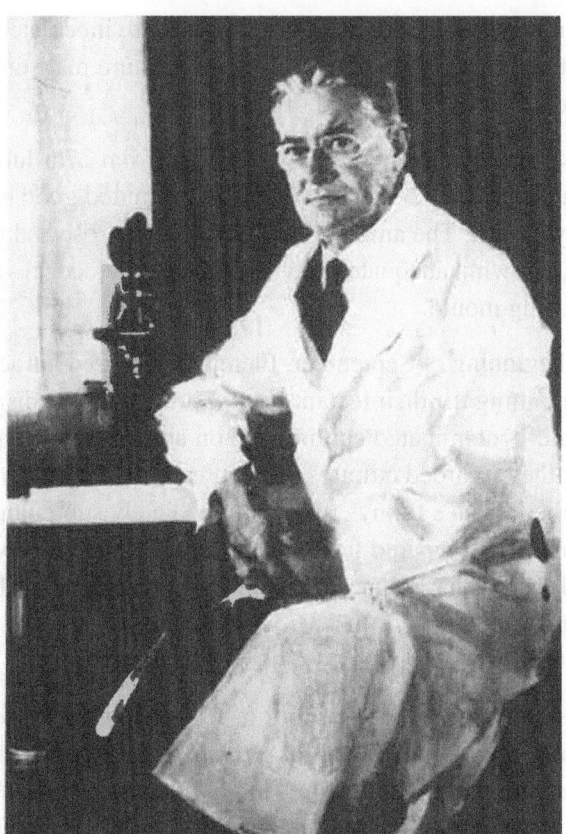

Figure 8.5
Portrait of Howard Florey (by Cedric Deane, 1962, in the entrance hall of the Sir William Dunn School of Pathology, Oxford).

Fleming's 1929 paper ends with the suggestion that penicillin 'may be an efficient antiseptic for application to, or injection into, areas infected with penicillin-sensitive microbes'. The possibility of using penicillin sytemically in man was not considered.

Fleming's interest in penicillin was restricted almost entirely to its use as a selective agent for the culture of the penicillin-resistant species, *Haemophilus (Bacillus) influenzae* – a delicate micro-organism which was grown extensively by Fleming in the production of vaccines. He was, however, occasionally persuaded to use his crude penicillin 'mould juice' on the infected eyes or in the paranasal sinuses of his colleagues (Selwyn, 1980). In 1929 he also encouraged some rather abortive attempts by his junior staff to extract and purify penicillin. Some further studies of the fungal product carried out elsewhere in the University of London by P. W. Clutterbuck, R. Lovell and H. Raistrick were published in 1932, and by R.D. Reid in the U.S.A. in 1935. But only slight progress was made, and the introduction of Prontosil and

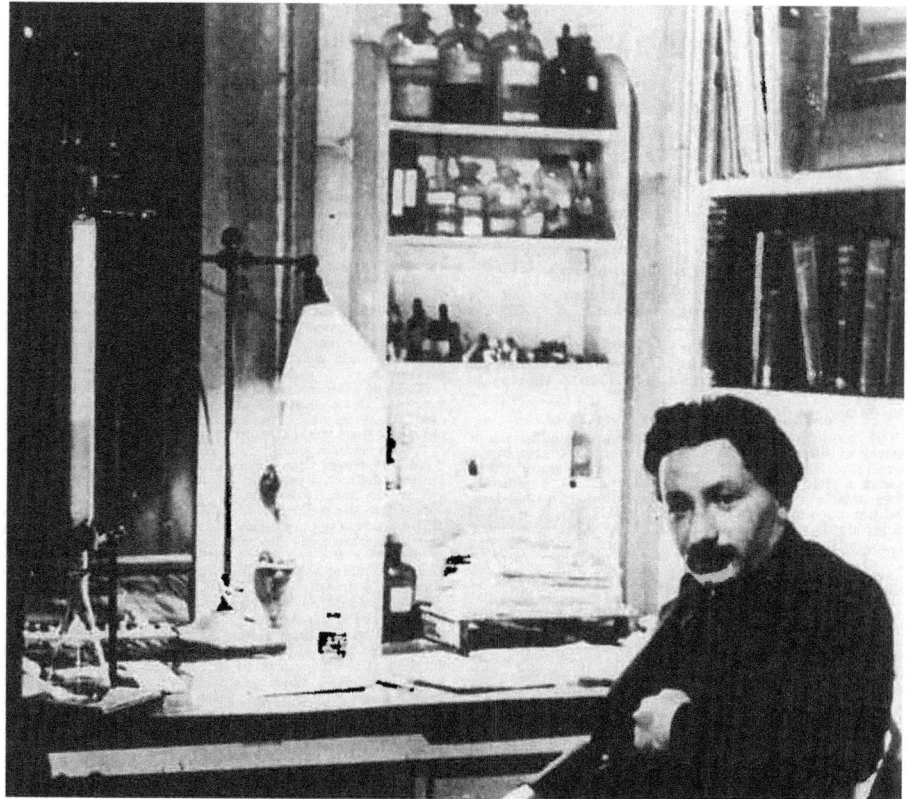

Figure 8.6

Ernst Chain in the Sir William Dunn School of Pathology, Oxford (about 1945). The alumina column on the left was used for purifying penicillin.

its active principle, sulphanilamide, in 1935 further reduced the minimal interest that existed in penicillin.

8.2.3 The work of Florey's group in Oxford (1938–1942)

Penicillin as a chemotherapeutic agent became a reality at the Sir William Dunn School of Pathology in the University of Oxford 13 years after Fleming's original observation of 1928. Contrary to the popular account, this phase of the story began quietly in 1938 – one year before the outbreak of World War II. Howard Florey (Fig. 8.5), the Professor of Pathology at Oxford and his assistant, the biochemist Ernst Chain (Fig. 8.6), were interested in natural antibacterial substances. In 1937 Chain had elucidated the mode of action of lysozyme, which Fleming had discovered 15 years earlier. Chain then searched the literature for other bacteriolytic agents, and by chance he read Fleming's 1929 paper on penicillin. Because of the

THE LANCET]   [AUG. 16, 1941

ORIGINAL ARTICLES

FURTHER OBSERVATIONS ON PENICILLIN

E. P. ABRAHAM,*
D. PHIL. OXFD

A. D. GARDNER,
D.M. OXFD, F.R.C.S.

E. CHAIN,*
PH.D. CAMB.

N. G. HEATLEY,†
PH.D. CAMB.

C. M. FLETCHER,‡
M.B. CAMB., M.R.C.P.

M. A. JENNINGS,*
B.M. OXFD

H. W. FLOREY, M.B. ADELAIDE, F.R.S.

(The Sir William Dunn School of Pathology and the Radcliffe Infirmary, Oxford)

THE work on penicillin briefly reported by Chain and others (1940) is here presented in greater detail, and its further development to the stage of human therapy is described.

Growth of Penicillin-producing Mould

The mould will grow and produce penicillin on a variety of different media, but that used by Clutterbuck, Lovell and Raistrick (1932) is easy to prepare and gives as high a yield of penicillin as others containing peptone, horse-muscle digests, &c. This modified Czapek-Dox medium consists of: NaNO$_3$ 3 g., KH$_2$PO$_4$ 1 g., KCl 0·5 g., MgSO$_4$.7H$_2$O 0·5 g., FeSO$_4$.7H$_2$O 0·01 g., glucose 40 g., with water to 1 litre. Oxford tap-water has proved as good as distilled water for this purpose. Yeast-extract has usually been added to speed up the growth of the mould (details later).

The medium, sterilised by autoclaving, is sown with a spore suspension made by shaking up sterile water in a screw-capped bottle containing a slope on which the mould has grown and spored freely. Twenty-four hours after sowing a very delicate fluffy gauze-like growth can be seen with difficulty on the bottom of the vessel (at 24° C.). The growth becomes more voluminous during the next day and on the 3rd day, if the liquid layer is not more than 1 cm. thick, this reaches the surface of the medium and throws up dry white mycelium, usually in isolated foci, particularly around the sides of the vessel.

of development may be greater or less than that described, depending largely on the depth of the medium. A systematic study of the factors influencing penicillin-production was begun, but it could not be completed owing to the very numerous and often interdependent variables, and to the fact that the assay-method then in use could only detect large differences of titre. The following conclusions, however, could be drawn:

1. Penicillin production seems to take place over a wide range of oxygen tension. (The mould will not grow anaerobically.)

2. The mould grows satisfactorily at 24° C. At lower temperatures growth is delayed and as harvesting of the medium is carried out in the incubator higher temperatures have not been studied, 24° C. being about the upper limit of comfort. Fleming (1929) in his original description stated that the mould would not grow at 37° C. and this has been confirmed.

3. Crude attempts to change the pH of the medium or to maintain it at a constant value have not resulted in a noticeable increase in yield of penicillin, nor has the incorporation of ten times the normal amount of phosphate buffer.

4. The medium should not have a depth greater than 1·5–2 cm. If deeper than 2 cm. diffusion is visibly inadequate, for two distinct layers can be seen in it, the upper being yellow, the lower colourless.

5. When the medium is fit to be harvested it can be drawn off from under the mycelium and replaced with fresh medium in which more penicillin will form in about half the time required for the initial production. The medium can be changed several times in this way; with one batch it was changed 14 times.

6. The mould must be grown and the medium harvested and replaced under strictly sterile conditions since penicillin is destroyed by certain bacteria (Abraham and Chain 1940).

7. The addition of yeast-extract (Gladstone and Fildes 1940) accelerates the growth of the mould but does not affect the yield of penicillin. In large-scale growth we have always used yeast-extract; in starting a batch the medium is made up to contain 10% of it, but the medium used for replacement contains only 2½%. The accelerating effect of the yeast is not impaired by prolonged autoclaving at a high temperature. Marmite or malt extract have no effect on the rate of growth or on the yield of penicillin.

Figure 8.7

Title and opening section of the Oxford team's paper on the clinical use of penicillin in human infections (*The Lancet* 2, 177–189; 1941).

paper's erroneous description of a direct bacteriolytic effect, Chain decided to make a detailed study of penicillin!

To his surprise, Chain found that the Fleming strain of *Penicillium notatum* was available in an adjacent laboratory, where it had been used for several years in studies on bacteriophage. After a leisurely first year, the project gained momentum at the end of 1939 when Norman Heatley joined Florey and Chain. Within a few months, substantial quantities of concentrated and relatively pure penicillin had been used to cure experimental infections in mice. This work was reported in *The Lancet* on 24th August 1940 under the title *Penicillin as a Chemotherapeutic Agent* (Chain et al., 1940).

The original batches of penicillin at Oxford possessed pyrogenic activity. This was removed chromatographically by Edward Abraham, who joined the team in 1940; penicillin was now ready for use in human infections. This phase began on 12th February 1941, and the impressive early results were published in *The Lancet* on 16th August 1941 (Abraham et al., 1941).

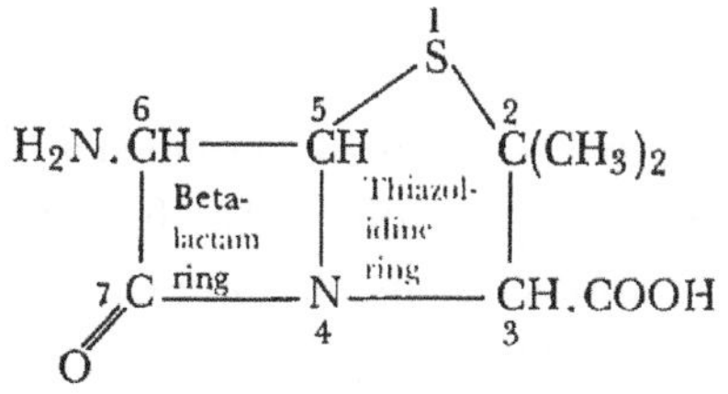

Figure 8.8
The penicillin 'nucleus' 6-APA.

The Oxford team's second Lancet paper (Fig. 8.7), modestly entitled *Further Observations on Penicillin,* can be regarded as the official inauguration of the Antibiotic Era. This work was ultimately recognised by the award of the Nobel Prize for Medicine in 1945 jointly to Florey, Chain and Fleming.

8.3 The development of penicillin and its derivatives

Back in 1941, however, enormous efforts were made in Oxford and then in some other British laboratories to produce penicillin for use in war casualities. Nevertheless, major progress was only made after the visit of Florey and Heatley to the U.S.A. in the latter half of 1941. Heatley remained for almost one year to guide the scaling up of penicillin production. This was initially carried out at the Northern Regional (Agricultural) Research Laboratory at Peoria, Illinois, where the original fungal strain was replaced by a mutant induced in a *Penicillium chrysogenum* strain from a mouldy canteloupe melon.

Subsequently, the remarkable co-operation of Merck and Co. and E.R. Squibb & Sons in 1942, joined later by other companies, led to the foundation of the modern pharmaceutical industry. Their large-scale deep fermentation technology was able to respond rapidly to the discovery of the further antibiotics – streptomycin in 1943 (announced in 1944), chloramphenicol in 1947, and the first tetracyclines between 1948 and 1953.

The first pure crystalline penicillin (sodium benzylpenicillin or 'penicillin G') was prepared by E.R. Squibb & Sons in 1943; but a further 14 years elapsed before J.C. Sheehan announced the total synthesis of the penicillin molecule.

In the same year, 1957, a discovery of enormous significance was made by a group at the Beecham Research Laboratories in Surrey, England. The members, including G.N. Rolinson, F.R. Batchelor and J.H.C. Nayler, under the guidance of Ernst Chain, found that if *Para*-aminobenzylpenicillin was produced by fermentation in the absence of side-chain precursors (which contain phenyl groups), they obtained an inactive molecule, 6-amino-penicillanic acid – 'the penicillin nucleus' (Fig. 8.8).

8.3.1 The semi-synthetic penicillins

Acylation at the C_6 position and insertion of novel side chains provided a potentially vast range of penicillin derivatives with widely differing properties. The first clinically important product of Beecham Research Laboratories was methicillin, which appeared in 1960 and had a bulky dimethoxyphenyl side chain that obstructed the hydrolytic action of staphylococcal penicillinase (β-lactamase). This destructive type of enzyme from bacteria had been originally described by Abraham and Chain as early as 1940, and by 1960 was responsible for penicillin-resistance in over 70% of 'hospital' strains of *Staph. aureus*. Orally available analogues of methicillin, including oxacillin and cloxacillin were introduced in 1962.

One year earlier, the first of the broad-spectrum semi-synthetic penicillins was announced. This was ampicillin, which contained an acyl-amino side chain, allowing penetration of the cell walls of many penicillin-resistant Gram-negative bacilli, including *Haemophilus influenzae* and *Salmonella typhi*. Ampicillin is an orally available antibiotic, which however has certain drawbacks such as relatively poor absorption from the intestine and vulnerability to most β-lactamases. Subsequent developments have been designed to correct these and other deficiencies (Selwyn, 1982). Thus carbenicillin introduced in 1967, followed by the ureido- series, including azlocillin and piperacillin, have particularly good activity against *Pseudomonas aeruginosa* and other 'problem' bacteria.

Since 1970 a wide variety of β-lactam antibiotics have been derived from micro-organisms other than *Penicillium* species – notably from the *Streptomyces* group of higher bacteria (Selwyn, 1983). All these compounds possess the β-lactam ring of penicillin (Fig. 8.8) attached to novel groupings instead of the thiazolidine ring. However, the biggest range of antibiotics has been derived from the cephalosporin nucleus, which was first identified in 1954.

8.4 The cephalosporins

In 1945 Giuseppe Brotzu, the Professor of Bacteriology at the University of Cagliari, in Sardinia, was carrying out a methodical search for antibiotic-producing micro-organisms in sewage draining into the sea (Fig. 8.9). He was motivated by the belief that such organisms must be responsible for eliminating typhoid bacilli from the local beaches, which were heavily polluted with infected sewage. Although dilution, ultra-violet radiation and other factors were probably responsible for this effect, Brotzu nevertheless did discover a mould – *Cephalosporium acremonium* – which had antibacterial activity against a wide range of species, including *Salmonella typhi*. Moreover, he apparently obtained good preliminary results with injections of a crude fungal extract in patients suffering from typhoid and a variety of other infections (Selwyn, 1980).

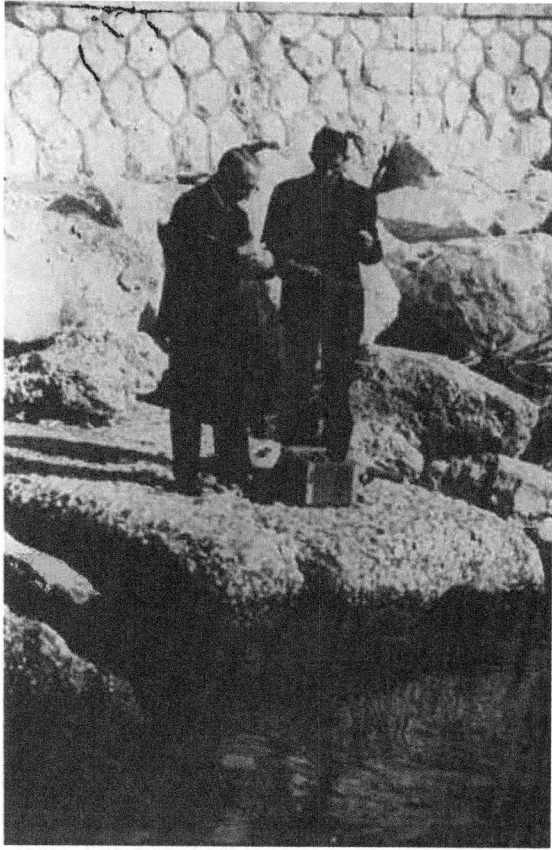

Figure 8.9
Giuseppe Brotzu (left) with an assistant, collecting sewage-rich water samples at Su Siccu beach, Cagliari, Sardinia.

Brotzu's findings were published privately in 1948 in an article simply entitled *Ricerche su di un nuovo antibiotico* (Brotzu, 1948).

No further progress was made until Brotzu sent this article and a culture of his mould to Sir Howard Florey at Oxford, where a decade earlier *Penicillium notatum* had been at a similar early stage. Within a year, Edward Abraham of the original penicillin team (Fig. 8.10) working with H.S. Burton had found that at least two antibiotics were produced by the mould. One was a narrow-spectrum steroid compound ('cephalosporin P') resembling fusidic acid, which was isolated 14 years later. The second was the broad-spectrum agent responsible for Brotzu's results. This was initially referred to as 'cephalosporin N', but was subsequently identified as a penicillin ('N').

The discovery of the first true cephalosporin was the result of serendipity, as Edward Abraham described in a lecture in 1974 (Abraham, 1974):

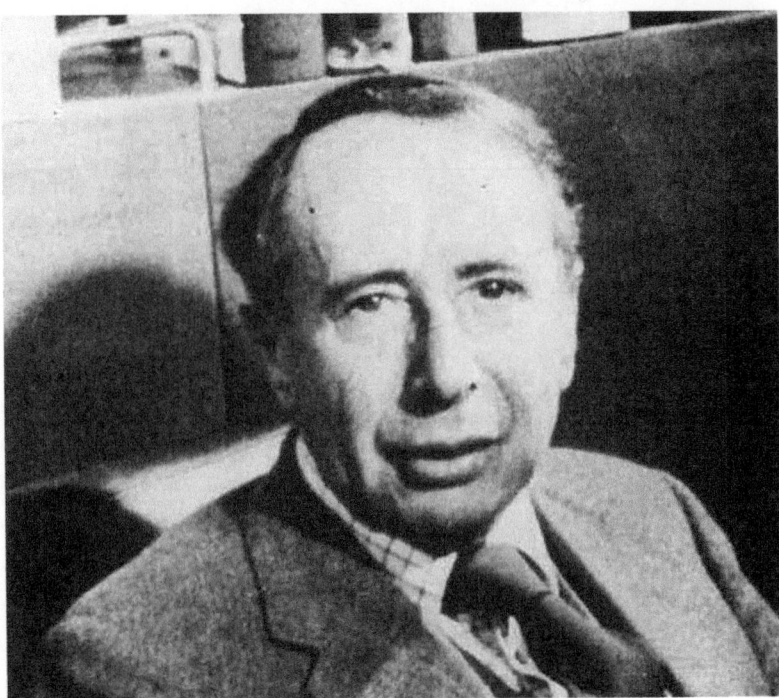

Figure 8.10
Edward Abraham in his Oxford office in 1974.

'Cephalosporin P and penicillin N were the only antibiotics which we detected by antibacterial assay of culture filtrates and crude extracts of the Sardinian *Cephalosporium* sp., but a third antibiotic was discovered in a purely academic study of the chemistry of penicillin N. In 1953, during an experiment designed to isolate the penillic acid of penicillin N in a pure form from partially purified penicillin N itself, Newton and I observed that the penillic acid was followed from an ion exchange column by a second substance which had a characteristic ultraviolet absorption spectrum. This substance named cephalosporin C, was isolated as a sodium salt in crystalline form. It was subsequently shown to have antibacterial activity, but the latter was too low for it to have been detected by antibacterial assay, at that time, in fermentation fluids. It thus seems unlikely that cephalosporin C would have been discovered in a conventional screening program. Its detection was, in fact, a totally unexpected bonus from our decision to put the finishing touches to the evidence for the structure of penicillin N.'

The announcement of their newly isolated antibiotic was made by Guy Newton and Edward Abraham (1955) in a paper entitled *Cephalosporin C, a New Antibiotic containing Sulphur and d-α-Aminoadipic Acid.* Although the antibiotic possessed relatively low activity against susceptible bacteria, its high degree of resistance to staphylococcal β-lactamase made it particularly interesting. Florey showed that it was non-toxic to mice in high doses intravenously and was effective against experimental infections.

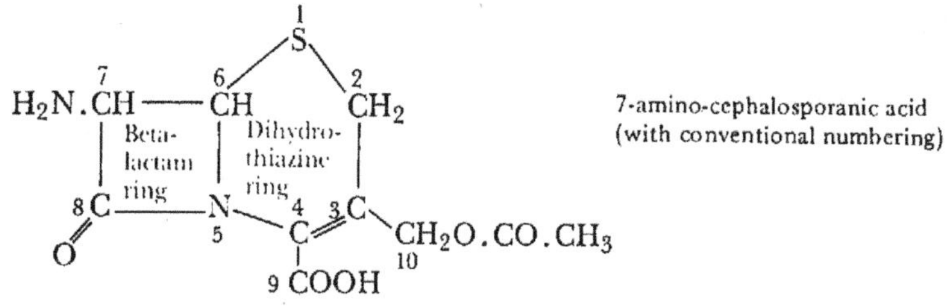

Figure 8.11
The cephalosporin 'nucleus' 7-ACA.

Poor yields from the original mould and difficulties in extracting the hydrophilic antibiotic retarded further progress. Fortunately, a higher-yielding mutant was isolated in 1957 at the British Medical Research Council's Antibiotic Research Station in Somerset, England. Sufficient cephalosporin C had been produced at Glaxo Laboratories by 1959 to enable Abraham and his colleagues, including Dorothy Hodgkin, at Oxford to determine the structure of the antibiotic which they reported in 1961 (Abraham and Newton, 1961; Hodgkin and Maslen, 1961).

The antibiotic would undoubtedly have been introduced for clinical use in the early 1960's for the treatment of staphylococcal infections if methicillin and, subsequently, comparable semi-synthetic penicillins had not made their appearance by that time.

Fortunately, the Oxford team had already established that the 'cephalosporin nucleus', 7-amino-cephalosporanic acid (7-ACA), which is represented in Fig. 8.11, was a rich source of active derivatives. Thus, 7-ACA was comparable with the penicillin nucleus, 6-ACA, but had the potential advantage that substituents could readily be introduced at the 3-carbon as well as at the 7-carbon (which is equivalent to the 6-carbon of 6-APA).

The first two semi-synthetic cephalosporins for clinical use were the injectable derivatives cephalothin and cephaloridine, which were introduced in 1964. The oral antibiotic cephalexin appeared in 1967, followed by cephradine and other 'first generation' cephalosporins. The 'second-generation' drugs, cefuroxime, cefamandole and cefoxitin were introduced in 1978 (Selwyn, 1980).

Since then a remarkable range of 'third-generation' cephalosporins has appeared, including cefotaxime, ceftazidime and the entirely synthetic agent latamoxef. Possessing the unusually low toxicity of penicillin and other β-lactam agents, the new cephalosporins have increased resistance to destruction by β-lactamases and an extended spectrum of activity against Gram-negative bacilli – including, to a varying extent, *Pseudomonas aeruginosa*. However, generally there has been a simultaneous loss in activity against Gram-positive bacteria, particularly *Staphylococcus aureus*.

The antibacterial panacea is therefore still awaited; but it may be not very far away.

Acknowledgements

The following figures are reproduced by kind permission of St. Mary's Hospital Medical School (Fig. 8.3), the Editor of *The British Journal of Experimental Pathology* (Fig. 8.4), The Sir William Dunn School of Pathology (Fig. 8.5 and 8.6), the Editor of *The Lancet* (Fig. 8.7), and Glaxo Laboratories (Fig. 8.9).

References

Abraham, E.P., 1974. Develop. Industr. Microbiol. 15, 3–15.

Abraham, E.P., Chain, E., Fletcher, C.M., Florey, H.W., Gardner, A.D., Heatley, N.G., Jennings, M.A., 1941. Lancet 2, 177–189.

Abraham, E.P., Newton, G.G.F., 1961. Biochem. J. 79, 377–393.

Brotzu, G., 1948. Lav. Ist. Igiene Cagliari 1, 1–11.

Chain., E., Florey, H.W., Gardner, A.D., Heatley, N.G., Jennings, M.A., Orr-Ewing, J., Sanders, A.G, 1940. Lancet 2, 226–228.

Fleming, A., 1922. Proc. R. Soc. B 393, 306–317.

Fleming, A., 1929a. Br. J. Exp. Pathol. 10, 226–236.

Fleming, A., 1929b. A System of Bacteriology in Relation to Medicine, Vol. 2, Chapt. 1, Privy Council (Medical Research Council), His Majesty's Stationery Office. London.

Florey, H.W., 1949. Antibiotics: A Survey of Penicillin, Streptomycin, and Other Antimicrobial Substances from Fungi, Actinomycetes, Bacteria and Plants, 1. Oxford University Press, London.

Hare, R., 1970. The Birth of Penicillin. George Allen & Unwin, London.

Hodgkin, D.C., Maslen, E.N., 1961. Biochem. J. 79, 393–402.

Macfarlane, G., 1984. Alexander Fleming: The Man and the Myth. Chatto and Windus, London.

Newton, G.C.F., Abraham, E.P., 1955. Nature (London) 175, 548.

Roberts, W., 1874. Phil. Trans. R. Soc, London 164, 457–477.

Sanderson, J.B., 1871. In: 13th Report of the Medical Officer of the Privy Council (John Simon), Appendix 5, Studies in contagion, Her Majesty's Stationery Office, London, pp. 48–69.

Selwyn, S., 1979. J. Antimicrob. Chemother. 5, 249–255.

Selwyn, S., 1980. In: The Beta-Lactam Antibiotics: Penicillins and Cephalosporins in Perspective, Chap. 1. Hodder and Stoughton, London, pp. 1–55.

Selwyn, S., 1982. J. Antiraicrob. Chemother. 9 (Suppl B), 1–10.

Selwyn, S., 1983. In: *Chemotherapeutic Strategy,* (Edwards, D.I., Hiscock, D.R., Eds.), MacMillan, Basingstoke and London.

Townend, B.R., 1943. Lancet 2, 653.

Tyndall, J., 1876. Phil. Trans. R. Soc., London 166, 27–63.

Commentary on The antibiotic explosion by H. Boyd Woodruff and Richard W. Burg

Karen Bush

Indiana University, Bloomington, IN, United States

H.B. Woodruff and R. Burg's 1986 historical review of antibiotic development was written from the perspective of scientists at Merck who had experience in both academic and pharmaceutical drug discovery programs (Woodruff and Burg, 1986). Burg was a fermentation specialist; Woodruff was a celebrated industrial microbiologist whose extensive experience in early antibiotic identification, under the direction of Selman Waksman at Rutgers, was used as the basis for Merck's successful antimicrobial natural product program (Bennett et al., 2017). This review article, coming on the downswing from the "Golden Age" of antibiotic drug discovery of the 1950s and 1960s (Davies, 2006), provided an excellent overview of the initial research accomplishments in antibiotic drug discovery, with resulting successes in both human and agricultural antibiotics.

Unsurprisingly, the authors strongly supported the screening of natural products as an effective approach to the identification of new antimicrobial agents, an approach that historically had been highly successful. This point of view prevailed for several decades. With the rapid development of robotic high throughput screening methodology in the 1990s, natural product screening to identify novel antibiotics was an obvious application (Wu et al., 1997). Many major pharmaceutical companies developed biological assays to screen thousands of soil, marine, and plant extracts to look for unusual biological activities, not only antimicrobial (Deschamps et al., 2007). However, the results of these screening campaigns were not highly successful, with many known β-lactams and tetracyclines rediscovered by multiple groups. No novel antibiotics based on new natural product-derived structures have been approved for human use since daptomycin (2003), a lipopeptide natural product abandoned by scientists at Lilly in the late 1980s and later developed by Cubist (Tally and DeBruin, 2000). As a result, most large companies discontinued natural product research by the early 21st century. This does not mean we have given up on natural products. Dozens of reports appear every year describing the antibacterial properties of products produced from soil samples, but most of

Discoveries in Pharmacology, Volume 3, Hemodynamics and
Immune Defense.
DOI: https://doi.org/10.1016/B978-0-443-18442-0.00006-9

these compounds are unsuitable for medicinal use due to unfavorable physical properties or toxicities to human cells. An important exception recently described by the Lewis laboratory was the discovery of teixobactin, a natural product emerging from a novel screening procedure of unculturable environmental bacteria (Ling et al., 2015). This unusual depsipeptide has a dual mechanism of action, by binding to highly conserved motifs of lipid II and lipid III, precursors of peptidoglycan, and cell wall teichoic acid, respectively. As a result, teixobactin exhibits a very low frequency of resistance selection (Ling et al., 2015; Lloyd et al., 2020), although genomic analyses have identified an early indicator of resistance (Gunjal et al., 2020). Several medical chemistry groups have synthesized teixobactin analogs with more favorable pharmacological and synthetic properties than the original molecule, but none of the teixobactin has entered clinical trials (Gunjal et al., 2020). Because most of the "low-hanging fruit" in the natural products world was already identified at the time of the original review, Woodruff and Burg recognized that future agents would eventually rely on synthetic modifications to improve the antibacterial spectrum of the natural antibiotics. Indeed, today, the majority of new antibacterial agents are synthetic, or semi-synthetic, derivatives of known chemical classes. However, new synthetic scaffolds introduced since the 1986 review have also led to effective antimicrobial agents in the fluoroquinolone, oxazolidinone, diazabicyclooctane, and boronic acid classes. The two latter classes include novel β-lactamase inhibitors developed in combination therapies to protect previously approved β-lactam antibiotics susceptible to hydrolysis by recently emerged β-lactamases.

In the 1986 review, the authors mentioned antimicrobial resistance (AMR) only briefly. However, AMR had been a concern of the infectious disease community even before the clinical use of penicillin (Abraham and Chain, 1940). Both academic and pharmaceutical scientists recognized these problems shortly after penicillin resistance in the staphylococci rapidly emerged in England and the United States in the mid-1940s (Medeiros, 1997). The "explosion" of the novel, chemically differentiated, antibacterial agents available by the mid-1980s, as described by Woodruff and Burg (Woodruff and Burg, 1986), resulted in the emergence of alarming clinical resistance in both gram-positive and gram-negative pathogens. Organisms such as methicillin-resistant *Staphylococcus aureus*, vancomycin-resistant enterococci, extended-spectrum β-lactamase-producing enteric bacteria, and carbapenemase-producing gram-negative pathogens are now recognized by the Center for Disease Control as serious or urgent antibiotic resistance threats (CDC, 2019). In 2019, AMR was estimated to be associated with 5 million deaths globally (Antimicrobial Resistance Collaborators, 2022). Unfortunately, many patients in this population were affected by multidrug resistance (MDR) to at least two agents from different antibiotic classes identified before 1990.

As a result of AMR concerns, antibiotics are used much more frequently in combinations to treat infections caused by MDR pathogens. In 1986, the only Food and Drug Administration (FDA)-approved combination drugs were trimethoprim-sulfamethoxazole (1981); the first carbapenem, imipenem, which required protection by cilastatin, a renal dehydropeptidase

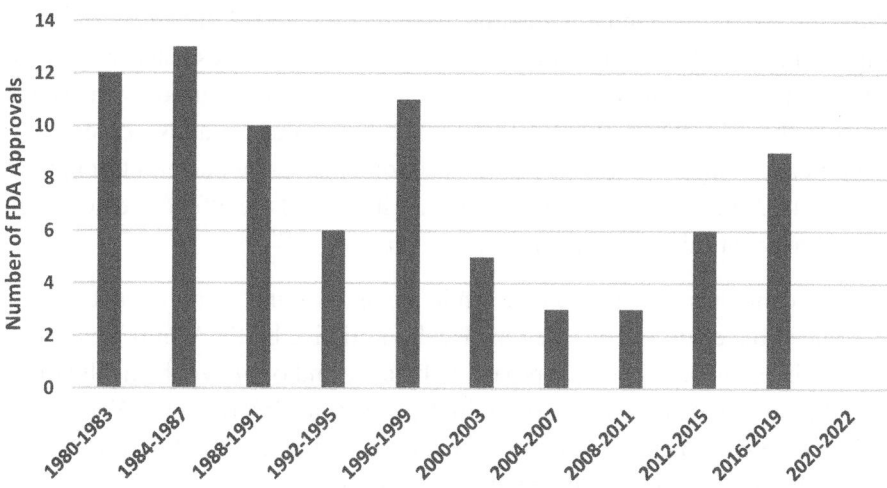

Figure 9.1

The number of approvals by the Food and Drug Administration for systemic antibacterial drugs from 1980 to 2022. (From: Powers, 2011; Butler et al., 2022; Chahine et al., 2022.)

inhibitor (1985); and the first β-lactamase inhibitor combinations, amoxicillin-clavulanic acid (1984), and ampicillin-sulbactam (1986). Curiously, the latter two, which are currently among the most highly prescribed fixed combinations drugs (Bortone et al., 2021), were not mentioned by Woodruff and Burg. This trend of using combination therapy continues, partially as a result of the explosion of novel β-lactamases that travel on plasmids carrying MDR genetic factors (Bush, 2018); four of the last eight FDA-approved systemic agents to treat MDR gram-negative infections have been β-lactamase inhibitor combinations.

Regulatory approvals of systemic antimicrobial agents reached a peak in the mid-1980s, hit a low point, and then rebounded in the time period 2012–2019 (Fig. 9.1). Part of the decrease in the early 21st century was due to an increase in regulatory stringency during the review of new drug marketing applications (Echols, 2011). Increased hurdles regarding both efficacy and toxicity of new agents led to the rejection of antibiotics that previously might have sailed through the approval process. After a brief decade exhibiting the resurgence of new drugs to combat MDR infections, however, it appears that new antibiotic approvals are sliding downward again, as there have been no new systemic antibacterial drugs approved since 2019. Large pharmaceutical companies are once again exiting the field of infectious disease discovery and development, and small companies are struggling to find investors willing to bring their novel molecules to the market.

In addition to the increased regulatory requirements, a contributing factor to the decline in interest in antibiotic development has been an emphasis on antibiotic stewardship and a dearth of commercial sales for new agents. For example, the Infectious Disease Society of America and the Clinical Laboratory Standards Institute have recommended that many of the newly approved agents be placed in reserve for use only against the most resistant pathogens, in spite of their potent activity and proven efficacy to treat infections caused by many MDR gram-negative pathogens (IDSA, 2022; CLSI, 2023). This guidance aims to preserve the utility of current antibiotics and to reduce the selection of resistant bacteria through overuse of the older agents. Although this is a laudable goal, it has had the effect of discouraging the development of new antimicrobial agents (Schulz et al., 2019).

Antibiotic stewardship has also been a concern in the agricultural area. In an attempt to lower the risk of AMR in the environment, the One Health initiative by the World Health Organization supports an integrated, unifying approach to balance and optimize the health of people, animals, and the environment (WHO, 2017). In the 1980s, as described by Woodruff and Burg, antibiotics were used extensively for both human and agricultural purposes to not only prevent or cure disease in food-producing animals but also as growth promoters in livestock (Woodruff and Burg, 1986). This is another area that has seen a great change in direction. Today, both the United States and the European Union are severely limiting antibiotic use in agriculture, especially antimicrobial agents used for human therapy. The FDA now requires veterinary approval for the use of any medically important antibiotics and prohibits their use for growth production or feed efficiency (FDA, 2019). Effective in January 2022, the EU expanded their previous limitations, and now not only prohibits the use of antibiotics for growth promotion in livestock but also bans them for disease prevention (Wallinga et al., 2022).

Thus, the explosion of antibiotics in the 1980s, and, later in the 20-teens, will likely not be repeated in the near future. However, resistant organisms will continue to emerge, in spite of the best-designed stewardship programs. New agents will still be needed to combat these pathogens, and a new explosion of antibiotics may be anticipated.

References

Abraham, E.P., Chain, E., 1940. An enzyme from bacteria is able to destroy penicillin. Nature 146, 837.

Antimicrobial Resistance Collaborators, 2022. Global burden of bacterial antimicrobial resistance in 2019: a systematic analysis. Lancet North Am. Ed. 399 (10325), 629–655. https://doi.org/10.1016/S0140-6736(21)02724-0.

Bennett, J.W., Eveleigh, D., Goodman, R.M., 2017. H. Boyd Woodruff (1917-2017): pioneer in antibiotics and industrial microbiology. Science 356 (6336), 381. https://doi.org/10.1126/science.aan39.

Bortone, B., Jackson, C., Hsia, Y., Bielicki, J., Magrini, N., Sharland, M., 2021. High global consumption of potentially inappropriate fixed dose combination antibiotics: analysis of data from 75 countries. PLoS One 16 (1), e0241899. https://dx.doi.org/10.1371/journal.pone.0241899.

Bush, K., 2018. Past and present perspectives on β-lactamases [Review]. Antimicrob. Agents Chemother. 62 (10), e01076. –01018 https://dx.doi.org/10.1128/AAC.01076-18 .

Butler, M.S., Gigante, V., Sati, H., Paulin, S., Al-Sulaiman, L., Rex, J.H., Fernandes, P., Arias, C.A., Paul, M., Thwaites, G.E., Czaplewski, L., Alm, R.A., Lienhardt, C., Spigelman, M., Silver, L.L., Ohmagari, N., Kozlov, R., Harbarth, S., Beyer, P., 2022. Analysis of the clinical pipeline of treatments for drug-resistant bacterial infections: despite progress, more action is needed. Antimicrob. Agents Chemother. 66 (3), e0199121. https://doi.org/10.1128/aac.01991-21.

CDC, 2019. Antibiotic Resistance Threats in the United States. U.S. Department of Health and Human Services, Atlanta, GA. www.cdc.gov/DrugResistance/Biggest-Threats.html.

Chahine, E.B., Dougherty, J.A., Thornby, K.A., Guirguis, E.H., 2022. Antibiotic approvals in the last decade: are we keeping up with resistance? Ann. Pharmacother. 56 (4), 441–462. https://doi.org/10.1177/10600280211031390.

CLSI, 2023. Performance Standards for Antimicrobial Susceptibility Testing, thirty-third ed. Clinical and Laboratory Standards Institute, Wayne, PA CLSI Supplement M100.

Davies, J., 2006. Where have all the antibiotics gone? Can. J. Infect. Dis. Med. Microbiol. 17 (5), 287–290. https://doi.org/10.1155/2006/707296.

Deschamps, J.D., Gautschi, J.T., Whitman, S., Johnson, T.A., Gassner, N.C., Crews, P., Holman, T.R., 2007. Discovery of platelet-type 12-human lipoxygenase selective inhibitors by high-throughput screening of structurally diverse libraries. Bioorg. Med. Chem. 15 (22), 6900–6908. https://ovidsp.ovid.com/ovidweb.cgi?T=JS&CSC=Y&NEWS=N&PAGE=fulltext&D=med6&AN=17826100.

Echols, R.M., 2011. Understanding the regulatory hurdles for antibacterial drug development in the post-Ketek world. Ann. N. Y. Acad. Sci. 1, 153–161. http://ovidsp.ovid.com/ovidweb.cgi?T=JS&CSC=Y&NEWS=N&PAGE=fulltext&D=medl&AN=22191531.

FDA. (2019). Veterinary feed directive (VFD). https://www.fda.gov/animal-veterinary/development-approval-process/veterinary-feed-directive-vfd. (Accessed 14 October 2022).

Gunjal, V.B., Thakare, R., Chopra, S., Reddy, D.S., 2020. Teixobactin: a paving stone toward a new class of antibiotics? J. Med. Chem. 63 (21), 12171–12195. https://doi.org/10.1021/acs.jmedchem.0c00173.

IDSA. (2022) IDSA guidance on the treatment of antimicrobial-resistant gram-negative infections: version 2.0. https://www.idsociety.org/practice-guideline/amr-guidance-2.0/. (Accessed 17 October 2022).

Ling, L.L., Schneider, T., Peoples, A.J., Spoering, A.L., Engels, I., Conlon, B.P., Mueller, A., Schäberle, T.F., Hughes, D.E., Epstein, S., Jones, M., Lazarides, L., Steadman, V.A., Cohen, D.R., Felix, C.R., Fetterman, K.A., Millett, W.P., Nitti, A.G., Zullo, A.M., Chen, C., Lewis, K., 2015. A new antibiotic kills pathogens without detectable resistance. Nature 517, 455–459.

Lloyd, D.G., Schofield, B.J., Goddard, M.R., Taylor, E.J., 2020. De novo resistance to Arg_{10}-teixobactin occurs slowly and is costly. Antimicrob. Agents Chemother. 65 (1), 16. https://dx.doi.org/10.1128/AAC.01152-20.

Medeiros, A.A., 1997. Evolution and dissemination of β-lactamases accelerated by generations of β-lactam antibiotics. Clin. Infect. Dis. 24, S19–S45. https://doi.org/10.1093/clinids/24.Supplement_1.S19.

Powers, J., 2011. Need new antibiotics. In: Reviving the Pipeline of Life-Saving Antibiotics: Exploring Solutions to Spur Innovation. Washington, DC. https://www.pewtrusts.org/-/media/legacy/uploadedfiles/phg/content_level_pages/issue_briefs/aippipelineproceedings9webpdf.pdf.

Schulz, L.T., Kim, S.Y., Hartsell, A., Rose, W.E., 2019. Antimicrobial stewardship during a time of rapid antimicrobial development: potential impact on industry for future investment. Diagn. Microbiol. Infect. Dis. 95 (3), 114857. https://dx.doi.org/10.1016/j.diagmicrobio.2019.06.009.

Tally, F.P., DeBruin, M.F., 2000. Development of daptomycin for gram-positive infections. J. Antimicrob. Chemother. 46 (4), 523–526. https://doi.org/10.1093/jac/46.4.523.

Wallinga, D., Smit, L.A.M., Davis, M.F., Casey, J.A., Nachman, K.E., 2022. A review of the effectiveness of current US policies on antimicrobial use in meat and poultry production. Curr. Environ. Health Rep. 9, 339–354. https://doi.org/10.1007/s40572-022-00351-x.

WHO. (2017). One health. https://www.who.int/news-room/questions-and-answers/item/one-health.

Woodruff, H.B., Burg, R.W., 1986. The antibiotic explosion. In: Parnham, M.J., Bruinvels, J. (Eds.), Discoveries in Pharmacology, 3. Elsevier Science Publishers B. V., pp. 303–351.

Wu, P., Daniel-Issakani, S., LaMarco, K., Strulovici, B., 1997. An automated high throughput filtration assay: application to polymerase inhibitor identification. Anal. Biochem. 245 (2), 226–230. https://ovidsp.ovid.com/ovidweb.cgi?T=JS&CSC=Y&NEWS=N&PAGE=fulltext&D=med4&AN=9056217.

The antibiotic explosion

H. Boyd Woodruff and Richard W. Burg

Contents

Disclaimer: The original text that follows is reproduced from the first edition and carries errors and omissions from it. The editors and publisher agreed to retain them and honor the original authors and challenges they had to deal with in publishing back in those times.

Discoveries in Pharmacology, Volume 3, Hemodynamics and Immune Defense.
DOI: https://doi.org/10.1016/B978-0-443-18442-0.00069-0
© 1986, Elsevier Science Publishers B.V.

9.1 Introduction

An explosion is a rapid and spectacular expansion. That definition is descriptive of the effect on microbiological research of the report issued in 1940 of the successful use of crude penicillin in curing systemic bacterial infections of man (Abraham et al., 1941). Research microbiologists who had studied microbial associations but who had failed to appreciate the practical consequences of the antibacterial actions that they had observed revised their experiments to search for specific antibacterial products. Chemists shifted their attention from the synthesis of analogues of sulphanilamide to the isolation of pure antibiotics. A result was the discovery within the first 20 years of 437 previously unrecognized chemical entities which were deemed worthy of discussion in an encyclopedia published in 1961 (Korzybski and Kurylowicz, 1961).

Very soon, the explosion made it necessary for catalogues to be prepared to establish order among the many new antibacterial substances which appeared in the literature. The substances were antibiotics, chemical compounds of varied structures and diverse biological properties. A paperback volume assembled by Spector (Spector, 1956) initially proved useful. It was followed by many compendiums, each larger and of increased usefulness for the complex field, culminating in the ten-volume CRC Handbook of Antibiotic Compounds, published in 1980 (Berdy, 1980). Specialized indices also have received wide usage, especially the Pfizer *Handbook of Microbial Metabolites* (Miller, 1961) and the *Index of Antibiotics from Actinomycetes,* presently consisting of two editions (Umezewa, 1967 and 1978), with continuations which list recently published antibiotic structures as addenda in monthly issues of the *Journal of Antibiotics.*

Within a few years after the initiation of the explosion, new scientific journals were introduced for publication of the many articles covering all phases of research with antibiotics. Noteworthy are the *Journal of Antibiotics* started in Japan, which has become international in scope, and *Antimicrobial Agents and Chemotherapy,* a publication of the American Society for Microbiology. Furthermore, several serial annual volumes were started and have continued yearly, some appearing for more than thirty years. Each volume contains chapters dealing with specialized aspects of antibiotic research. Thus, the antibiotic explosion is characterized by both the large number of new chemical compounds isolated and by the thousands of pages of published scientific data describing them.

9.2 Historical implications

An explosion may be controlled or uncontrolled. The second can cause uncountable damage, for example the result following an inadvertent spark in a munitions dump or the failure to control a nuclear reactor. In contrast, controlled explosions are used widely for the benefit of mankind: in road building, in preparing ground for new construction, in the mining of coal and minerals. For safety, controlled explosions often are set in motion by applying flame to a long fuse. As the flame moves forward along the fuse it smolders, occasionally flashing a bright spark, but nothing of consequence happens until a final spark ignites the explosive charge. In like manner, a long trail of research can be identified, progressing stage by stage from the earliest days of bacteriology to the critical flash of the Florey et al. announcement of the curative value of penicillin. (Crellin, 1980; Florey et al., 1949; Lechevalier and Solotorovsky, 1965; Waksman, 1975).

Historians frequently trace the initiation of antibiotic research to the early masters of bacteriology. In so doing they tend to belittle the impact of the true innovators of the antibiotic field – Florey, Chain, Dubos, Waksman, Burkholder, Duggar, Abraham and others. Indeed, in the light of present knowledge, the statements of the early masters are interesting. Those well-known scientists predicted the future with surprising accuracy. Noteworthy is a statement of Pasteur in 1877 who spoke of one microbe producing an antiseptic effect in attacking another. After finding that mixtures of aerobic soil microorganisms interfered with the growth of the anthrax bacterium in vitro and also when the bacterial mixtures were inoculated into animals, Pasteur with his characteristic lack of modesty proclaimed that his experiments 'justify perhaps the greatest hopes for therapeutics'. Nine years later the clinical application of the principles of antagonism had progressed to the use of pure cultures. Cantini used the word 'bacteriotherapy' in describing his studies. He employed a pure culture, which he called *Bacterium termo,* initially to interfere with the progression of skin lesions of *Mycobacterium tuberculosis* and later, with some success, he infused the living bacterium into lungs of tubercular patients, temporarily interrupting progression of the disease.

The word antibiosis also entered the language early, in 1889, only a decade following Lister's extensive studies which established the value of antisepsis in surgery. Interestingly, it was the words of literary-minded experimentalists which were most descriptive of the ideas of the time. It would be difficult today to improve upon a statement of John Tyndall, the noted 19th century British natural philosopher and director of the Royal Institution. In a letter to Thomas Huxley he wrote: 'The most extraordinary cases of fighting and conquering between the bacteria and the penicillium have been revealed to me'. Neither Fleming's report of the finding of the pencillin-producing mould nor Florey's statements concerning penicillin as the product are as expressive in describing the antibiosis phenomenon.

Gosio's success in 1896 in isolating the antibiotic mycophenolic acid as a pure crystalline substance seems to have been ignored. The tide of interest of leading scientists of the time was shifting to immunology rather than chemotherapy. The spark was flaming out in spite of the brilliance of its early flashes. But it was not quite extinguished. Even the great proponent of the importance of host resistance mechanisms, Metchnikoff, noted a repressive effect of a *Pseudomonas* culture on a vibrio. Then in 1899, Emmerich and Low not only observed a similar phenomenon, they acted upon it. They compounded an ointment from the bacteriotoxic substances present in old cultures of *Pseudomonas aeruginosa* that was marketed as a topical preparation for use against infections. The product, pyocyanase, was used widely, especially in Germany, for many years. Others of the early masters also became interested in therapeutic applications, but their studies usually ended with a demonstration in a laboratory animal. Their sparks died out without influencing man. Thus, in 1897, Duchesne used extracts of *Penicillium glaucum* successfully in treatment of diseased laboratory animals. But others were more creative. The Belgian workers Gratia and Dath, in 1924, discovered that actinomycetes had lytic activity, dissolving certain Gram-positive pathogens, and they used such extracts in the topical therapy of human infections, as did Fleming five years later in applying filtrates of his *Penicillium notatum* to skin infections.

Promising as the statements which accompanied the above research were, they, like the occasional sparks which arise from a smoldering fuse – flashes of brilliance to be sure, but having little lasting influence – were inadequate to set in motion a true explosion. The reason was not lack of insight. The time was not right. As in a controlled explosion, the tinder must be reached before initiation of the explosion, so in these early days of microbiology significant steps of chemical purification had not been applied to appropriate antibiotics to permit systemic chemotherapy of severe life-threatening infections, the necessary event to ignite the antibiotic explosion.

The discovery of the antibacterial activity of the synthetic dye prontosil in 1932, and its subsequent use as a therapeutic agent against bacterial infections, closely followed by the identification of sulphanilamide in 1935 as the active entity, set the stage for the antibiotic era. Ehrlich's search for a magic bullet, a non-toxic drug specific in killing pathogenic microbes without harm to man, in which most scientists had lost faith, was justified.

9.3 Major discoveries

9.3.1 Tyrothricin – a planned discovery

The entry of the antibiotic tyrothricin on the scene excited popular imagination. The sulpha drugs had been introduced to medicine and had reduced the fear of 'blood poisonings' due to pathogenic cocci, as well as the great threat of pneumococcal pneumonia. More miracles were expected. The report of the discovery at the prestigious Rockefeller Institute of a new natural antibacterial derived from a soil microorganism was welcomed by the news media. Newspaper articles and magazine reports soon appeared detailing the facts of the discovery, and overstating its promise.

The scientific community was also excited because of the exquisite planning which led to the discovery. Rene Dubos, an immigrant from France, because of an interest in ecology, had studied in Selman A. Waksman's section of soil microbiology at Rutgers University. He proved to be a creative student. Atypically for a Ph.D. graduate from an agricultural college, in 1927 he entered the field of medical research at the Rockefeller Institute. Within the first few years he recognized that the pathogenicity of *Diplococcus pneumoniae* (the name used at the time) could be attributed to its polysaccharide capsule which protected it from attack by normal host-resistance mechanisms. Dubos and his associate Avery, later of DNA fame, reasoned that if the capsule could be removed enzymatically the microbe would become susceptible to phagocytosis and its pathogenicity would be lessened. None of the available carbohydrases were effective, so Dubos called upon his past experience in soil microbiology and set up enrichment cultures. He repeatedly added isolated pneumococcal capsular material to soil. For the rare soil microorganism among the millions present per gram of soil able to cleave the capsule, thereby releasing fermentable sugars, the capsule became a nutrient. Capsule hydrolyzers multiplied. Eventually, Dubos succeeded in isolating a hydrolyzer in pure culture and from it obtained the desired enzyme (Dubos and Avery, 1931).

His thesis proved correct. *Diplococcus pneumoniae* freed of its capsule by enzymatic action was no longer a pathogen. It was unable to cause disease in mice, even with massive inocula.

Dubos then made the extension for which he deserves great credit, a forerunner of his many accomplishments, for which he was greatly honoured in later life. If enrichment of the soil with the capsule of a pathogen would lead to multiplication of a capsule-hydrolyzing soil microbe, why would not enrichment of soil with a living pathogen lead to multiplication of a pathogen-killing soil microbe? He made the approach, succeeded, and from his pure cultures of pathogen-killing soil microbe obtained its antibacterial complex, tyrothricin (Dubos, 1939). Tyrothricin was later split into two pure antibacterial substances, one bacteriostatic and the other bactericidal, which Dubos and his co-worker named gramicidin and tyrocidin (Dubos and Hotchkiss, 1941).

Attempts were made to use Dubos and Hotchkiss' two substances to treat human infections, but toxicity interfered. In the end, the most important applications were as topical preparations, some of which are marketed today more than 40 years after the discovery. Of great importance for the future of the field, tyrothricin interested leaders of the pharmaceutical industry, who developed large-scale fermentations for growth of the soil microbe *Bacillus brevis* and techniques for extraction of the pure antibiotic from large quantities of bacterial broths. Thus the American pharmaceutical industry was prepared to accept the next major antibiotic development, penicillin, with minimal hesitation when it was offered. An important by-product, also, was the activity of Dubos' professor, Selman Waksman, as a consultant. He advised Merck & Co., Inc. on the production of tyrothricin. Therefore, Waksman, also, was prepared to recognize the importance of penicillin when its properties were published and to believe that the time was right to initiate a broader-based search for additional microbially produced antibacterials.

9.3.2 Penicillin

The facts associated with the discovery of penicillin and a description of its impact on medicine are described in the preceding chapter. The penicillin story also has been told previously from many viewpoints, scientifically in a 1094 page report written by its developers (Clarke et al., 1949) and historically by major participants in its rediscovery (Florey and Abraham, 1951). Of particular interest are lectures prepared by Ernst Chain, the Nobel Prize co-awardee for its rediscovery, as well as by American, European and Japanese workers in the field (Chain, 1980; Helfand et al., 1980; Ettlinger, 1980; Yagisawa, 1980). By the end of the 1939–1946 World War, an event that by the needs created markedly accentuated antibiotic developments and their therapeutic applications, penicillin had become well established world wide as a safe, pre-eminent therapy for infections caused by Gram-positive bacteria, as well as for the Gram-negative *Neisseria* species.

Typical of the impact of penicillin, even at the beginning, was Selman Waksman's reaction at Rutgers University upon reading the first report from Oxford University of the in vivo efficacy of penicillin. Rushing into the laboratory, copy of the 1941 *Lancet* issue* in hand, he excitedly interrupted the senior author's attempts to probe a problem in soil microbiology. 'Woodruff, he said, 'Drop everything. See what these English have done with a mould. I know the actinomycetes will do better.' Truly, the Oxford research was the spark which set the antibiotic explosion in motion. At Rutgers University, at Yale, at Illinois, in laboratories in Holland, Switzerland, even in war-torn Japan and Germany, scientists reacted. The search for more and better natural products was under way.

9.3.3 The antibiotics of the streptomycetes

Once it became recognized that the antimicrobial actions expressed by microbes growing in association could have practical implications, microbiologists attacked the problem with vigor, each emphasizing his favourite microbe. As tinder, they had become ignited. The antibiotic explosion began.

At the Agricultural Experiment Station of Rutgers University, a state-supported institution in New Jersey, U.S.A., Prof. Selman A. Waksman and a graduate student, Jackson W. Foster, had reported their observations on microbial associations in a paper under the general title *Associative and Antagonistic Effects of Microorganisms* (Waksman and Foster, 1937). That the possibility for practical clinical application was present in soil microbes but was unrecognized throughout Waksman's early career becomes clear from Waksman's own words, taken from an early paper published in 1923 written in association with Robert L. Starkey

---

* E. Chain, H.W. Florey, A.D. Gardner, N.G. Heatley, M.A. Jennings, J. Orr-Ewing and A.G. Sanders (1941) Lancet *ii*, 226–228.

who was to serve for many years as Waksman's associate in research at Rutgers University. 'Certain actinomycetes produce substances toxic to bacteria as illustrated by the fact that around an actinomyces colony upon a plate a zone is found free from fungus and bacterial growth' (Waksman and Starkey, 1923). How similar this description is to Fleming's observation made six years later. Waksman also failed to take full advantage of a grant received in pre-penicillin days from the National Tuberculosis Association to study destruction of *Mycobacterium tuberculosis* organisms in the soil, nor did Waksman attempt to explain the death of *M. tuberculosis* occurring in a culture tube containing a mould contaminant which he had received from the New Jersey Agricultural Experiment Station poultry pathologist. (The same person later provided Waksman and his graduate students with a culture tube containing one of the original producers of streptomycin.)

As noted, following Dubos' discovery of tyrothricin, Waksman's attention shifted from mere descriptions of the associations to consideration of the antimicrobial factors themselves. Then, with the report of the clinical effectiveness of penicillin, Waksman's approach shifted wholeheartedly to the search for more and better antibacterial agents. It is interesting to see the resultant change in direction of Waksman's printed words. In an article published only a few months after the Oxford University report, in the November 1940 issue of *Scientific Monthly,* titled *Microbes in a Changing World,* he stated 'We are finally approaching a new field of domestication of microorganisms for combatting the microbial enemies of man and of his plants and animals' (Waksman, 1940).

As Waksman's first student to work under the new objective, the senior author of this chapter was requested by him to attempt isolation of a penicillin mimic from the streptomycetes, the group of filamentous bacteria which were the life-long topic of Waksman's research. Following Dubos' lead, soil enrichment procedures were used. Living *Escherichia coli* cells were added repeatedly to soil and after several weeks the enriched soil was searched by varied techniques for the presence of *E. coli*-lysing streptomycetes (Waksman and Woodruff, 1940). Today we realize that the enrichment procedures employed in the early antibiotic searches were not needed. Dubos' recovery of an antibiotic-producing bacillus can be duplicated easily by plating unenriched soils (Stokes and Woodward, 1942) (Fig. 9.1). Actinomycin, the product obtained from the *E. coli*-enriched soil, although capable of killing *E. coli* at high concentrations, fails to lyse it. The great enrichment of bacteriophage which occurred in the soil pots receiving living *E. coli* cells probably explains the lytic action observed at the time the actinomycin-producer *Actinomyces antibioticus* was isolated. In fact the enrichment caused no increase in proportion of antibiotic producers present in the author's soil pots, both the antibiotic- and non-antibiotic-producing microorganisms of the soil having multiplied at the same rates following enrichment (Woodruff and Waksman, 1960). Nevertheless, the idea that enrichment would prove useful was the incentive for setting up the experiments to search for new antibacterials and in fact the search succeeded. Products never before seen from microbes were isolated. Some were bactericidal, rapidly killing a wide range of microorganisms.

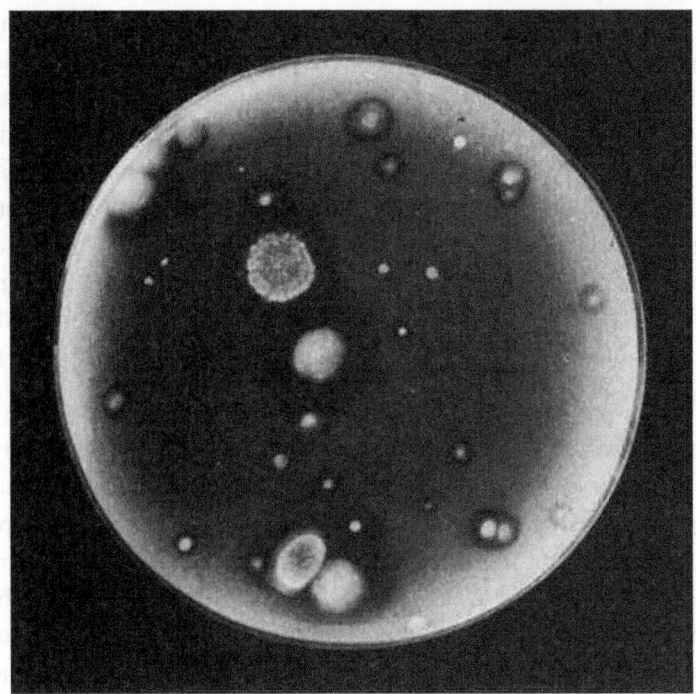

Figure 9.1

Demonstration of antibiotic production by soil microorganisms. An appropriate dilution of soil was added to a petri dish which was flooded with nutrient agar seeded with a sensitive indicator bacterium. Antibiotic producing strains of soil microorganisms are surrounded by clear areas in which growth of the indicator organism has been inhibited.

Actinomycin, the first pure antibacterial agent obtained from the genus *Streptomyces,* is among the most active antibacterials ever recognized (Waksman and Woodruff, 1941). Unfortunately it is not selective in its action. It proved highly toxic for animals as well as for bacteria. Therefore, it was unsuited for chemotherapy. Long afterward one of the actinomycins found utility as an anti-neoplastic agent, an extension of the value of microbiologically produced natural products which is beyond the scope of this chapter (see Chapter 8 for a discussion of anticancer agents).

That a product with such wide range of activity could be obtained from a microorganism without it being lethal for the producing streptomycete interested Waksman greatly. He believed the phenomenon of antibiosis would prove to be general, that many similar products would be found by continued screening. He decided a class name should be adopted for the phenomenon. He encouraged his students in varied seminars to make suggestions but finally selected a name of his own choosing, antibiotic, without realizing that a foreign-language equivalent word existed. Waksman clearly stated the definition for antibiotic: 'a chemical substance produced by a microorganism which in dilute solution has the capacity to inhibit or even to destroy other microorganisms' (Waksman, 1953). The definition has become accepted by scientists and laypersons alike. Dr. Waksman has received credit for it and is recognized as one of the great pioneers of the antibiotic field (Fig. 9.2).

Waksman was correct in believing that many more antibiotics would be found. The second discovered in his laboratory was streptothricin, the topic of the senior author's thesis (Waksman and Woodruff, 1942). Purified streptothricin was curative for bacterial infections in laboratory animals. It was active in laboratory animals even against the highly resistant *Brucella abortus,* the bacterium of undulant fever. Plans were made for large-scale production and construction of a factory was started. Then streptothricin failed in practical trials in man due to delayed toxicity.

Shortly thereafter streptomycin was discovered by Waksman and his graduate students (Schatz et al., 1944). Two producing cultures, strains of *Streptomyces griseus,* were isolated

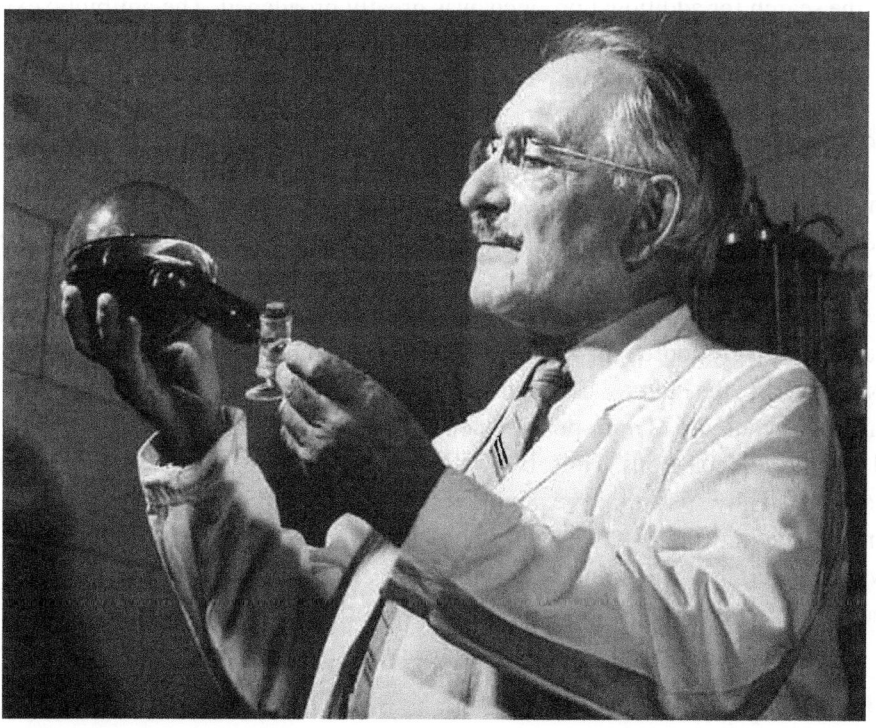

Figure 9.2
Dr. Selman A. Waksman, professor of soil microbiology at Rutgers University in New Jersey, U.S.A., photographed at the time of receipt of the Nobel Prize following the discovery of streptomycin. Waksman was an early pioneer in research on soil streptomycetes and the first to investigate them systematically for the production of antibiotics.

almost similtaneously. The first came from the expected source of the species, the soil. The second was obtained from a highly unlikely place, the throat of a chicken undergoing posting in the university pathology laboratory, a clear lesson that one should not arbitrarily eliminate any source as inappropriate for discovery of microbial products of value. Streptomycin proved to be extremely promising in early laboratory studies, including in vivo evaluations, sufficiently so that it was accepted by a pharmaceutical company for development. Fortunately, the manufacturing techniques devised for streptothricin before its clinical failure were directly applicable to streptomycin, so the developmental progress was rapid. The real thrust toward clinical application, however, occurred when William Feldman and Corwin Hinshaw of the Mayo Clinic observed that streptomycin was effective in curing tuberculosis in guinea pigs (Feldman and Hinshaw, 1945). Manufacture of streptomycin was started immediately in the U.S.A. and soon spread to production in over a dozen countries of the world. Streptomycin proved to be the beginning of the demise of the white plague, so long feared by mankind. Waksman received many accolades for the discovery of streptomycin, including a Nobel Prize. With the realization of the increasing potential for application of antibiotics in medicine, the search for additional products was greatly broadened. The antibiotic explosion was fully in progress.

9.3.4 Bacitracin

Somewhat surprisingly, the next major development arose from a class of microorganisms which over the years has proven rather unproductive as a source of useful antibiotics, that is the Eubacteriales, or common bacteria. Miss Balbina Johnson in New York City recovered an antibiotic-producing strain of *Bacillus subtilis* from a leg wound of a young patient, Margaret Tracy, again an unlikely source for a non-pathogen (Johnson et al., 1945). An antibiotic product was isolated from the culture. Understandably, it was named bacitracin. It proved effective against infections caused by Gram-positive cocci, with the special characteristic that it seldom produced allergic side reactions. Thus, bacitracin became a preferred product for treatment of infections of sensitive tissues, for example it is used in ophthalmology and for skin and mucous membrane infections. It is not sufficiently safe for wide-scale systemic use, but its discovery taught research microbiologists that antibiosis is not the property of a few species among the many microbes of the world, but is characteristic of microbes as a whole.

9.3.5 The aminocyclitols

Today, with thousands of natural products isolated, approximately 2% of which show some activity in vivo, and with tens of thousands of semi-synthetic derivatives prepared, nearly all of which have some in vivo activity, it is extremely difficult to discover new antibiotics of value. It is interesting to note, therefore, the ease with which success was achieved in the early days. It would seem that for years scientists had cast their eyes downward, searching the ground for the rare piece of undamaged fruit, not bothering to raise their eyes to the trees overhead. Then, when Florey and his group did so, others with organizing skills did so too, and, like the ripe apples, pears and peaches which abound in their natural environment, the actinomycins, streptomycin, chloramphenicol, the tetracyclines, bacitracin all were ripe for the picking and were easily and quickly found.

In view of the above, it is instructive to note the recollections of Hubert Lechevalier, who as a student with Waksman at Rutgers University discovered the second and third antibiotics from the Waksman laboratories to reach the marketplace and earn royalties to support further research at the University, the aminocyclitol neomycin and the polyene candicidin (Lechevalier, 1980). Lechevalier describes his thesis work thus: 'It was a silly-simple project: collect soil samples, plate them out, isolate actinomycetes, test them for antibiotic activity against non-pathogenic strains of mycobacteria and hope you will find something that will be active against the pathogenic strains. I collected four soil samples, isolated 172 actinomycetes, and found four strains which had outstanding antibiotic activity. Further work revealed that one of these produced a basic, water-soluble antibiotic to which Dr. Waksman assigned the name neomycin'. Neomycin was, in fact, a broad-spectrum antibacterial agent, much broader in in vitro activity than the somewhat chemically related earlier discovery, streptomycin.

Candicidin, much different in structure from earlier discoveries, was an antifungal substance not active against bacteria. It was discovered with equal ease. Lechevalier reports, 'The professor of mycology, Dr. Conrad M. Haenseler, also had an interest in finding antibiotics active against the agent of Dutch Elm Disease. As I had done for Dr. Waksman, I also isolated for Dr. Haenseler a series of actinomycetes, but it was one of the remaining three strains from the screen which had yielded neomycin which was most active against fungi. From it I isolated the heptaene, candicidin'. Thus, from as few as 172 actinomycetes isolated, two products of clinical value were obtained.

That substances found so easily would not be an exclusive discovery made at only one institution is not surprising. In fact, nearly simultaneous discoveries have been the rule rather than the exception with the commercially useful products obtained in the authors' laboratories. Note the finding of cycloserine at the Pfizer and the Merck laboratories, novobiocin at Upjohn and Merck, cephamycin C at Lilly and Merck. Similarly, Yukimasa Yagasawa, long time editor of the *Journal of Antibiotics,* reports that a substance named streptothricin B was reported in 1948 by Hamao Umezawa in Japan a few months prior to the Waksman and Lechevalier publication on neomycin (Yagasawa, 1980). The products proved to be the same. Neomycin became the product of commerce, however. Japan, still in the throes of war-time recovery, had placed its limited resources on production of the proven antibiotics penicillin and streptomycin to meet the overwhelming needs of its ill and starving population and could not afford to pursue new products of uncertain value.

However, by 1950, the Ministry of Education of Japan could offer grants in support of new antibiotic research. That support has continued since and Japan has become a leader in antibiotic discoveries. Hamao Umezawa has proven highly successful, first in the Institute of Health of Japan, later in a special institute attached to Tokyo University. He has opened the door to further aminocyclitol research, having discovered the kanamycins (Umezawa et al., 1957), antibiotics with improved safety over neomycin, explained the loss of effectiveness of aminocyclitol antibiotics occasionally seen in the clinic as an enzymatic inactivation by enzymes present in resistant pathogens, and he has pioneered in the development of semisynthetic derivatives of the aminocyclitols as a solution to the resistance problem.

The history of the development of the aminocyclitols emphasizes the value of a purely biological approach to antibiotic discovery. Success in discovery of new antibiotics had become so easy that research on their source, the microbe, had been neglected. One merely had to plate soils and take what was offered. With narrow-spectrum antibiotics produced by nearly 50% of soil isolates, broad-spectrum by 10%, a few soil platings would offer a lifetime of research opportunities. The weakness of the approach was shown by research workers who as part of their graduate studies had been introduced to the *Micromonospora,* a genus of filamentous bacteria seldom recovered from soil platings but very rich in lake bottom muds. From *Micromonospora* spp. a previously unknown antibiotic, an aminocyclitol, was isolated (Weinstein et al., 1963). It was named gentamicin, the *mi* in the name dictated by the official naming agencies of the U.S.A. and the World Health body to differentiate it from the antibiotics of the true *Streptomyces* which were entitled to use my, as in mycin. Gentamicin has become an ultimate-spectrum drug, one chosen when clinical needs are severe and when the toxicities which are associated with the aminocyclitols, vestibular and otic damage and renal toxicities, can be tolerated by the seriously ill patient.

9.3.6 The broad-spectrum antibiotics

To this point, the antibiotics available for oral administration were not truly broad spectrum in activity. Each had its speciality application. An idea was becoming established that specificity in spectrum is an essential characteristic of useful antibiotics, necessary for safety and for lack of toxicity to the host animal cell; that products which killed a broad spectrum of bacteria would be lethal to animal cells, too, due to lack of specificity of action. The error of the notion was soon exposed – first with the discovery of chloromycetin, later named chloramphenicol, by Paul Burkholder of Yale University (Ehrlich et al., 1947) closely followed by its independent discovery by David Gottlieb and associates (1948) at the University of Illinois and by Umezawa et al. (1948) in Japan. Chloramphenicol has a very broad spectrum of activity. It is efficiently absorbed following oral dosage and at first appeared to be very nontoxic.

Chloramphenicol became the major product of the Parke-Davis Co., which profited greatly from receipt of the exclusive license under its U.S. patent. Later, the use of chloramphenicol dropped precipitously due to its association with a rarely occurring but fatal form of aplastic anemia and the company suffered adversities. The fact had not been recognized fully that the antibiotic explosion was a continuing conflagration, in which good products would be replaced repeatedly by better products and that emphasis should be placed on the search for them. Clearly, as had been expected by some, chloramphenicol was not the end of the line.

Discovery of the next class of broad-spectrum antibiotics, the tetracyclines, still in wide use today, can be attributed to a group of scientists, the mycologists and the plant pathologists, who played a very important part in the early history of antibiotic development, but whose research specialities have been largely neglected in the written record. An extensive survey of many chemicals for antimicrobial activity was conducted in England by the mycologists Wilkins and Harris (1942). Although the substances tested were synthetic chemicals, not antibiotics, failing to meet the definition requirement of production by a microbe, Wilkins and Harris' techniques for screening were borrowed by many microbiologists and formed a basis for the early antibiotic screens. The mycologist R. Weindling of Cornell University, with the objective of curing fungus infections of plants, searched for an antifungal antibiotic and found activity present in a culture of *Trichoderma.* As early as 1934 he obtained gliotoxin (Weindling, 1934). The fact that gliotoxin proved too toxic for human use denied him the adulation and place in history achieved by Fleming, by Florey and Chain, and by Waksman.

It was, however, another mycologist, Dr. Benjamin Duggar, a celebrated professor at the University of Wisconsin, who refused to accept the limitations of retirement and directed his post-retirement years at a practical objective, the discovery of an antibiotic active against both Gram-positive and Gram-negative bacteria, who deserves credit for organizing the group effort at the Lederle Research Laboratories which led to discovery of the first tetracycline, chlortetracycline, a product of *Streptomyces aureofaciens* (Duggar, 1948). Several of the Lederle staff who assisted Duggar were University of Wisconsin graduates and easily fell into the revered professor-student relationship which led to efficiency in operation and the notable success. The tetracyclines proved even more valuable than initially anticipated. They were effective against a wide range of Gram-positive and Gram-negative bacteria. In addition, efficacy in diseases of man extended to the wall-less mycoplasma, which are completely resistant to the β-lactam antibiotics, and to various pathogens often classified as large viruses because of their requirement for living animal cells within which to multiply.

As noted previously, useful antibiotics were rather easily discovered in the early days, and the tetracyclines were no exception. One of the major problems we have faced in setting up screening programmes for Merck & Co., Inc. has been the frequency of rediscovery of tetracyclines and the waste of time spent on their purification until their identity was proven. It is instructive to note, however, that Selman Waksman, the world-wide authority on the genus *Streptomyces,* and a budding antibiotic specialist in the years 1948–1954 when chlortetracycline, oxytetracycline and tetracycline were discovered, with his large staff of assisting graduate students failed to discover the tetracyclines.

The reason for Waksman's failure eventually was discovered, his screening technique. In contrast to Duggar's approach, which was an impatient search for the earliest expression of antibiotic activity, Waksman and his staff were more patient, waiting up to two weeks of incubation prior to reading cross-streak plates. His experience had shown that prolonged incubation led to continued accumulation of streptomycin and of the aminocyclitol antibiotics, so that with adequate incubation even minor producers among the soil population could be detected. But with tetracyclines, his approach was a failure. Tetracyclines are susceptible to inactivation in alkaline conditions. During the prolonged incubation, the gradually increasing pH resulting from breakdown of media proteins by the cultures led to destruction of all tetra-cycline antibiotic present and to failure of detection. So Waksman and his students missed the tetracycline class of antibiotics, a group which far outstripped streptomycin and neomycin in frequency of usage and in range of diseases cured.

The lesson, of course, is clear. Antibiotic discovery is not the province of any one specialty scientist, microbiologist, mycologist, chemist or physicist. The keys to success are an ap-propriate source of the microbes to be investigated to provide variety, and the efficacy of the screening methods employed to detect activity. Creativity is the essential factor, and creativity of the discoverers is amply demonstrated by the listing in Table 9.1 , drawn from the 1983 edition of the Physicians' Desk Reference, a compendium of properties of all antibiotics approved by the U.S. Food and Drug Administration judged to be important and offered for sale during that year (Huff, 1983).

9.3.7 The cephalosporins

The cephalosporins have become the most widely used and most important of the antibiotics. They are closely related to the penicillins, sharing an identical mode of action and identity in biosynthetic pathway, except for the final steps which involve a ring expansion from the five-member thiazolidine to the six-member δ-dihydrothiazine. Both types of antibiotics contain the four-member β-lactam ring at the reactive site, capable of an irreversible binding reaction leading to inactivation of the enzymatically catalyzed cross-linking of the bacterial cell wall, the result of such inactivation being death of the bacterial cell. The β-lactam ring also is the target of penicillinases and cephalosporinases and its hydrolysis by such enzymes leads to loss of antibiotic activity. In an attempt to overcome the susceptibility to destructive enzymes, thousands of chemical modifications of the cephalosporins have been made. The most impor-tant characteristic of the cephalosporin group, both natural isolates and semisynthetic deriva-tives, which has led to widespread clinical use, is the ability of the cephalosporins to penetrate the outer membrane of a great variety of pathogens, reaching the cell wall formation site with lethal action. The result is an exceptionally wide spectrum of antibiotic action compared with

Table 9.1: U.S.-FDA approved clinically significant antibiotics.

Antibiotic	Type*	Formulation**
The penicillins		
Original		
Penicillin G	N	im, iv,
Penicillin V	N	O
Limited spectrum		
Cloxacillin	S	o
Dicloxacillin	S	o
Methacillin	S	im, iv
Nafcillin	S	im, iv, o
Oxacillin	S	im, iv, o
Medium spectrum		
Amoxicillin	S	o
Ampicillin	S	im, iv, o
Bacampicillin	S	o
Cyclocillin	S	o
Hetacillin	S	o
Broad spectrum		
Azlocillin	S	Iv
Carbenicillin	S	im, iv, o
Mezlocillin	S	im, iv
Piperacillin	S	im, iv
Ticarcillin	S	im, iv
The cephalosporins		
Medium spectrum		
Cefaclor	S	o
Cefadroxil	S	o
Cefazolin	S	im, iv
Cephalexin	S	o
Cephalothin	S	im, iv
Cephapirin	S	im, iv
Cephradine	S	im, iv, o
β-Lactamase resistant		
Cefamandol	S	im, iv
Cefotaxime	S	im, iv
Cefoxitin	S	im, iv
Moxalactam	S	im, iv
Aminocyclitols		
Amikacin	S	im, iv
Gentamicin	N	im, iv, t
Kanamycin	N	im, iv, o
Neomycin	N	o, t
Tobramycin	N	im, iv
Tetracyclines		
Chlortetracyline	N	t
Demeclocycline	N	o
Doxycycline	S	o

(continued on next page)

Table 9.1: U.S.-FDA approved clinically significant antibiotics—cont'd

Antibiotic	Type*	Formulation**
Methocycline	S	o
Minocycline	S	iv, o
Oxytetracycline	N	im, iv, o
Tetracycline	N	im, iv, o, t
Macrolides		
Erythromycin	N	o, t
Troleandomycin	S	o
Special target		
Bacitracin	N	t
Capreomycin	N	im
Chloramphenicol	N	o, t
Clindamycin	S	im, iv, o, t
Colistin	N	im, iv, o.
Cycloserine	N	o
Gramicidin	N	t
Lincomycin	N	im, iv, o
Polymyxin B	N	im, iv, t
Rifampin	S	o
Spectinomycin	N	im
Vancomycin	N	iv, o
Antifungals		
Amphotericin B	N	iv, o, t
Candicidin	N	t
Griseofulvin	N	o
Nystatin	N	o, t
Antiviral		
Viradine	N	im, iv

* N = natural isolates; S = semi-synthetic origin.

** im = intramuscular; iv = intravenous; o = oral; t = topical, including optic forms.

a more limited spectrum of antibacterial activity of the other major class of β-lactams, the penicillins.

The cephalosporins are also interesting as examples of serendipity in antibiotic research. As early as 1948, when the primacy of antibiotics for treatment of infectious disease was just becoming fully recognized by the medical profession, the cephalosporin-producing microorganism was first isolated in Sardinia, Italy. The culture was obtained from the sea, near a sewage outfall, an unlikely site for the aerobic mould, a species of *Cephalosporium*. However, it was many years before the first antibiotic product of the mould, a cephalosporin modified semisynthetically, reached the marketplace (cf. p. 297).

The cephalosporin-producing mould was obtained because Professor G. Brotzu assumed on the basis of prior publications that antibiosis might play a role in the death of pathogens during the purification of sewage. He acted on the belief, searched the sewage outfall, isolated an antibiotic-producing mould, and used a crude antibiotic-containing extract made from it to treat infections of man, including intestinal diseases. He described his studies in detail in a journal of minor circulation (Brotzu, 1948). His report was eventually brought to the attention of the Oxford University workers who were experienced in research on penicillin. They isolated two antibiotics from Brotzu's *Cephalosporium* sp., a sterol named cephalosporin P and penicillin N, a product previously obtained by others from a different species of *Cephalosporium* which had been named synnematin (Gottshall et al., 1951). This latter antibiotic explained the favorable clinical results obtained with crude concentrates by Brotzu. In spite of their activity in vivo, neither of the two antibiotics was judged sufficiently interesting, compared with the semisynthetic penicillins which had become available, to justify a major developmental effort. But five years after the initial culture isolation in 1953, Abraham and Newton at Oxford became intrigued by an ultraviolet-light-absorbing eluate obtained from an ion exchange column. They purified it and were surprised to find that it also had antibacterial activity. The level of potency was too low for it to have been detected in in vitro screening of the fermentation broth nor for it to have played any part in Brotzu's successful clinical studies with products obtained with his culture. Chemical analysis showed the eluate to contain a substance with β-lactam structure, therefore isolation was justified and was performed. Even more important, the substance was resistant to penicillinases. Its structure proved to be similar to penicillin N, but with an expanded thiazolidine ring and added acetyl side chain (Abraham and Newton, 1961). After much struggling, sufficient material was accumulated to prove activity in vivo and, based on analogy with the penicillins, biosynthetic approaches to modify the 7-β side chain appeared justified. Approaches to side-chain exchange which were successful with the penicillins failed and it was not until workers at the Lilly Research Laboratories succeeded in developing a chemical procedure for efficient side-chain removal that the full potential of the cephalosporins was realized (Morin et al., 1962).

Of the thousands of cephalosporin derivatives synthesized, ten have received approval by the U.S. Food and Drug Administration and have reached major status in the marketplace (see Table 9.1). Others are still being synthesized and evaluated in the clinic. The widespread clinical use of the cephalosporin-type antibiotics placed major demands upon fermentation facilities, especially because yields of the native precursor, cephalosporin C, obtained from species of *Cephalosporium* were very low. The problem was solved by development of a chemical technique for ring expansion, opening the well-developed and inexpensive penicillin fermentation process to exploitation for the purpose of producing cephalosporins.

The varied cephalosporins produced biosynthetically are not replicates. They differ from one another in important ways. Some are well absorbed following oral dosage. Others require parenteral administration. Some are relatively sensitive to cephalosporinases, others relatively resistant. Some are relatively narrow in spectrum but include problem infections such as methicillin-resistant staphylococci. Others have activity against anaerobes. The end result is a wider clinical usage of the cephalosporins than for any other class of antibiotic.

Discoveries in the cephalosporin field did not end with success in side-chain exchange and an inexpensive route of synthesis from penicillin. A new class of antibiotic was found independently in two pharmaceutical houses using two different screening approaches. Lilly Laboratory research workers were emphasizing products potentially useful in overcoming plant pathogens (Nagarajan et al., 1971). The Merck & Co. Inc. staff searched for specific inhibitors of cell wall synthesis (Stapley et al., 1972). The products discovered were present in culture filtrates of streptomycetes, not of moulds. Surprise was genuine therefore, when after isolation from the streptomycete broths and purification it was found that the compounds had the cephalosporin ring structure. They were, however, cephalosporins with an important difference, a difference so significant that a new name was created, cephamycin. The cephamycins have a methoxyl group in the 7-α position on the β-lactam ring. Associated with it is strong resistance to cephalosporinases and penicillinases. Side-chain exchange of a natural cephamycin led to antibiotics with broader antibacterial spectrum. Notable is the replacement of the alpha-aminoadipic acid natural side chain with a thienyl group, yielding cefoxitin with desired biological properties. Cefoxitin is now marketed world wide (Woodruff et al., 1975).

Molecular models demonstrate the basis for the stability of the cephamycins against destructive enzymes. The bulk of the methoxyl group provides steric hindrance against enzymatic attack, but it does not interfere with binding of cephamycins to the penicillin-binding proteins of the cell which is the essential preliminary step to the blockade of the cell wall formation process. Among the thousands of cephalosporin modifications previously created by chemists, including those at the β-lactam site, no one had considered favourably introduction of a 7-α methoxyl, possibly because no one expected that steric hindrance could be sufficiently selective to offer a blockade against an undesirable enzyme while retaining activity against the second essential one. As has happened so often in the past, the microbe proved to be a good teacher for the scientist.

9.3.8 Other antibiotics

The search for additional antibiotics has continued on a worldwide scale and has been highly successful. Microbes are capable of accumulating a great variety of organic substances, some with remarkable specificity of action. An interesting example is fosfomycin, the first substance containing a C-P bond isolated from a bacterium (Hendlin, et al., 1969; Woodruff et al., 1975). Fosfomycin is a small molecule of 138 daltons. It reacts covalently with pyruvyltransferase, the enzyme responsible for the first branch point of cell wall formation. The enzyme is inactivated by fosfomycin, leading to death of the bacterial cell. Otherwise, fosfomycin appears to be inert chemically, inhibiting no known step of mammalian metabolism, therefore it is exceptionally safe and nontoxic. Fosfomycin also has the exceptional property of being actively transported into bacterial cells by two transport mechanisms, to the point that concentrations within the bacterial cell reach 20 to 50 fold the external level, a factor which markedly accentuates its killing power. One system, that normally responsible for α-glycerol phosphate transport, is constitutive; the other, which transports glucose-6-phosphate, is adaptive. Transport systems are readily lost by mutation and, because such loss leads to resistance, the in vitro estimates of antibiotic activity of fosfomycin are complicated by the high frequency of occurrence of resistant colonies.

Science generally is considered an activity based on established facts, not swayed by political or personal opinion. Surprisingly, therefore, the history of antibiotic development shows evidence of national favouritism. Fosfomycin is widely used in Southern European countries, South America and Japan, not approved or little used in the U.S. or Northern Europe. An explanation can be the broad-based acceptance of parenteral administration of drugs by populations of the former areas of the world, the preference for oral administration in the latter. The macrolide antibiotics however, provide a more direct example of favouritism. These compounds, inhibitors of bacterial-protein synthesis, which are relatively nontoxic, orally absorbed, and highly effective against staphylococci, streptococci, and mycoplasma, have become favourites of pediatricians. Their acceptance in the U.S. arose from developmental activities of a consortium of four middlewestern pharmaceutical companies, which followed their initial discovery by McGuire et al. (1952). Later, other macrolides were discovered, noteworthy being spiramycin by Pinnert-Sindico et al. (1955) in France and leucomycin by Hata et al. (1953) in Japan. Spiramycin and leucomycin have become major products in their countries of origin, relegated to minor places elsewhere.

The answer, obviously, is that microbes are so fruitful in the antibiotics they produce that we presently have a superabundance of antibiotics to meet human needs. Questions have been raised whether it will always be so. The capacity of pathogens to become resistant to antibiotics, either by release of destructive enzymes, by loss of transport mechanisms, by alteration of binding sites, by exclusion or by other mechanisms, either as mutational events or through interchange of DNA fragments, is so efficient that fear has been expressed repeatedly throughout the forty-year history of antibiotic development that mankind eventually will be returned to the state of uncontrolled infections.

There is a dichotomy of approaches to the problem. Some advocate the discovery of antibiotic products of broader and broader spectrum, with new mechanisms of action, able to persist against all known resistance mechanisms, as the ultimate approach. An antibiotic recently approved for clinical use which approaches this objective is imipenem, used as a combination of a semisynthetic derivative of the natural streptomycete antibiotic thienamycin, modified to improve chemical stability, with a synthetic enzyme inhibitor designed to prevent enzymatic destruction of the antibiotic within the body (Norby et al., 1983).

A contrasting approach is to search for narrow-spectrum antibiotics designed to meet specific needs. Good examples are the monobactams (Sykes et al., 1982), compounds initially discovered as products of bacteria obtainable only from a unique ecological niche in the state of New Jersey, which through total synthesis have become broadened to a wide range of candidates, the more interesting of which are presently under clinical investigation. It is not possible at present to predict which approach will be most productive, but at present the capabilities of microbiologists to bring forth new products appear to exceed the rate at which pathogenic microbes learn to cope with them.

9.3.9 Chemical variations

Because the structures of antibiotics are varied and complex, they have presented interesting challenges to those interested in synthesis. The early expectation that chemical synthesis would supplant microbial fermentation as the primary commercial source of antibiotics has proven true for only a few, notably chloramphenicol, cycloserine and fosfomycin. Other antibiotics have been synthesized, but each has presented exceptional challenges to the synthetic chemist and costs have made commercial manufacture prohibitive.

Synthetic chemistry has, however, had far-reaching impact on the field. Early in research on penicillin it became apparent that different penicillins were produced by the same culture grown under different conditions. The product produced in America in large fermentors containing corn steep liquor as a nutrient was crystallized relatively easily after adequate purification, whereas that produced in the country of origin, England, proved more difficult to purify and to crystallize. Until it was recognized that multiple products were being made, great confusion existed in attempts to establish the chemical structure of penicillin. The same laboratory which had discovered the yield-enhancing properties of corn steep liquor, the Northern Regional Research Laboratory of the U.S. Department of Agriculture, solved the problem by noting that phenylacetic acid added to the fermentor directed the synthesis toward the American-type product, with significant further advances in yield (Moyer and Coghill, 1947). Crystallization was accomplished by Squibb research workers (Wintersteiner et al., 1949) and with it and studies with labelled precursors (Behrens, 1949) came proof that the added phenylacetic acid had been incorporated into the penicillin side chain and that the product being produced in the American fermentors was benzylpenicillin.

Benzylpenicillin became the product of commerce. Research workers at the Lilly Laboratories made the important extension that alternate precursors could be fed to the culture in place of phenylacetic acid, yielding other side-chain-substituted end products (Behrens et al., 1948). Penicillin V, produced with phenoxyethanol supplementation, proved important. Its acid stability made it a preferred form for oral therapy since, differing from benzylpenicillin, little destruction occurred due to stomach acidity.

The production of the preferred forms of antibiotics other than penicillin, accomplished by approaches different from precursor addition, has considerable commercial importance. With streptomycin, for example, either the impotent mannosidostreptomycin or the desired strep-tomycin is accumulated in culture broth dependent on the action of a natural enzyme, mannosidase, released by the streptomycin-producing actinomycete as it undergoes lysis at the end of the fermentation. A key step in streptomycin manufacture is to encourage such lysis at the proper moment in the fermentation to achieve maximal yield (Woodruff and McDaniel, 1954). With tetracycline, mutant cultures were found to accumulate a demethylated variant, also biologically active (McCormick et al., 1957). The variant has become a primary product of commerce.

That success in research which was recognized by the award of a Nobel Prize should not be attributed to a flash of good fortune but was characteristic of the creativity of the man was proven by Ernst Chain's second major demonstration, in association with the research staff of the Beecham Company, that the side chain of penicillin could be removed efficiently by enzymatic action, then be replaced at will by simple acetylation reactions (Chain, 1971). Thus a simple approach was opened to synthesis of thousands of β-lactam derivatives. Its significance is demonstrated by the fact that of the 28 penicillins and cephalosporins approved by the U.S. Food and Drug Administration and appearing in the Physicians' Desk Reference, only 2 are natural fermentation products; 26 have been prepared through side-chain exchange to improve their properties (Table 9.1). The level of effort expended by chemists in gaining the 26 is difficult to measure, but significant. It is generally recognized that over 40000 semi-synthetic derivatives have been made, those with desirable properties or believed to be potentially useful as precursors for further synthetic action having been protected by patents.

Today, the discovery of a new antibiotic which opens a new field of application is cause for much celebration by the biologists involved. It is, however, merely taken as the starting point for further synthetic activities by chemists. An example is the anthelmintic and insecticide antibiotic, avermectin, far superior in its natural state to any product synthesized by man in potency, spectrum and selectivity in its mode of action (Burg et al., 1979; Woodruff and Stapley, 1982). Yet, the product introduced to the market throughout the world was not aver-mectin, but ivermectin, a semi-synthetic derivative with improved safety index (Chabala et al., 1980).

9.4 The mode of action of antibiotics

Success in therapy of infections of man is the primary objective of antibiotic research and justifies the extensive laboratory and clinical efforts that have been expended. Secondary objectives also have far-reaching significance. Studies on the mode of action of antibiotics have had great impact on basic science (Gale et al., 1981). Initially these studies were undertaken as purely scientific endeavours. They explained the selective activity of the clinically useful antibiotics in attacking bacterial cells without harm to animal cells. The targets of the clinically useful antibiotics which have been identified are unique components of bacteria, not present in animal cells. Examples are the bacterial cell wall whose synthesis is blocked by the β-lactam antibiotics and by non-β-lactam products such as ristocetin, vancomycin, cycloserine and fosfomycin; the 70 S ribosome involved in bacterial protein synthesis whose function is blocked by chloramphenicol and the macrolide antibiotics; the selective bacterial membrane which allows the antibiotic streptomycin to penetrate to its target within the cell; and, in the case of rifampin, the pathway of bacterial DNA synthesis. The discovery of specific targets and manipulation of their formation or activity through appropriate antibiotic supplementation has led to a new order of knowledge concerning structure and biochemical activity of bacterial cells. These sub-explosions in basic science which have spread from the parent antibiotic explosion have penetrated many fields ranging from genetics to taxonomy. Especially promising for the future is the new field of biotechnology, in which microbes have become the manufacturing systems for animal or plant products after an appropriate interchange of genetic materials has been accomplished (Abelson, 1983). The new field could not exist in its present state of development without the use of antibiotics as selective agents to aid in sorting out the desired genetic hybrids from unchanged antibiotic-sensitive parents.

9.5 Allied fields of science

Somewhat more prosaic, but equally significant for its practitioners, are the gains in engineering science made in meeting requirements for optimal production of antibiotics. Ernst Chain has stated that the development of the rotating oxygen electrode in his laboratory was forced upon his staff by the necessity of measuring dissolved oxygen levels in penicillin fermentors while fermentations were in progress without breaking sterility barriers (Chain, 1980). In fact, the science of bioengineering was created by the need to develop the skills necessary to control factors critical for optimal antibiotic yields in factory-scale fermentors (Bartholomew et al., 1950). In a similar vein, the need to evaluate many nutrients simultaneously at varied concentrations has led to advances in statistical techniques. The observation that mutation of antibiotic-producing cultures could lead to increases in productivity led to a new investigation of mutagens and optimal methods for their application, a highly successful endeavour, which has increased yields of some antibiotics by more than ten thousand times (Fig. 9.3).

9.6 Pharmacology

Details of pharmacology of clinically useful antibiotics have been discussed in thousands of scientific papers and are summarized repeatedly in annual volumes and, as well, have provided subject matter for many books. Because the requirements established by government regulatory bodies throughout the world for approval of an antibiotic for marketing are rather rigid, the data presented in such publications show similarity in methods employed and in procedures for statistical evaluation of results. The Japanese authorities require that pharmacological data be published before granting permission to market. As a result, the special supplemental volumes containing such data published as addenda to the journal *Chemotherapy* (Japan) provide convenient sources of full information for any antibiotic sold in that country, although somewhat difficult to use because of general unfamiliarity of most scientists with the Japanese language. Among items commonly presented in such publications are the in vitro properties, including antibacterial spectra and absolute potencies, the effect of pH on antibacterial potency, the stability in body fluids and at body temperature, a listing of inactivating agents including the binding effect of serum, and the synergistic and antagonistic effects observed in combination with other antibiotics or other medicinals likely to be administered during the process of chemotherapy.

Knowledge concerning the fate of an antibiotic following administration by various routes obviously is critical to success in therapy. Some antibiotics require systemic administration. They are too poorly absorbed following oral administration to provide suitable chemotherapeutic action. Parenteral dosage by intravenous drip is normally the choice for seriously

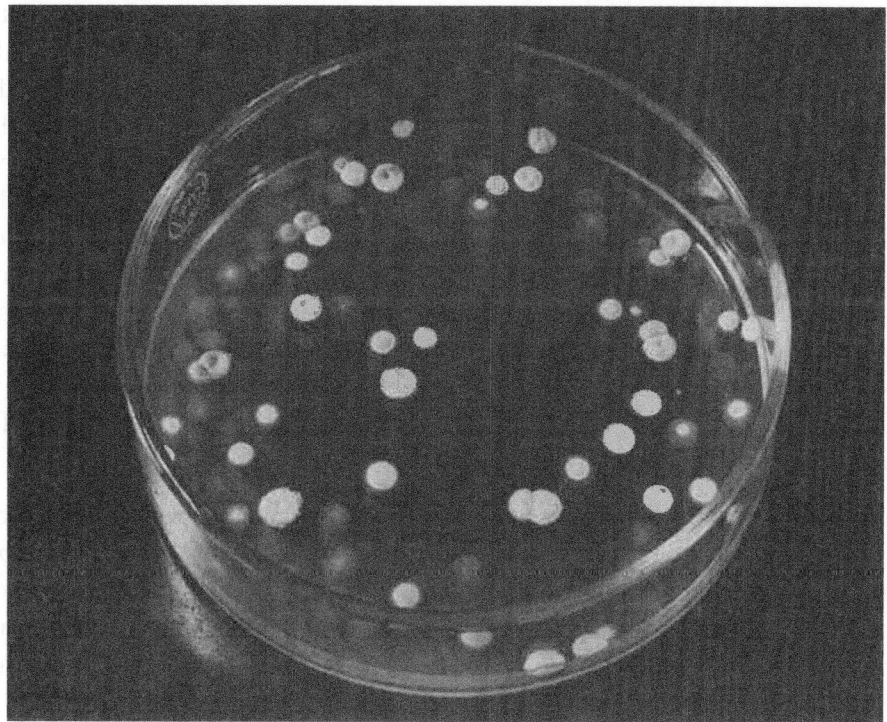

Figure 9.3
Petri dish containing colonies of a streptomycin-producing strain of *Streptomyces griseus* grown from spores exposed to a mutagen. Morphological variations induced by the mutagen are evident. Physiological changes, including increases in antibiotic production, also occur.

ill patients because of the advantage it offers for fine control of dosage and the ability to maintain relatively constant blood and tissue levels. Intramuscular injection can be used for follow-up therapy. It provides high peak levels of antibiotic following dosage, an advantage for bactericidal agents. In fact, a single intramuscular dose may be adequate for treatment of highly susceptible pathogens, for example the single-shot penicillin treatment for gonorrhoea. Normally, however, the cycling blood level and potential for pain and tissue damage resulting from intramuscular dosage are considered to be disadvantages of the method.

For some antibiotics such as streptomycin and cefoxitin the oral route of administration remains unsatisfactory. For others, chemical modification, formulation to offer protection against gastric acid, or even use of the unmodified antibiotic itself may prove suitable to provide adequate blood levels following oral dosage. Peak blood levels generally appear an hour or more after oral dosage. The oral route permits long-term therapy to be given to ambulatory patients, and it is widely used for the less acute infections.

Blood levels of an antibiotic are usually measured intermittently and provide an effective assessment, in association with in vitro antibacterial data, of the potential for successful therapy. The half-life of the blood level is usually quoted as a condensation of the more extensive blood level values. The half-life is, of course, dependent upon many factors, of which the site and mechanism of excretion are especially important. Most antibiotics are excreted via the kidney, but the parameters of excretion, either by tubular secretion or glomerular filtration, and whether or not reabsorbed, are important determinants of the type of blood level curves observed. Some antibiotics, for example macrolides, are largely secreted in the bile and appear in the faeces, where they may be destroyed or persist and be partially reabsorbed. Metabolism of antibiotics may occur in the body. In such cases the metabolites may have little antibacterial activity. It is common, therefore, to use microbiological assays to assess blood levels. If chemical assays are employed, it is essential to establish that the method used measures only the biologically active forms of the antibiotic. For example, little biologically active chloramphenicol is found in body excreta. Chloramphenicol is mostly converted to the biologically inactive glucuronide prior to elimination.

Infections may be localized in the brain, in bone, or at other sites in which the free blood level provides an inaccurate measure for predicting therapeutic effects. In such cases, prior experimentation with animals usually is used as the guide to select the preferred antibiotic for specific types of infections. It is necessary to perform the studies with infected animals. For example, the penicillins and cephalosporins fail to pass the meninges into the brain of uninfected animals, but often are effective in curing disease due to penetration through the inflamed tissue. In the case of osteomyelitis or endocarditis, it may be impossible to achieve adequate local levels of an antibiotic for assured therapy. In such cases, mixtures of antibiotics with synergistic action can be employed to heighten the antibacterial effect to a level of adequacy.

Characteristic aspects of antibiotic therapy are the problems of bacterial persistence and bacterial resistance. That these problems would occur with antibiotics which are bacteriostatic in action is not surprising. Elimination of infective organisms from the body usually is accomplished by continuing therapy until the bacteriostatically inhibited microbes are removed by the normal host defense mechanisms. Unexpectedly, persistence of bacteria during short-term therapy has proven equally to be a problem with bactericidal antibiotics. In the case of some cidal antibiotics, for example streptomycin, the failure may be traced to inability of the antibiotic to penetrate into animal cells. Bacteria located therein are able to reinitiate infection once the streptomycin has been excreted from the body. With other types of antibiotics, notably those which act by preventing cell wall formation, wall-less L-forms may persist, regenerating to normal pathogens when the antibiotic is no longer present. In all cases, best therapeutic results are obtained with prolonged antibiotic therapy, simultaneously accentuating aspects of host resistance by favourable patient management.

The problem of resistant strains can be severe. Enzymes exist in many bacteria which are capable of destroying antibiotics. Such strains are normally resistant and may proliferate in a hospital environment if a single antibiotic is overused or adequate cleanliness is not observed. Especially serious is the capability of the DNA template which directs destructive enzyme synthesis to be located in plasmids which multiply independently of the bacterial nucleus and which are capable of transfer from cell to cell, even from non-pathogens to pathogens. The best preventative for spread of such resistant organisms in a closed environment has proven to be constantly vigilant hospital chemotherapy committees who demand the practice of antibiotic rotation, give careful attention to selection of the appropriate antibiotic to match the identified infective microorganism, insist upon prescribed procedures for cleanliness, and screen hospital personnel to detect carriers of resistant organisms, providing for their treatment or requiring their isolation from patients.

9.7 Toxicity

It is a presumption of antibiotic practice, due to selectivity of action, that clinically employed antibiotics will not be toxic. Those antibiotics which are not selective will have failed animal toxicity evaluations and will have been rejected by their discoverers or by government regulatory authorities. In practice, however, this theoretical situation is seldom achieved. Often, certain tissues of the body prove to have high sensitivity to an antibiotic. Such is the case with the vestibular and cochlear apparatus in their high sensitivity to streptomycin and to aminocyclitol antibiotics, leading to permanent vertigo or hearing loss after prolonged treatment, or the problem of aplastic anaemia associated with chloramphenicol. In other instances, violent allergic responses, sometimes fatal, may occur. Anaphylactic reactions occur rarely, noteworthy with the penicillins. Much less severe rashes and pruritus occur with relatively higher frequency with some antibiotics, notably ampicillin. The above forms of toxicity are usually associated with man, not clearly predictable from animal experimentation. Other forms of toxicity, damage to liver cells or to the kidney, haemolysis, etc., can be assessed in laboratory animals and form part of the data collected and reported to governmental regulatory authorities at the time of filing a new drug application.

A further unfavourable response, which may or may not be classified as toxicity, is the change in normal microbial flora of the body associated with antibiotic therapy and the symptomology resulting from it. The effect may be relatively minor, a few days of diarrhoea, or may result in an irritating but rather easily controlled overgrowth by intestinal fungi. However, on occasion, the effect can be severe, even fatal, if not recognized and treated promptly; examples are intestinal coccal overgrowths in infants receiving oral doses of broad-spectrum tetracycline antibiotics, and the pseudomembranous colitis caused by overgrowth of toxin-producing *Clostridium difficile* following therapy with clindamycin.

The important factor to remember is that use of an antibiotic requires a medical judgment, a balance of desired therapeutic effect against the potential for an unfavourable reaction. When need is evident, antibiotics truly are miracle drugs. They cure infections long considered untreatable. They never should be employed in absence of need as defined by clinical judgment.

9.8 Antibiotics in agriculture

The major impact of the antibiotic explosion has been on human health. As with most explosions, there have been extensions into other areas. Although antibiotics have been used for the control and cure of diseases in animals in much the same way that they have been used in man, an accidental discovery led to a new and unexpected use for antibiotics and, ultimately, to the search for new fermentation products for use exclusively in agriculture.

9.8.1 Growth permittants

There had been earlier published observations that antibacterial agents, including sulphonamides and streptomycin, stimulated the growth of animals (Moore et al., 1946). However, the significance of these observations was evidently not apparent to the investigators because they were not pursued.

The observation which ultimately led to commercial application was a classical example of serendipity – the discovery of the unexpected while investigating an unrelated phenomenon. Thomas Jukes, E.L.R. Stokstad and coworkers at Lederle Laboratories were studying the 'animal protein factor', a dietary component required for the growth of chicks fed a strictly vegetable diet. The factor was present in sources of animal protein such as liver extract and sardine meal. Investigators at the research laboratories of Merck & Co., Inc. had shown that pure vitamin B-12 replaced the animal protein factor (Ott et al., 1948). While searching for a more convenient source of the factor, the investigators at Lederle assayed in chicks the dried fermentation mash of *Streptomyces aureofaciens*. The chicks grew more rapidly and to a greater final weight than chicks whose diet was supplemented with liver extract or purified vitamin B-12 (Stokstad et al., 1949). Microbiological assay of the *S. aureofaciens* preparation indicated that it contained 0.4 to 1.0 μg of vitamin B-12 per gram, but the chick assay indicated that it contained about 4 μg/g. They concluded, logically enough, that the 'animal protein factor' consisted of vitamin B-12 plus some factor as yet unidentified.

The unidentified factor was soon shown to be the antibiotic chlortetracycline, which produced essentially the same growth response in chicks as the dried *S. aureofaciens* mash (Stokstad and Jukes, 1950a). The growth-enhancing activity was quickly confirmed in turkeys (Stokstad and Jukes, 1950b) and pigs (Jukes et al., 1950). The commercial implications of this discovery were not overlooked by these investigators or by their company.

The stimulation of growth and improvement of feed efficiency was soon found with oxytetracycline, bacitracin and penicillin. Thus began the era of antibiotic feed additives for farm animals. The fermentation products that are approved for use as feed additives in the U.S. are listed in Table 9.2. Some additional products that are used for the treatment of diseases, usually by parenteral or topical administration, are listed in Table 9.3.

The amount of antibiotic required for growth enhancement is significantly lower than that which must be used for the cure of bacterial infections. Chlortetracycline is fed to swine

Table 9.2: Fermentation products used as feed additives (Taken from Leidahl, 1983).

Name	For use in* Poultry	Swine	Cattle	Sheep	Use level Growth (g/ton)	Disease (g/ton)
Bacitracin	G,F,D,E	G,F,D	G,F,D		4–50	50–500
Bambermycins	G,F	G,F			1–4	
Chlortetracycline	G,F,D,E	G,F,D	G,F,D	G,F,D	10–50	50–400
Erythromycin	G,F,D,E	G,F	G,F		4.6–18.5	92.5–185
Hygromycin B	A	A				8–12
Lasalocid	C		G,F		10–30	68–113
Lincomycin	G,F	D			2–4	40–100
Monensin	C		G,F		5–30	90–110
Neomycin	D	D	D	D		70–140
Novobiocin	D					200–350
Nystatin	D					50–100
Oxytetracycline	G,F,D,E	G,F,D	G,F,D	G,F,D	5–50	50–500
Penicillin G	G,F,D	G,F,D			2.4–50	50–100
Streptomycin**	G,F,D,E	G,F,D			12–18.75	75
Tylosin	G,F,D	G,F,D			4–50	100–1000
Virginiamycin	G,F	G,F,D			5–20	25–100

* G = growth; F = feed efficiency; D = disease treatment; E = egg production; A = anthelmintic and C = coccidiostat.
** Used only in combination, e.g. with penicillin G. ***Liver abscesses.

Table 9.3: Fermentation products used topically or parenterally in animals.*

Name	Activity	Type
Amoxicillin	antibacterial	semi-synthetic penicillin
Ampicillin	antibacterial	semi-synthetic penicillin
Bacitracin	antibacterial	peptide
Cephapirin	antibacterial	semi-synthetic cephalosporin
Chloramphenicol	antibacterial	
Chlortetracycline	antibacterial	tetracycline
Cloxacillin	antibacterial	semi-synthetic penicillin
Dihydrostreptomycin	antibacterial	aminocyclitol
Erythromycin	antibacterial	macrolide
Gentamicin	antibacterial	aminocyclitol
Griseofulvin	antifungal	grisan
Hetacillin	antibacterial	semi-synthetic penicillin
Ivermectin	anthelmintic, ectoparasiticide	semi-synthetic avermectin
Panmycin	antibacterial	aminocyclitol
Lincomycin	antibacterial	
Neomycin	antibacterial	aminocyclitol
Novobiocin	antibacterial	
Nystatin	antifungal	polyene
Oxytetracycline	antibacterial	teracycline
Penicillin G	antibacterial	natural penicillin
Polymyxin B	antibacterial	peptide
Spectinomyciri	antibacterial	aminocyclitol
Tetracycline	antibacterial	tetracycline
Thiostrepton	antibacterial	
Tylosin	antibacterial	macrolide
Zeranol	growth promotant	semi-synthetic resorcylic acid lactone

*The list of compounds, except for ivermectin, is taken from Aronson, 1983.

at 10 to 50 g/ton of feed for improvement of growth and feed efficiency. The treatment of disease requires 100 to 200 g/ton. Antibiotics that are fed at low levels to enhance growth and improve feed efficiency are called 'growth permittants'.

The use of growth permittants has led to a revolution in the raising of animals for food. For example, the administration of 70 to 80 mg of chlortetracycline per day per head of cattle leads to an average 6% increase in weight gain and 4% increase in feed efficiency (U.S. Office of Technology Assessment, 1979). This enables the production of more meat at a lower cost. It has also permitted a more intensive method of raising animals.

The mechanism by which antibiotics exert their growth-enhancing effect is not known. It is generally assumed that they must act on the intestinal flora. Among the theories proposed are the prevention of a subclinical infection, inhibition of toxin-producing organisms, elimination of microorganisms that compete for essential nutrients, and the reduction of ammonia production in the intestinal tract and in litter. Growth permittants are more effective in young animals and under suboptimal growth conditions such as dirty or crowded housing or low-energy feeds.

The feeding to animals of antibiotics that are also used in man has become extremely controversial. There is little doubt that feeding subtherapeutic levels of antibiotics is conducive to the selection of antibiotic-resistant microorganisms. Moreover, antibiotic resistance is frequently carried on cytoplasmic genetic elements called plasmids, and these plasmids often carry resistance factors for several different antibiotics. Even more serious is the fact that plasmids can be transferred from one bacterium to another, even between different species and genera. Strains of *Salmonella typhimurium* which contain plasmids bearing multiple antibiotic resistance have been isolated from farm animals, farm workers and hospital patients. One study has provided evidence that the plasmids from *S. typhimurium* strains isolated from animals and humans were often identical or nearly identical (O'Brien, et al., 1982).

Farm animals have long been considered to be a significant source of intestinal infections of humans. It has been anticipated that antibiotic-resistant bacteria derived from animals could also initiate infections, but firm epidemiological proof has been lacking. A recent publication clarifies the situation (Holmberg et al., 1984). The authors report that an antibiotic-resistant *Salmonella* which caused serious disease in humans in several geographically distinct areas of the U.S.A. was derived from beef products obtained from a single farm on which cattle had been fed subtherapeutic levels of chlortetracycline and that animals on an adjacent farm had died due to salmonellosis caused by the same strain. The evidence presented included isolation of *Salmonella newport* with the identical antibiotic resistance pattern and identical R plasmid content from 18 patients and from a calf dead from salmonellosis. An interesting aspect is the fact that most of the patients who became seriously ill were themselves using antibiotics at the time of illness.

Some countries, including the United Kingdom, have curtailed the use of antibiotics as growth permittants that are used in human medicine and the pressure for a similar ban is great in the U.S. This has prompted a continuing search for new antibiotics for use exclusively in animal health. The new antibiotics must be structurally unrelated to those used for human medicine so that cross resistance is not a problem. Two antibiotics, virginiamycin and the bambermycins, have been licensed in the U.S. for enhanced growth and increased feed efficiency of chickens and pigs (Table 9.2). Summarized data from field trials (Council for Agricultural Science and Technology, 1981) indicate that bambermycins may be less effective than most of the other antibiotics used as growth permittants while virginiamycin is competitive in its effects in both chickens and swine. The data indicate that chlortetracycline, especially fed in combination with sulphamethazine and penicillin (ASP-250), the most commonly used feed additive for enhancement of growth and feed efficiency, is superior to all other antibiotics.

Attempts to find new and more effective antibiotics for use as growth permittants are continuing and several new antibiotics are in various stages of development. This effort, in a significant way, contributes to the antibiotic explosion.

9.8.2 Growth promotants

Growth permittants act indirectly to enhance growth. Compounds which act directly by some physiological effect are called growth promotants. The more effective anabolic agents have oestrogenic activity. The most effective growth promotant, used widely for many years, is the synthetic oestrogen diethylstilboestrol. However, the compound has carcinogenic action, and its use in animals destined for human consumption has been banned in the U.S. and much of the rest of the world.

One fermentation product is used as a growth promotant. Zearalenone, while not an antibiotic, is included in this discussion since it is produced by a microorganism and is an example of the logical extension of the antibiotic explosion.

The discovery of the resorcylic acid lactones, of which zearalenone is a member, is an example of the importance of investigating thoroughly an unusual phenomenon (Hidy et al., 1977). A number of observations had been reported in the midwestern U.S. of oestrogenic effects (vulvular enlargement and mammary gland stimulation) in swine that had been fed moldy corn. The isolation of the fungus *Gibberella zeae* (the perfect stage of *Fusarium roseum 'graminearum'*) from the corn and characterization of the oestrogenic activity extracted from it was a cooperative effort of the Purdue University Agricultural Experiment Station and Commercial Solvents Corp.

Early fermentations were performed on grain in static incubation (similar to the early methods of producing penicillin), but this required 6 or 7 weeks of incubation, and isolation of the activity was difficult. Later, surface cultures using a synthetic medium on vermiculite as a support were used, but the fermentation still required 4 to 5 weeks. Eventually, a mutant strain of *G. zeae* was isolated which produced zearalenone in submerged fermentations. This was a major breakthrough, and production became commercially feasible. The yield was improved to greater than 32 g/liter in a two-week fermentation.

A large number of analogues of zearalenone have been studied for their efficacy and safety. A reduction product, zearalanol (or zeranol), was ultimately selected for commercial development. Unlike diethylstilboestrol and oestrogenic steroids, zearalanol appears to be lacking in carcinogenic activity. Zearalanol is administered in the form of an implant pellet (placed under the skin of the ear) to beef cattle and feedlot lambs. It has 30 to 50% of the growth and feed efficiency enhancement of diethylstilboestrol.

9.8.3 Coccidiostats

The vast majority of the antibiotics that have been discovered fail in practical application and remain little more than laboratory curiosities. Among the numerous reasons for failure are narrowness of antibacterial spectrum, lack of activity in vivo, toxicity, and chemical or metabolic instability. An antibiotic that appeared destined for the curio shelf because it exhibited the first three of these reasons for failure was monensin. Because of the persistence of the researchers at Eli Lilly and Company, it has become one of the most important antibiotics for use in animal health.

Monensin, produced by *Streptomyces cinnamonensis,* was initially picked as a lead with weak activity against *Bacillus subtilis, Micrococcus luteus, Staphylococcus aureus* and *Neurospora crassa,* but it lacked antibacterial activity in mice, and its LD_{50} was about 44 mg/kg (oral) in mice (Haney and Hoehn, 1968). It is the habit of pharmaceutical researchers to test new compounds as widely as possible. Monensin controlled powdery mildew on beans at 3.2 parts per million and it was cytotoxic to HeLa cells and murine clone NCTC 1742 cells at < 0.1 μg/ml. It was chosen for isolation on the basis of this antitumour activity. The purified compound proved to be inactive after extensive antitumour testing in animals.

Lilly had initiated an anticoccidial screen in chicks, and monensin was shown to be active. Because the fermentation yields were extremely low, heated discussions ensued between the agricultural products marketing and research groups as to whether a suitably priced commercial product could be obtained. The challenge was met by the microbial physiologists and isolation chemists, and the yield was soon increased sufficiently to suggest that a commercially feasible product was indeed possible (Stark et al., 1968).

Monensin controls infections by the six species of *Eimeria (E. acervulina, E. brunetti, E. maxima, E. mivati, E. necatrix* and *E. tenella),* the parasitic protozoa that cause mortality and morbidity in chickens. At 110 g/ton (0.0121%), it significantly reduces mortality, coecal and intestinal lesions and production of oocysts. It also improves weight gain and feed efficiency (Shumard and Callender, 1968).

In the early 1960's, Henry Lardy of the Enzyme Institute, University of Wisconsin, and a Lilly consultant, often received new antibiotics from Lilly for testing in his mitochondrial energy systems. Monensin was submitted for testing, and it was found to have a number of specific effects on mitochondrial metabolism, including the specific inhibition of the uptake of alkali metal cations (Estrada-O. et al., 1968). Burton Pressman, a former colleague of Lardy, had discovered the ion-transport properties of a number of antibiotics and had coined the term 'ionophore' to describe these compounds (Pressman et al., 1967). Pressman showed that monensin was also an ionophore and helped to explain the effects noted in Lardy's tests.

Monesin belongs to the family of polyether ionophores which are characterized by a chain of tetrahydrofuran and tetrahydropyran rings and a terminal carboxyl group. Their three-dimensional structures present an oxygen-rich, hydrophilic internal region and a hydrocarbon-rich lipophilic exterior. The carboxyl group forms a salt with sodium and/or potassium, and the internal oxygens complex with the cation to form a neutral lipophilic salt which passes readily through the plasma membrane of cells. This ability to transport cations across the cell membrane prevents the sodium/potassium pump from maintaining the usual high intracellular concentration of potassium. Their antibacterial activity can be reversed by increasing the potassium concentration of the medium to the point that the necessary high internal potassium level of the cells is attained.

A number of other antibiotics belonging to this class had been discovered earlier than monensin. Three of these, nigericin, X-206 and dianemycin, were also tested by the Lilly group and found to have coccidiostat activity (Shumard and Callender, 1968). The revelation that antibiotics of this type have coccidiostat activity led to an explosion of ionophores. The number in the literature now exceeds 40, most being discovered in Japan. Predictably, all have coccidiostat activity to a greater or lesser degree, and some are being developed as new coccidiostats.

One of the ionophores, X537A, which had been discovered much earlier, (Berger et al., 1951) is now licensed as a coccidiostat in the U.S. It was named lasalocid. It is different from most of the other ionophores in being able to complex with divalent cations such as Ca^{2+} and Mg^{2+} as well as with monovalent cations. This is possible because the lasalocid molecule is small enough that there is space for two molecules to combine with a single divalent cation to form a neutral complex.

There are other antibiotics that can complex with cations to form lipid-soluble salts. One interesting group consisting of two members, boromycin and aplasmomycin, contains boron as part of the molecule. They form neutral complexes with monovalent cations and have coccidiostat activity. Two other groups are the macrotetralides (nonactin, monactin, dinactin, trinactin and tetranactin) and the cyclic depsipeptides (valinomycin and enniatin). The former are cyclic compounds containing four tetrahydrofuran rings and the latter are cyclic peptides. They are neutral compounds and thus form positively charged complexes with cations. Although they lack coccidiostat activity, one compound, tetranactin, is being developed as an insecticide.

9.8.4 *Rumen additives*

The story of monensin does not end with its development as a coccidiostat. Ruminants have long been believed to be inefficient. They convert energy-poor cellulose-containing vegetation such as grass into animal protein. The rumen is actually an anaerobic fermentation vessel in which some microorganisms hydrolyze the cellulose and others produce methane and short-chain fatty acids, primarily acetate, propionate and butyrate. The fatty acids are utilized by the ruminant for energy and for protein synthesis, while the methane is a waste product. If methane production could be suppressed, there would be more carbon and energy available to the ruminant. Moreover, if fatty-acid formation were shifted toward propionate, which is gluconeogenic, still more energy and carbon would become available for protein synthesis.

The Agricultual Research Division of Eli Lilly and Company was interested in products to improve growth and/or feed efficiency in ruminants. An in vivo screen to detect effects of compounds on the volatile fatty-acid ratio in the rumen fermentation was devised. Monensin was one of the first compounds found to be active in this screen. Methane production was slightly reduced, and propionate was increased as much as 75% with concomitant decrease in acetate and butyrate (Richardson et al., 1974).

Subsequent testing in sheep and cattle demonstrated that monensin was effective in increasing feed efficiency about 10% (Perry et al., 1976). Monensin has been approved by the F.D.A. for use in feedlot cattle for improved feed efficiency. It has also been approved for increased rate of weight gain in cattle on pasture.

9.8.5 Anthelmintic agents

One antibiotic has long been used as an anthelmintic agent in swine and chickens. Hygromycin B was isolated from fermentation broth of *Streptomyces hygroscopicus* by workers at the Lilly Research Laboratories (Mann and Bower, 1958). Although it has activity against both Gram-positive and Gram-negative bacteria and some fungi its activity is too weak for it to be therapeutically useful. However, as is the custom of pharmaceutical researchers, it was tested against a variety of other organisms. It was inactive against *Trichomonas vaginalis, Toxoplasma* sp., *Trypanosoma equiperdum, Trypanosoma gambiense* and *Eimeria tenella*. It did exhibit activity in vitro against *Leptospira pomona,* in vitro and in vivo against *Entamoeba histolytica* and in vivo against *Borrelia novyi, Syphacia obvelata* and *Aspicularis tetraptera.*

It was the activity against the two oxyurid nematodes, *S. obvelata* and *A. tetraptera* that was the most interesting. When incorporated into the diet at 0.05% and fed for 7 days, hygromycin B reduced the worm burden of these two species by 99 and 91%, respectively. A small trial in pigs indicated that hygromycin B fed at 2 g per 100 lb of feed was effective in reducing the egg count in faeces of *Metastrongylus* sp., *Oesophogostomum* sp., *Trichuris suis* and *Strongyloides ransomi. Ascaris lumbricoides* eggs were reduced somewhat. There were very few *Metastrongylus, Hyostrongylus, Strongyloides, Trichuris ox Ascaris* worms in the pigs at the termination of the experiment although the *Oesophogostomum* sp. counts were high and there were numerous lesions caused by these nematodes (Goldsby and Todd, 1957; McCowen et al., 1957).

Hygromycin B was the first fermentation product to find commercial use as an anthelmintic. Moreover, it exhibited a broader spectrum of activity and was safer to use than the other anthelmintics available at that time. It is licensed for use in the U.S. as a feed additive against *Ascaris galli, Heterakis gallinae* and *Capillaria obsignata* in chickens and against *Ascaris suis, Oesophogostomum dentatum* and *Trichuris suis* in swine. The use level is 8–12 g/ton for chickens and 12 g/ton for swine (Leidahl, 1983).

The discovery of a substance useful in farm animals is favoured by the availability of an in vivo screening procedure using small laboratory animals. At Merck Sharp & Dohme Research Laboratories, fermentation broths were screened for coccidiostat activity using mice infected with *Eimeria vermiformis*. Although it was an effective assay, the one compound that showed great promise and was the subject of intensive effort for nearly a year had to be abandoned when a patent on the same compound was issued to Eli Lilly and Company. Such are the travails of research!

Although the mouse assay had been unsuccessful for finding a new coccidiostat, it proved efficient enough to encourage use in an analogous assay to search for anthelmintic activities. Previously used in vitro screens for anthelmintics had proven to be too nonspecific and detected numerous metabolic poisons. A mouse assay was expected to be more selective for anthelmintic agents as it had been for coccidiostats.

The pinworms 5. *obvelata* and *A. tetraptera*, which had successfully detected the anthelmintic activity of hygromycin B, have been favourite parasites for the testing of anthelmintics in the laboratory, but the infections are difficult to control and spontaneous remissions are common. The nematode *Nematospiroides dubius* was selected for the Merck assay because of the greater reproducibility of the infection. Faecal pellets from infected mice were examined microscopically for eggs, and, if they were absent, the small intestine was examined for worms. As in the coccidiostat assay, the fermentation products were mixed with the feed and freeze-dried. Most of the cultures that showed anthelmintic activity were very toxic and did not appear to be worth pursuing further. It was almost immediately evident that nontoxic anthelmintic agents would be more difficult to find than coccidiostats.

Cultures freshly isolated from soil provided the major source for screening. Culture collections were also utilized. One large collection had been obtained from the Kitasato Institute in Tokyo, Japan. All of these cultures were grown for the anthelmintic assay. In a group of 50 Kitasato cultures was one bearing the number OS-3153. This culture had been isolated from a soil sample collected in Kawana, Ito City, Shizuoka Prefecture, Japan. Although the mouse which received the diet containing the OS-3153 product was free of eggs and worms, it had consumed only 13 of the 25 g of feed provided and weighed only 14 g. Since the mice normally weighed 18 to 20 g when put on test and about 28 g when the test was terminated, it was evident that OS-3153 was either unpalatable or toxic.

This culture was regrown on the original medium and on a second unrelated medium in order to confirm its activity. The mouse which received OS-3153 grown on the original medium ate all of the diet but weighed only 15 g. More significant was the absence of eggs and worms. The mouse receiving OS-3153 grown on the second medium died before the termination of the experiment. Thus, of the first three mice to receive OS-3153, one died and the other two had lost weight. Because anthelmintic activity associated with toxicity had been encountered previously, there was little cause for excitement for the moment.

The culture was grown again, this time on a larger scale to provide sufficient material to test at more than one level. Broth was titrated in serial 2-fold dilutions from 50 ml down to 6.2 ml per 25 g of feed. In this experiment, there was little sign of toxicity. The mice ate all of the diet, and the mouse receiving the highest level weighed 22 g and the others weighed 25 to 29 g. There were no eggs or worms in any of the mice. There was great jubilation in the laboratory when the results of this test were reported. This was the first time that more than one level (let alone four) of a fermentation product had exhibited anthelmintic activity accompanied by near normal weight gain. It was only after considerably more screening that we began to realize how fortunate we had been. In over 100,000 cultures screened, this was the only non-toxic anthelmintic discovered.

Cultures obtained in the anthelmintic screen that became candidates for chemical isolation of their active components were assigned sequential 'product numbers' by the junior author of this chapter. At this time, there were two candidates awaiting assignment, a coccidiostat and the anthelmintic. The next two numbers in the series were 75 and 76. It was decided to give the anthelmintic culture a special blessing by designating it C-076 in honor of the U.S. bicentennial year 1976 which was only a few months away.

Events moved quickly after that. The culture was determined to be a new species of *Streptomyces* and was named *S. avermitilis*. Roughly translated, the name means the *Streptomyces* capable of separating from worms. The fermentation yield was improved by medium optimization and isolation of a superior strain (Burg et al., 1979). The anthelmintic activity was isolated (Miller et al., 1979) and identified as a family of eight closely related 16-membered ring lactones, each bearing a disaccharide side chain (Albers-Schönberg et al., 1981). The compounds, named avermectins, exhibited remarkably broad activity against at least eight families of nematodes: Filariidae, Oxyridae, Trichinellidae, Trichuridae, Heterakidae, Metastrongylidae, Trichostrongylidae and Strongylidae (Egerton, et al., 1979). They lacked activity against trematodes and cestodes, however.

In contrast to the other compounds that have been discussed in this section, where the utility in agriculture was a secondary discovery, the discovery of the avermectins provides an example of 'seek and ye shall find'. In fact, the avermectins lack activity against bacteria and fungi and could only have been detected by their activity against an animal species. It would not necessarily have had to be a helminth since it was soon discovered that the avermectins possessed potent activity against insects (Ostlind, et al., 1979) ticks (Wilkins, et al., 1981) and mites (Wilkens, et al., 1980). The direct search for an anthelmintic agent had provided an unexpected bonus.

The avermectins are among the most potent therapeutic agents known. Avermectin B_{1a} the most effective anthelmintic among the eight members, controls all the nematodes when administered orally or parenterally in a single $100 \mu g/kg$ dose. It controls *Ancylostoma caninum* in dogs given a single 3 to $5 \mu g/kg$ oral dose (Egerton et al., 1979). It has also proven effective in eliminating the microfilariae of *Dirofilaria immitis* (canine heartworm) when administered to dogs at 50 or $100 \mu g/kg$, although it appears to be ineffective against the adult worms (Blair and Campbell, 1978).

The first avermectin to be marketed is a semisynthetic derivative, 22,23-dihydroavermectin B_{1a} (Chabala et al., 1980). It is somewhat less active than the parent compound but was determined to possess twice the safety factor. The compound has been named ivermectin. At $200 \mu g/kg$, it controls the nematode parasites of sheep, cattle and horses; in addition, it also controls fly, tick and mite ectoparasites.

Ivermectin may also prove useful in human medicine. Early trials have shown that it can eliminate the microfilariae of *Onchocerca volvulus* when administered orally at $50 \mu g/kg$ (Aziz et al., 1982). *O. volvulus* is the cause of river blindness (onchocerciasis) a serious disease in certain parts of Africa.

In studies on the mode of action of the avermectins, it was observed that nematodes became paralyzed. They were neither rigid nor flaccid but maintained normal muscle tone and moved when irritated. It was shown that avermectin blocks transmission between interneuron(s) and excitatory motoneurons in the ventral nerve cord of *Ascaris* (Kass et al., 1980). In studies on lobster opener and stretcher neuromuscular junction preparations, it was concluded that avermectin B_{1a} acts on the GABA [γ-aminobutyric acid] ergic synapse and lowers resistance of the muscle membranes by causing an increase in chloride ion permeability (Mellin et al., 1983).

9.8.6 Plant diseases

The antibiotic explosion has had a great impact on animal husbandry. However, it has had a lesser effect on the control of plant diseases even though the early antibiotic literature is replete with numerous trials of antibiotics for that use (Goodman, 1959). Plant pests have been controlled for the most part by inorganic salts and synthetic chemicals. The reason for this is largely economic. Fermentation products are more expensive to produce than the synthetic chemicals (Leben and Keitt, 1954).

A few antibiotics have been developed for the control of bacterial and fungal diseases of plants (Thomson, 1982). Streptomycin is used for fireblight of apple and pear (*Erwinia amylovora*), walnut blight (*Xanthomonas juglandis*), bacterial spot of tomato and pepper (*Xanthomonas vesicatoria*), and tobacco wildfire (*Pseudomonas tabaci*). Oxytetracycline is used for bacterial spot of peaches as well as for fireblight of pears. It is also the only treatment for lethal yellows disease of palms, a particularly devastating disease which threatens the coconut industry in many parts of the world.

Both streptomycin and oxytetracycline act systemically. This trait is especially useful because it provides a complete cure of the bacterial infections. Oxytetracycline is applied by injection for the control of pear decline and lethal yellows disease.

Cycloheximide is used as a foliar fungicide, especially on turf grasses and ornamentals. It is effective against cherry leaf spot (*Cocomyces hiemalis*), 'fading out' of turf (*Curvularia lunata*), melting out (*Helminthosporium* sp.) and powdery mildew of roses (*Sphaerothera pannosa* var. *rosa*).

Five antifungal antibiotics are used in Japan. Three, kasugamycin, blasticidin S and validamycin, are used for the control of rice blast. Polyoxin is used for rice sheath blight but more often for diseases of fruits and vegetables. It inhibits the synthesis of chitin, an important constituent of the cell walls of many fungi. Piomycin is used for the control of fungal diseases of fruits and vegetables.

The use of synthetic chemicals as pesticides has raised environmental concerns. As was discussed in relation to the use as feed additives of antibiotics used in human medicine, the objections raised are certainly valid. However, it is necessary to weigh the risk/benefit factors. In many instances, the risks have been considered too great. An example is the banning of DDT which had been a highly effective insecticide. Unfortunately, it tended to accumulate in the food chain and endangered the survival of many species of birds of prey because it inhibited the deposition of egg shell calcium carbonate. The development in many insects of resistance to DDT was becoming a serious problem so the banning of DDT was not as calamitous as it would otherwise have been.

The environmental issue has encouraged the search for alternate pesticides. Fermentation products and other natural products offer certain advantages. They are usually biodegradable so that they do not accumulate in the environment. The fact that they already occur naturally offers a certain psychological advantage to their use. They often have modes of action which are entirely unexpected.

One fermentation product which has been used as an insecticide and miticide is tetranactin. This is one of the macrotetrolide ionophores. A nucleoside antibiotic, nikkomycin, which inhibits chitin synthetase, is being considered for use as an insecticide. The cuticle of insects consists of chitin and inhibition of its synthesis leaves an insect vulnerable after it moults.

Two additional fermentation products that are being investigated for possible use as insecticides and miticides are the milbemycins and the avermectins. The milbemycins were discovered prior to the avermectins and patented as acaricides. They are structurally similar to the avermectins, possessing the same 16-membered lactone and spiroketal ring system. However, they lack a hydroxyl at the 13-position and thus the disaccharide side chain of the avermectins. They also bear a variety of other substituents. The absence of the disaccharide substituent may account for their lack of antihelminthic activity although one, milbemycin D, which has an isopropyl substituent at position 25 as in the 'small b'-avermectins is an exception.

The avermectins, which had been found to control insect, mite and tick ectoparasites of animals, are also being tested for possible use in controlling similar plant pests (Putter et al., 1981). Avermectins B_{1a} and B_{2a} are the most effective for this purpose. Avermectin B_{1a} applied as a foliar spray exhibits an LD_{90} of 0.02 to 0.03 ppm against the 2-spotted spider mite (*Tetranychus urticae*) on bean plants. Avermectin exhibits excellent persistence and is lethal to the 2-spotted spider mite for up to one month after application to bean leaves at 0.5 to 1.0 ppm. Avermectin B_{1a} is also effective against a variety of insect pests among the Coleoptera, Diptera, Homoptera, Hymenoptera, Isoptera, Lepidoptera and Orthoptera. In a bait formulation applied at a level of about 120 mg per hectare, avermectin B_{1a} was found to halt egg production of the queen of the red imported fire ant (*Solenopsis invicta*). The queen appears to become permanently infertile so that avermectin offers a means of controlling this pernicious pest. The avermectins are also effective against plant parasitic nematodes. Avermectin B_{2a} appears to be especially effective in this regard. When incorporated into soil at a level of 160 to 240 g per hectare, it controls the rootknot nematode *Meloidogyne incognita* in greenhouse tests.

9.9 Non-antibiotic pharmacologically active fermentation products

That microorganisms are virtuoso chemists is undisputed. The wide variety of structures found among the antibiotics attests to that. Whether these compounds are produced by design or by chance – in a manner analogous to a million apes typing for eternity and reproducing all of the world's literature (plus a few new masterpieces) along with a preponderance of nonsense – is disputed. It is easy to rationalize the production of antibiotics as providing a competitive advantage in a soil crowded with microorganisms vying for the limited nutrients. However, there are other compounds produced by microorganisms that are more difficult to understand. Perhaps the detection procedures that have been used select for the 'masterpieces' and miss the 'nonsense'. In other words, what microorganisms appear to produce may be more the result of what is sought than of their actual synthetic capabilities.

The ability of microorganisms to produce antibiotics has received the most attention since infectious diseases were the most serious health problem and the methods available for the detection of antibiotics are sensitive and selective. Moreover, in vivo models are available for follow-up tests that require only small amounts of material.

Until recently, the ability of microorganisms to produce compounds effective in the treatment of physiological diseases has received little attention. This is largely the result of the lack of simple in vitro assays to detect such compounds. In the last decade, however, the situation has changed dramatically. The biochemical lesions responsible for a wide variety of physiological disorders have been identified, largely through the study of the modes of action of agents effective in treating those diseases. Examples are atherosclerosis, associated with high serum cholesterol which can be reduced by the use of inhibitors of 3-hydroxy-3-methylglutaryl-CoA reductase (HMG-CoA reductase), the key enzyme in the pathway of cholesterol biosynthesis; rheumatoid arthritis, the symptoms of which can be ameliorated by inhibitors of prostaglandin synthesis; hypertension, which can be reduced by inhibitors of catecholamine synthesis, blockers of α- and β-adrenergic receptors, inhibitors of renin which produces angiotensin I, inhibitors of angiotensin-converting enzyme which produces the hypertensive peptide angiotensin II and blockers of calcium uptake; gastric ulcers, which can be treated by antagonists of the histamine-H_2 receptor to lower gastric acid secretion and by inhibitors of pepsin; and various psychological disorders, which can be treated by antagonists of neuroreceptors.

The production of enzyme inhibitors by microorganisms has only become evident in recent years, beginning with the pioneering work of Hamao Umezawa of the Institute of Microbial Chemistry, Tokyo, Japan (Umezawa, 1973). A list of some of the more interesting enzyme inhibitors is compiled in Table 9.4. Some of these compounds have helped to provide greater insight into the biochemistry of the enzymes inhibited, but a few may have important clinical applications. Leupeptins have some anti-inflammatory activity (Aoyagi et al., 1969). Bestatin, one of the more extensively studied inhibitors discovered at the Institute of Microbial Chemistry, is an 'immunomodulator' (Umezawa, 1980). In an oral dose as low as 0.1 μg, bestatin enhances delayed-type hypersensitivity to sheep erythrocytes in mice. Bestatin was found to inhibit tumour growth in mice. In clinical studies in cancer patients, bestatin was found to increase the percent of thymus derived lymphocytes (T-cells), which are usually suppressed in cancer patients, and to have antitumour activity. Pepstatin, an extremely potent inhibitor of pepsin, may be useful in the treatment of gastric ulcers.

Compactin was first discovered as a rather uninteresting antifungal compound produced by *Penicillium brevicompactum* (Brown et al., 1976). Somewhat later, it was discovered independently as a potent inhibitor of HMG-CoA reductase and designated ML-236B, a product of *Penicillium citrinum* (Endo et al., 1976). HMG-CoA reductase produces mevalonic acid, a key intermediate in the synthesis of cholesterol, and the Sankyo group demonstrated that ML-236B exhibited activity in vivo in inhibiting the synthesis of cholesterol.

Table 9.4: Enzyme inhibitors.

Fermentation product	Enzymes inhibited	Pharmacological activity
Amastatin	aminopeptidase A	
Antipain	papain, trypsin	
Bestatin	aminopeptidase B, leucine aminopeptidase	immunomodulator
Chymostatin	chymotrypsin	
Elasnin	human granulocyte elastase	
Elastatinal	pancreatic elastase	
Leupeptin	papain, cathepsin B, thrombokinase	anti-inflammatory
Pepstatin	pepsin, proctase B, cathepsin D, renin	gastric ulcer
Fusaric Acid	dopamine β-hydroxylase	hypotensive
Oudenone	tyrosine hydroxylase	hypotensive
Dopastin	dopamine β-hydroxylase	
Esterastin	esterase	
Forphenicine	alkaline phosphatase	
Diketocoriolin B	(Na^+,K^+)-ATPase	immunomodulator
Panosialin	sialidase, trypsin, plasmin, pepsin	
Siastatin	sialidase (bacterial)	
Coformycin	adenosine deaminase	
Compactin	HMG CoA reductase	hypocholesterolemic
Mevinolin	HMG CoA reductase	hypocholesterolemic

An even more potent inhibitor of HMG-CoA reductase was isolated by Endo from *Monascus ruber* and named monacolin K (Endo, 1979). Again there was an independent discovery of this same compound, this time at Merck Sharp & Dohme Research Laboratories. The producing organism was still another fungus, *Aspergillus terreus,* and the compound was named mevinolin (Alberts et al., 1980). Both ML-236B and mevinolin have been tested and found to lower blood cholesterol in man. Mevinolin is being used clinically to lower the blood cholesterol in people with familial hypercholesterolemia. This genetic defect shortens the lives of these people. The males, especially, develop severe atherosclerosis and suffer myocardial infarcts at an early age. Thus, the compassionate use of mevinolin for these people is well justified.

Another compound nearly relegated to the curio shelf was discovered in the laboratories of Sandoz, Ltd., Basel, Switzerland, as a rather weak antifungal agent. Cyclosporin A is a cyclic undecapeptide produced by *Cylindrocarpon lucidum* and *Trichoderma polysporum.* J.F. Borel and coworkers at Sandoz found that cyclosporin A was a potent immunosuppressant (Borel et al., 1976). When administered orally to mice immunized with sheep erythrocytes, it depressed the appearance of both direct and indirect plaque-forming cells in their spleens. At 200 mg/kg administered daily for 10 days, it more than doubled skin allograft survival in mice. It also doubled the survival time in mice and rats to graft vs. host disease induced by the administration of foreign spleen cells. It was active against experimental allergic encephalomyelitis and adjuvant arthritis in rats, although inactive in acute inflammatory assays such as carrageenin foot oedema. It was found to inhibit the multiplication of lymphocytes in vitro at a concentration which was two orders of magnitude lower than the level that is cytotoxic to other cells. This specificity of activity against lymphocytes was also observed in vivo.

Cyclosporin A, in clinical trials, has shown great promise and stands to revolutionize the field of organ transplants. The one-year survival rate for liver grafts, an especially difficult organ to transplant, was 35% with traditional immune suppressant therapy. This rate has increased to 65 to 70% with the use of cyclosporin A. The survival rate of kidneys transplanted from mismatched cadavers has increased from only 50% to over 80% with the use of cyclosporin A. Although it is mildly and reversibly hepatotoxic and nephrotoxic in rats (Farthing et al., 1980), it is surprisingly non-toxic in clinical use. About 10 to 15% of the patients have elevated blood creatinine levels, a sign of nephrotoxicity.

Cyclosporin is being investigated for the treatment of autoimmune disease such as uveitis which, in severe cases, leads to blindness. It also shows potential as an antiparasitic agent against schistosomiasis and malaria (Kolata, 1983).

9.10 The promise of the future

Few of the early participants in antibiotic research expected the antibiotic explosion to continue unchecked for fifty years. Millions of microbes have been screened to detect antibiotics, but the expected decay due to redundance in detection has not occurred because creative research has led to introduction of new highly-selective ultra-sensitive screening techniques. Simultaneously, great advances have been made in the efficiency of chemical approaches to antibiotic identification and structure determination. Whether the antibiotic explosion continues like a controlled nuclear reaction or will flame out within forthcoming years is dependent on continuation of creativity in approach. Biotechnology offers new approaches to evaluate. The targets for natural-product activity are being widened continually through development of simplified enzymatic and tissue culture screens which are indicative of chronic disease states. Those active in the field continue to be challenged and are optimistic. They anticipate success. It appears probable that forthcoming years will bring need for further expansion of our antibiotic indices, going beyond the present ten-volume limit, and that physicians and agricultural scientists will be offered an ever-widening range of natural-product structures with which to treat the ills of mankind, his domestic animals and his plant food sources. At present, the antibiotic explosion continues actively in progress. Its future is in the hands of the basic and applied scientists of the world.

Acknowledgements

The authors are indebted to Miss Matilda Heisch for her skillful editing of the manuscript, to Mrs. Ellen Volante for her timeless typing through numerous revisions and to Dr. Robert Hamill of Lilly Research Laboratories for providing us with unpublished information behind the discovery and development of monensin.

References

Abelson, P.H., 1983. Science 219, 611–746.

Abraham, E.P., Chain, E., Fletcher, C.M., Gardner, A.D., Heatley, N.G., Jennings, M.A., Florey, H.W., 1941. Lancet ii, 177–188.

Abraham, E.P., Newton, G.G.F., 1961. Biochem, J 79, 377–393.

Albers-Schonberg, G., Arison, B.H., Chabala, J.C., Douglas, A.W., Eskola, P., Fisher, M.H., Lusi, A., Mrozik, H., Smith, J.L., Tolman, R.L., 1981. J. Am. Chem. Soc. 103, 4216–4221.

Alberts, A.W., Chen, J., Kuron, G., Hunt, V., Huff, J., Hoffman, C., Rothrock, J., Lopez, M., Joshua, H., Harris, E., Patchett, A., Monaghan, R., Currie, S., Stapley, E., Albers-Schönberg, G., Hensens, O., Hirschfield, J., Hoogsteen, K., Leisch, J., Springer, J., 1980. Proc. Natl. Acad. Sci. U.S.A. 77, 3957–3961.

Aoyagi, T., Miyata, S., Nanbo, M., Kojima, F., Matsuzaki, M., Ishizuka, M., Takeuchi, T., Umezawa, H., 1969. J. Antibiot. 22, 558–568.

Aronson, C.E. (Ed.), 1983. Veterinary Pharmaceuticals and Biologicals 1982/1983. Veterinary Medicine Publishing Co., Edwardsville, Kansas, pp. 4/1 to 4/31.

Aziz, M.A., Diallo, S., Diop, I.M., Lariviere, M., Porta, M., 1982. Lancet ii, 171–173.

Bartholomew, W.H., Karow, E.O., Sfat, M.R., Wilhelm, R.H., 1940. Ind. Eng. Chem. 42, 1801–1815.

Behrens, O.K., 1949. In: The Chemistry of Penicillin, (Clarke, H.T., Johnson, J.R., Robinson, R., Eds.), Princeton University Press, Princeton, NJ, pp. 659–679.

Behrens, O.K., Corse, J., Edwards, J.P., Garrison, L., Jones, R.G., Soper, Q.F., van Abeele, F.R., Whitehead, C.W., 1948. J. Biol. Chem. 175, 793–809.

Berdy, J., 1980. CRC Handbook of Antibiotic Compounds, 10. CRC Press, Boca Raton, Florida.

Berger, J., Rachlin, A.I., Scott, W.E., Sternbach, L.H., Goldberg, M.W., 1951. J. Am. Chem. Soc. 73, 5295–5298.

Blair, L.S., Campbell, W.C., 1978. J. Helminthol. 52, 305–307.

Borel, J.F., Feurer, C., Gubler, H.U., Stähelin, H., 1976. Agents Actions 6, 468–475.

Brotzu, G., 1948. The Works of the Institute of Hygiene of Cagliari (Lavori dell' Instituto d' Ipiene di Cagliari), Cagliari. Italy.

Brown, A.G., Smale, T.C., King, T.J., Hasenkamp, R., Thompson, R.H., 1976. J. Chem. Soc. Perkin 1165–1170 I 1976.

Burg, R.W., Miller, B.M., Baker, E.E., Birnbaum, J., Currie, S.A., Hartman, R., Kong, Y.-L., Monaghan, R.L., Olson, G., Putter, I., Tunac, J.B., Wallick, H., Stapley, E.O., Oiwa, R., Omura, S., 1979. Antimicrob. Agents Chemother. 15, 361–367.

Chabala, J.C., Morzik, H., Tolman, R.L., Eskola, P., Lusi, A., Peterson, L.H., Woods, M.F., Fisher, M.H., Campbell, W.C., Egerton, J.R., Ostlind, D.A., 1980. J. Med. Chem. 23, 1134–1136.

Chain, E., 1971. Proc. R. Soc, Ser. B 179, 293–319.

Chain, E., 1980. In: Parascandola, J. (Ed.), The History of Antibiotics, A Symposium. American Institute of the History of Pharmacy, Madison, WI, pp. 15–29.

Clarke, H., Johnson, J., Robinson, R., 1949. The Chemistry of Penicillin. Princeton University Press, Princeton, NJ, p. 1094.

Council for Agricultural Science and Technology (1981) Antibiotics in Animal Feeds, Report No. 88, Ames, Iowa, pp. 28 and 32.

Crellin, J., 1980. In: Parascandola, J. (Ed.), The History of Antibiotics, A Symposium. American Institute of the History of Pharmacy, Madison, WI, pp. 5–13.

Dubos, R.J., 1939. Proc. Soc. Exptl. Biol. Med. 40, 311–312.

Dubos, R.J., Avery, O.T., 1931. J. Exptl. Med. 54, 51–57.

Dubos, R.J., Hotchkiss, R.D., 1941. J. Exptl. Med. 73, 629–640.

Duggar, B.M., 1948. Ann. N.Y. Acad. Sci. 51, 177–181.

Egerton, J.R., Ostlind, D.A., Blair, L.S., Eary, C.H., Suhayda, D., Cifelli, S., Reik, R.F., Campbell, W.C., 1979. Antimicrob. Agents Chemother. 15, 372–378.

Ehrlich, J., Bartz, Q.R., Smith, R.M., Joslyn, D.A., Burkholder, P.R., 1947. Science 106, 417–419.

Endo, A., 1979. J. Antibiot. 32, 852–854.

Endo, A., Kuroda, M., Tsujita, Y., 1976. J. Antibiot. 29, 1346–1348.

Estrada-O., S., Rightmire, B., Lardy, H.A., 1968. In: Antimicrobial Agents and Chemotherapy –1967, (Hobby, G.L., Ed.), American Society for Microbiology, Ann Arbor, MI, pp. 279–288.

Ettlinger, L., 1980. In: The History of Antibiotics, A Symposium, (Parascandola, J., Ed.), American Institute of the History of Pharmacy, Madison, WI, pp. 57–67.

Farthing, M.J.G., Clark, M.L., Pendry, A., Sloan, J., Alexander, P., 1980. Biochem. Pharmacol. 30, 3311–3316.

Feldman, W.H., Hinshaw, H.C., 1945. Proc. Staff Meet. Mayo Clinic. 20, 313–318.

Florey, H.W., Abraham, E.P., 1951. J. Hist. Med. 6, 302–317.

Florey, H.W., Chain, E., Heatley, N.G., Jennings, M.A., Sanders, A.G., Abraham, E.P., Florey, M.E., 1949. Antibiotics, I. Oxford Univ. Press, London, pp. 1–73.

Gale, E.F., Cundliffe, E., Reynolds, P.E., Richmond, M.H., Waring, M.J., 1981. The Molecular Basis of Antibiotic Action, 2nd edn. John Wiley & Sons, New York, NY, p. 646.

Goldsby, A.I., Todd, A.C., 1957. North Am. Vet. 38, 140–144.

Goodman, R.N., 1959. In: Antibiotics, Their Chemistry and Non-Medicinal Uses, (Goldberg, H.S., Ed.), D. Van Nostrand Company, Inc., Princeton, NJ, pp. 322–448.

Gottlieb, D., Bhattacharyya, P.K., Anderson, H.W., Carter, H.E., 1948. J. Bacteriol. 55, 409–417.

Gottshall, R.Y., Roberts, J.M., Portwood, L.M., Jennings, J.C., 1951. Proc. Soc. Exptl. Biol. Med. 76, 307–311.

Haney, M.E., Jr., Hoehn, M.M., 1968. In: Antimicrobial Agents and Chemotherapy –1967, (Hobby, G.L., Ed.), American Society for Microbiology, Ann Arbor, MI, pp. 349–352.

Hata, T., Sano, Y., Ohki, M., Yokohama, Y., Matsumae, A., Ito, S., 1953. J. Antibiotics Ser. A 6, 87–89.

Helfand, W.H., Woodruff, H.B., Coleman, K.M.H., Cowen, D.L., 1980. In: The History of Antibiotics, A Symposium, (Parascandola, J., Ed.), American Institute of the History of Pharmacy, Madison, WI, pp. 31–56.

Hendlin, D., Stapley, E.O., Jackson, M., Wallick, H., Miller, A.K., Wolf, F.J., Miller, T.W., Chaiet, L., Kahan, F.M., Foltz, E.L., Woodruff, H.B., Mata, J.M., Hernandez, S., Mochales, S., 1969. Science 166, 122–123.

Hidy, P.H., Baldwin, R.S., Greasham, R.L., Keith, C.L., McMullen, J.R., 1977. Adv. Appl. Microbiol. 22, 59–82.

Holmberg, S.D., Osterholm, M.T., Senger, K.A., Cohen, M.L., 1984. New. Eng. J. Med. 311, 617–622.

Huff, B.B., 1983. Physicians' Desk Reference, 3068 pp., Medical Economics Company, Inc., Oradell, NJ.

Johnson, B.A., Anker, H.S., Meleney, F.L., 1945. Science 102, 376–377.

Jukes, T.H., Stokstad, E.L.R., Taylor, R.R., Cunha, T.J., Edwards, H.M., Meadows, G.B., 1950. Arch. Biochem. 26, 324–325.

Kass, I.S., Wang, C.C., Walrond, J.P., Stretton, A.O.W., 1980. Proc. Natl. Acad. Sci. U.S.A. 77, 6211–6215.

Kolata, G., 1983. Science 221, 40–42.

Korzybski, T., Kurylowicz, W., 1961. Antibiotica. Veb Gustav Fischer Verlag, Jena, p. 1105.

Leben, C., Keitt, G.W., 1954. Agric. Food Chem 2, 234–239.

Lechevalier, H.A., 1980. In: The History of Antibiotics, A Symposium, (Parascandola, J., Ed.), American Institute of the History of Pharmacy, Madison, WI, pp. 113–123.

Lechevalier, H.A., Solotorovsky, M., 1965. Three Centuries of Microbiology, McGraw-Hill, New York, NY, pp. 429–492.

Leidahl, L. Ed., 1983. 1983 Feed Additive Compendium, 334 pp., The Miller Publishing Company, Minneapolis, MI.

Mann, R.L., Bromer, W.W., 1958. J. Am. Chem. Soc. 80, 2714–2716.

McCormick, J.R., Sjolander, N.O., Hirsch, U., Jensen, E.R., Doerschuk, A.P., 1957. J. Am. Chem. Soc. 79, 4561–4563.

McCowen, M.C., Callender, M.E., Brandt, M.C., 1957. In: Antibiotics Annual 1956–1957, (Welch, H., Marti-Ibanez, F., Eds.), Medical Encyclopedia, Inc., New York, NY, pp. 883–886.

McGuire, J.M., Bunch, R.L., Anderson, R.C., Boaz, H.E., Flynn, E.H., Powell, H.M., Smith, J.W., 1952. Antibiot. Chemother. 2, 281–283.

Mellin, T.N., Busch, R.D., Wang, C.C., 1983. Neuropharmacology 22, 89–96.

Miller, M.W., 1961. The Pfizer Handbook of Microbial Metabolites, McGraw-Hill, New York, NY, pp. 772.

Miller, T.W., Chaiet, L., Cole, D.J., Cole, L.J., Flor, J.E., Goegelman, R.T., Gullo, V.P., Joshua, H., Kempf, A.J., Krellwitz, W.R., Monaghan, R.L., Ormond, R.E., Wilson, K.E., Albers-Schönberg, G., 1979. Antimicrob. Agents Chemother. 15, 368–371.

Moore, P.R., Evenson, A., Lackey, T.D., McCoy, E., Elvehjem, C.A., Hart, E.B., 1946. J. Biol. Chem. 165, 437–441.

Morin, R.B., Jackson, B.G., Flynn, E.H., Roeske, R.W., 1962. J. Am. Chem. Soc. 84, 3400–3401.

Moyer, A.J., Coghill, R.D., 1947. J. Bacteriol. 53, 329–341.

Nagarajan, R., Boeck, L.D., Gorman, M., Hamill, R.L., Higgens, C.E., Hoehn, M., Stark, W.M., Whitney, J.G., 1971. J. Am. Chem. Soc. 93, 2308–2310.

Norby, S.R., Alestig, K., Bjornegård, B., Burman, L.Å., Ferber, F., Huber, J.L., Jones, K.H., Kahan, F.M., Kahan, J.S., Kropp, H., Meisinger, M.A.P., Sundelof, J.G., 1983. Antimicrob. Agents Chemother. 23, 300–307.

O'Brien, T.F., Hopkins, J.D., Gilleece, E.S., Madeiros, A.A., Kent, R.L., Blackburn, B.O., Holmes, M.B., Reerdon, J.P., Vergeront, J.M., Schell, W.L., Christenson, E., Bissett, M.L., Morse, E.V., 1982. New Eng. J. Med. 307, 1–6.

Ostlind, D.A., Ciffelli, S., Long., R, 1979. Vet. Rec. 105, 168.

Ott, W.H., Rickes, E.L., Wood, T.L., 1948. J. Biol. Chem. 174, 1047–1048.

Perry, T.W., Beeson, W.M., Mohler, M.T., 1976. J. Anim. Sci. 42, 761–765.

Pinnert-Sindico, S., Ninet, L., Preud'homme, J., Cosar, C., 1955. In: Antibiotics Annual 1954–1955, (Welch, H., Marti-Ibanez, F., Ed.), Medical Encyclopedia, New York, NY, pp. 724–727.

Pressman, B.C., Harris, E.J., Jagger, W.S., Johnson, J.H., 1967. Proc. Natl. Acad. Sci. U.S.A. 58, 1949–1956.

Putter, I., MacConnell, J.G., Preiser, F.A., Haidri, A.A., Ristich, S.S., Dybas, R.A., 1981. Experientia 37, 963–964.

Richardson, L.F., Raun, A.P., Potter, E.L., Cooley, C.O., Rathmacher, R.P., 1974. J. Anim. Sci. 39, 250.

Schatz, A., Bugie, E., Waksman, S.A., 1944. Proc. Soc. Exptl. Biol. Med. 55, 66–69.

Shumard, R.F., Callender, M.E., 1968. In: Antimicrobial Agents and Chemotherapy –1967, (Hobby, G.L., Ed.), American Society for Microbiology, Ann Arbor, MI, pp. 369–377.

Spector, W.S., 1956. Handbook of Toxicology, Vol. 2. Antibiotics. Saunders, Philadelphia.

Stapley, E.O., Jackson, M., Hernandez, S., Zimmerman, S.B., Currie, S.A., Mochales, S., Mata, J.M., Woodruff, H.B., Hendlin, D, 1972. Antimicrob. Agents Chemother. 2, 122–131.

Stark, W.M., Knox, N.G., Westhead, J.E., 1968. In: Antimicrobial Agents and Chemotherapy –1967, (Hobby, G.L., Ed.), American Society for Microbiology, Ann Arbor, MI, pp. 353–358.

Stokes, J.L., Woodward Jr., C.R., 1942. J. Bacteriol. 43, 253–263.

Stokstad, E.L.R., Jukes, T.H., 1950a. Proc. Soc. Exptl. Biol. Med. 73, 523–528.

Stokstad, E.L.R., Jukes, T.H., 1950b. Poultry Sci 29, 611–612.

Stokstad, E.L.R., Jukes, T.H., Pierce, J., Page Jr., A.C., Franklin, A.L, 1949. J. Biol. Chem. 180, 647–654.

Sykes, R.B., Parker, W.L., Wells, J.S., 1982. In: Trends in Antibiotic Research, (Umezawa, H., Demain, A.L., Hata, T., Hutchinson, C.R. (Eds.), Japanese Antibiotics Reserach Assoc., Tokyo, pp. 115–124.

Thomson, W.T., 1982. Agricultural Chemicals, Book IV, Fungicides, Thomson Publications, Fresno, CA, pp. 37–44.

Umezawa, H., 1967. Index of Antibiotics from Actinomycetes, Vol. I, University of Tokyo Press, Tokyo, pp. 940.

Umezawa, H., 1973. Pure Appl. Chem. 33, 129–144.

Umezawa, H. (1978) Index of Antibiotics from Actinomycetes, Vol. II, University of Tokyo Press, Tokyo, pp. 1466.

Umezawa, H., 1980. Biotechnol. Bioengineering 22, 99–110 Suppl. 1.

Umezawa, H., Tazaki, T., Kanori, H., Okami, Y., Fukuyama, S., 1948. Japan Med. J. 1, 358–363.

Umezawa, H., Ueda, M., Maeda, K., Yagishita, K., Kondo, S., Okami, Y., Utahara, R., Osato, Y., Nitta, K., Takeuchi, T., 1957. J. Antibiot. 10, 181–188.

U.S. Office of Technology Assessment. (1979) Drugs in Livestock Feed, Vol. I., p. 32, Technical Report, U.S. Government Printing Office, Washington, D.C.

Waksman, S.A., 1940. Sci. Monthly 51, 422–427.

Waksman, S.A., 1953. Am. Sci. 41, 8.

Waksman, S.A., 1975. The Antibiotic Era, University of Tokyo Press, Tokyo, pp. 224.

Waksman, S.A., Foster, J.W., 1937. Soil Sci 43, 69–76.

Waksman, S.A., Starkey, R.L., 1923. Soil Sci 16, 343–358 137–157, 247–268.

Waksman, S.A., Woodruff, H.B., 1940. J. Bacteriol. 40, 581–600.

Waksman, S.A., Woodruff, H.B., 1941. J. Bacteriol. 42, 231–249.

Waksman, S.A., Woodruff, H.B., 1942. Proc. Soc. Exptl. Biol. Med. 49, 207–210.

Weinstein, M.J., Luedemann, G.M., Oden, E.M., Wagman, G.H., 1963. In: Antimicrobial Agents and Chemotherapy –1963, (Sylvester, J.C., Ed.), American Society for Microbiology, Ann Arbor, MI, pp. 1–7.

Weindling, R., 1934. Phytopathology 24, 1153–1179.

Wilkins, C.A., Conroy, J., Ho, P., O'Shanny, W.J., Capizzi, T., 1981. In: Tick Biology and Control, (Whitehead G.B., Gibson, J.O., Eds.), Rhodes University, Grahamstown, South Africa, pp. 137–142.

Wilkins, C.A., Conroy, J.A., Ho, P., O'Shanny, W.J., Malatesta, P.F., Egerton, J.R., 1980. Am. J. Vet. Res. 41, 2112–2113.

Wilkins, W.H., Harris, G.C.M., 1942. Br. J. Exptl. Pathol. 23, 166–169.

Wintersteiner, O., Boon, W.R., Carrington, H.C., MacCorquodale, D.W., Stodola, F.H., Wachtel, J.L., Coghill, R.D., Risser, W.C., Philip, J.E., Touster, O., 1949. In: The Chemistry of Penicillin, (Clarke, H.T., Johnson, J.R., Robinson, R., Eds.), Princeton University Press, Princeton, NJ, pp. 106–143.

Woodruff, H.B., Kahan, F.M., Miller, A.K., Stapley, E.O., Wallick, H., 1975. In: Microbial Drug Resistance, (Mitsuhashi, S., Hashimoto, H., Eds.), University of Tokyo Press, Tokyo, pp. 539–559.

Woodruff, H.B., McDaniel, L.E., 1954. In: Industrial Fermentations, (Underkofler, L.A., Hickey, R.J., Eds.), Vol. II, Chemical Publishing Co., New York, NY, pp. 264–293.

Woodruff, H.B., Stapley, E.O., 1982. In: Trends in Antibiotic Research, (Umezawa, H., Demain, A.L., Hata, T., Hutchinson, C.R., Eds.), Japan Antibiotics Research Assoc., Tokyo, pp. 154–170.

Woodruff, H.B., Stapley, E.O., Wallick, H., Onishi, H.R., Zimmerman, S.B., Miller, A.K., Hendlin, D., 1975. In: Microbial Drug Resistance, (Mitsuhashi, S., Hashimoto, H., Eds.), University of Tokyo Press, Tokyo, pp. 409–424.

Woodruff, H.B., Waksman, S.A., 1960. Ann. N.Y. Acad. Sci. 89, 287–298.

Yagisawa, Y., 1980. In: Parascandola, J. (Ed.), The History of Antibiotics, A Symposium. American Institute of the History of Pharmacology, Madison, WI, pp. 69–90.

Index

Page numbers followed by "*f*" and "*t*" indicate figures and tables respectively.